The Child Surveillance Handbook

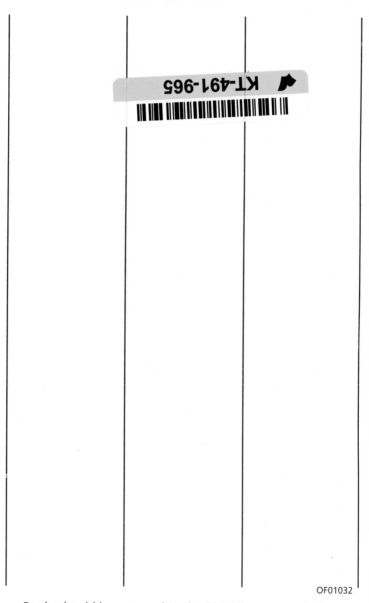

OF01032

Books should be returned to the SDH Library on or before
the date stamped above unless a renewal has been arranged

Salisbury District Hospital Library

Telephone: Salisbury (01722) 336262 extn. 4432 / 33
Out of hours answer machine in operation

The Child Surveillance Handbook

THIRD EDITION

DAVID HALL

JONATHAN WILLIAMS

and

DAVID ELLIMAN

Radcliffe Publishing
Oxford • New York

Radcliffe Publishing Ltd
18 Marcham Road
Abingdon
Oxon OX14 1AA
United Kingdom

www.radcliffe-oxford.com
Electronic catalogue and worldwide online ordering facility.

First Edition 1990
Second Edition 1994
Second Edition revised 1999

British Library Cataloguing in Publication Data

A catalogue record for this book is available from the British Library.

ISBN-13: 978 184619 109 1

Typeset by Pindar NZ, Auckland, New Zealand
Printed and bound by TJ International, Padstow, Cornwall, UK

Contents

Preface

The first edition of this book was published in 1990, a year after the publication of a major review of child health surveillance, *Health for All Children*[1] and aimed to offer a 'how to do it' guide that would complement the policy proposals set out in that review. This new edition, the third, has been extensively revised with much new material, based on new research and evolving government policy as set out in the most recent revision of *Health for All Children*.[2] For example, the tragic death of Victoria Climbié prompted much soul-searching about our approaches to child abuse, resulting in new legislation and procedures and a greater emphasis on developing the evidence base for child protection work. In 2008, the publication in England of an updated *Child Health Promotion Programme*[3] re-defined services for the under-5s, stressing that while the programme must be universal and available to all children, it should be adapted to the varying needs of individual families. Sophisticated parents who are expert in accessing information about children on the internet have very different needs from those of a young single mother who dropped out of school with no qualifications.

Twenty years ago, the main emphasis of child health surveillance programmes was the detection of abnormalities that are potentially disabling. This remains an important goal: health professionals must be familiar with the many different ways in which long-term disorders and disabilities can present. But increasingly we also recognise that the greatest burden of disadvantage, educational failure and wasted lives is due not to medical or biological disorders, but to adverse social and economic circumstances and the mental health problems that so often accompany them. That would be depressing were it not for the parallel increase in our understanding of what the underlying factors are and an increasing enthusiasm for applying this knowledge in new approaches to intervention.

In order to change the trajectory of children's lives, interventions often need to involve the whole family and the many other individuals who may be involved with a child's care. This, in turn, requires health professionals to increase their confidence and competence in working with parents as the key agents of change for their children.

We hope that this third edition of *The Child Surveillance Handbook* will help health professionals to develop their expertise in the many aspects of the new Child Health Promotion Programme. It offers an overview of current ideas about child development and family dynamics, both normal and atypical, and an accessible source of information about the many topics that are raised by parents. This book will be of particular value to health visitors, general practice trainees and early years staff. Paediatricians and child mental health staff who appreciate the importance of understanding child development (and we hope that applies to all of them!) will also find much of interest here.

David Hall
Jonathan Williams
David Elliman
January 2009

REFERENCES

1 Hall D. *Health for All Children.* Oxford: Oxford University Press; 1989.
2 Hall D, Elliman D, editors. *Health for All Children.* 4th ed. revised Oxford: Oxford University Press; 2006.
3 Department of Health. *Child Health Promotion Programme.* London: DH; 2008. Available at: www.dh.gov.uk/en/Publicationsandstatistics/Publications/DH_083645 (accessed 31 December 2008). NB: This is to be re-named in 2009 as the 'Healthy Child Programme'.

A NOTE ON REFERENCES AND FURTHER READING

This book does not attempt to justify every statement by comprehensive references to the literature, rather we have suggested recent reports and reviews available on the internet and, as far as possible, journals that are either accessible on-line free of charge or are likely to be available in the paediatric section of most UK hospital and community child health libraries. The URLs of internet resources do change but can often be located by a simple Google search.

When looking for relevant literature on the internet, start with Google as many reports, protocols and position statements are freely available – but follow the advice given for interpreting internet resources set out in page 33. For original papers, the easiest resources to use are Google Scholar (www.scholar.google.com) and the National Library of Medicine (www.ncbi.nlm.nih.gov/sites/entrez?db=pubmed).

If you are an NHS employee, you can obtain an ATHENS password from your medical librarian. This will allow you on-line access to many key publications, either directly or via the National Library for Health (www.library.nhs.uk).

WEB SITE FOR *THE CHILD SURVEILLANCE HANDBOOK*

Further information and links, including the additional material mentioned in Appendix 1, can be found at www.healthforallchildren.co.uk. This web site is updated from time to time with new material and links to recently published articles, reports, etc.

About the authors

David Hall
Emeritus Professor of Community
  Paediatrics, University of Sheffield
Honorary Professor of Paediatrics,
  University of Cape Town

Jonathan Williams
Consultant Child and Adolescent
  Psychiatrist, Barnet
Visiting Research Associate, Institute of
  Psychiatry
Honorary Consultant, Great Ormond
  Street Hospital for Children, London

David Elliman
Consultant in Community Child Health
Great Ormond Street Hospital for
  Children, London

Contributions and advice from:
Helen Bedford
Senior Lecturer in Children's Health
Institute of Child Health, London

Chung Chan
Locum Consultant Audiological Physician
The Royal National Hospital for Throat,
  Nose and Ear, London

Anne MacLean
Head of Dietetics
Yorkhill Hospital, Glasgow

Mirelle Martin
Specialist Midwife, Sheffield

Sue Peckover
Senior Research Fellow, University of
  Huddersfield

Mary Rudolf
Professor of Community Paediatrics,
  University of Leeds

Patrice Van Cleemput
Honorary Research Fellow, University of
  Sheffield

Acknowledgements

We acknowledge with thanks the following people who contributed to, or advised on, previous editions:

Gillian Baird
Professor of Paediatrics and Consultant Developmental Paediatrician, Guy's Hospital, London

Christine Bungay
Physiotherapist, Child Development Centre, St George's Hospital, London (retired)

Paul Calvert
Consultant Orthopaedic Surgeon, St George's Hospital, London (died 2004)

Emma C Cullingham
Community Dietician, Wandsworth

Ann Duizend
Health Visitor, Wandsworth

Alyson Elliman
Consultant in Sexual and Reproductive Healthcare, Croydon PCT

Sarita Fonseca
Consultant Community Paediatric Audiologist, St George's Hospital, London

Jenny Gallagher
Senior Lecturer in Dental Public Health, King's College London

Elizabeth Gordon
Consultant Urologist, St George's Hospital, London

Jacky Hayden
Dean of Postgraduate Medical Studies for the North Western Deanery
Previously, Regional Adviser in General Practice

Peter Hill
Professor of Child and Adolescent Psychiatry
Hospital for Sick Children, Great Ormond Street, London

Jean Pearson
Community Dietician, Nottingham

Anthony Williams
Reader in Child Nutrition and Consultant in Neonatal Paediatrics, St George's Hospital, London

Child health promotion programmes

DEFINING THE AIMS: WHAT ARE WE TRYING TO ACHIEVE?

Parents want their children to be healthy, happy and eventually self-supporting, but the perceptions of parents, children and professionals about what health and happiness mean do not always coincide. Healthcare programmes for individual young children and families aim to achieve:

- the promotion of optimal health, nutrition, development and emotional well-being;
- the prevention of illness, accidental injury and child abuse;
- the recognition and, if possible, elimination of potential problems affecting development, behaviour and education;
- the early detection of illness and abnormality, in order to offer investigation, treatment and support.

Children and young people put their aims rather differently. They have been grouped together under five main headings in *Every Child Matters*:[1]

- **being healthy**: enjoying good physical and mental health and living a healthy lifestyle;
- **staying safe**: being protected from harm and neglect;
- **enjoying and achieving**: getting the most out of life and developing the skills for adulthood;
- **making a positive contribution**: being involved with the community and society and not engaging in antisocial or offending behaviour;
- **economic well-being**: not being prevented by economic disadvantage from achieving their full potential in life.

In the 21st century, most children in industrialised countries are physically healthy and often the factors that stop them *feeling* healthy are in their family life and the world around them. Many more children are sad, anxious or afraid than suffer from organic illness. Abuse within the family, bullying by peers or teachers, lack of play and leisure space and facilities, discarded intravenous needles, dog mess and graffiti are the leading issues raised by children when asked about their main concerns. Mental health, emotional well-being, social relationships and the environment are as important in modern child health as physical disease or disability.

Governments are increasingly interested in community healthcare programmes because, in partnership with other agencies, they can reduce social exclusion and the inequalities within and between local communities. Child development attracts particular attention because of the potential for reducing long-term illness, educational failure, antisocial behaviour and crime by early interventions.[2] (*See* Boxes 1.1 and 1.5.)

BOX 1.1

'The nation [USA] has not capitalized sufficiently on the knowledge that has been gained from nearly half a century of considerable public investment in research on children from birth to age 5. In many respects, we have barely begun to use our growing research capabilities to help children and families negotiate the changing demands and possibilities of life in the 21st century.'

Until recently, community-based programmes for child health were known as 'child health surveillance programmes' and this term is still enshrined in UK practice, but it does not encompass the full range of 21st century preventive child health programmes. The term 'surveillance' focused attention on the identification of disorder and abnormality ('secondary prevention', *see* Figure 1.1), ignoring primary and tertiary prevention, and implied that child health depends on the constant vigilance of, and supervision by, health professionals.

Early detection of abnormalities is important, as described in Chapter 9, but it is just a small part of a modern programme[3] (*see* Figure 1.1). The term 'child health promotion' encapsulates a broader view of the overall aims and objectives and is clearly not just the responsibility of health professionals, but also of many other disciplines and agencies – for example, schools, social services, housing departments and voluntary organisations. The skills involved in providing information to parents about actions they can take, or avoid, to improve their children's health are considered in Chapter 2 – Communication and consultation.

WHAT DETERMINES HOW CHILDREN DEVELOP?

What matters most: a child's inherited nature (his genes) or the way he is brought up? This centuries-old debate – 'nature versus nurture' – is now outdated. The answer is that both are crucial. More importantly, they interact: different personalities and temperaments that can be recognised even in infancy produce different reactions from parents and other people who come into contact with the child.

Here is a brief summary of factors that determine how a child will turn out as an adult:

- **The genes s/he receives from the two parents.** In addition to the infinite variation of 'normal' genes there are genes that pre-dispose to developmental problems and disorders or behavioural syndromes. Some important characteristics of development and of long-term outcomes are now known to be quite strongly influenced by genes. This is true for hyperactivity, depressive illness and aggressive behaviour.
- **The child's experiences.** These have a powerful effect as well. For example, early exposure to social and conversational experiences supports brain development. Negative experiences also have long-term effects. Children who are exposed to violent, unpredictable early experiences subsequently react differently and in more extreme ways to stress and threat. It follows that the ability of parents to respond appropriately to the young child's needs

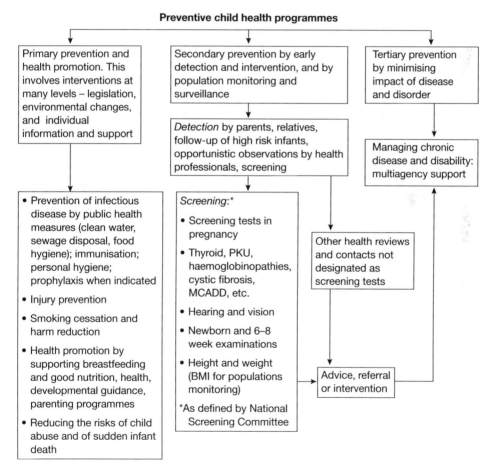

FIGURE 1.1 Diagram to show relationships between the terms used in preventive child health programmes. Primary prevention means preventing an event or disorder from occurring; secondary prevention means minimising its impact by early detection and intervention; tertiary prevention means managing or alleviating the problems caused by a disorder.[3] Reproduced with permission from BMJ Publishing Group.

is of crucial importance. Similarly, the quality of education, particularly – but certainly not exclusively – in the early years has a major influence on development.

▶ **Genes and experiences interact.** In one study, children with no genetic history of criminality had only a 3% chance of becoming criminals; if they had either a genetic risk or an environmental risk (for example, an adoptive parent who is a criminal or alcoholic) the risk rose to 9%, but exposure to both types of risk increased the figure to 40%. A child with a tendency to aggressive behaviour is more likely to grow up as a violent adult if his family and his neighbourhood tolerate violence. Infants with high scores on developmental testing at age two are more likely than those with low scores to do well at school and in adult life; but low scoring infants in middle-class families are more likely to do well than high scoring infants in poor families (*see* page 190). *See* Figure 1.2 for an illustration of how a gene that predisposes to depression may interact with maltreatment.

▶ **The timing of experiences.** This may be significant. The important issue of critical/sensitive periods is discussed on pages 50, 177.

▶ **Temperament.** This varies widely between children and affects both their learning style and the ways adults interact with them (*see* Chapter 3 – Mental health, temperament and behaviour).

▶ **Health of the mother during pregnancy.** This can affect the nutrition supply to the foetus and, in particular, to the developing brain. If the foetus is severely

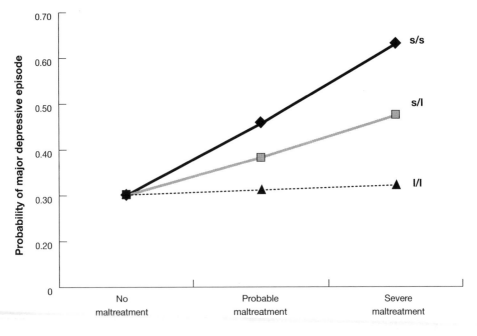

FIGURE 1.2 Some children (dotted line) carry a gene that protects them from the long-term depressive effects of abuse. However, they seem to have no special protection from other causes of depression. If children with a different genetic makeup (solid lines) are abused, they are much more likely to become depressed later in life. Reproduced from Caspi A, *et al.*[4] with permission from *AAAS*.

under-nourished for prolonged periods, brain development is likely to be affected.

▶ **Illness affecting the mother during pregnancy.** Alcohol abuse, infections or obstetric complications, for example, can cause injury to the developing brain.

▶ **Premature birth.** Very low birth weight babies have an increased risk of slower growth and of learning and behavioural difficulties even when there is no apparent brain damage.

▶ **Nutrition in infancy.** Children who experience prolonged severe malnutrition during infancy are likely to have reduced learning abilities (*see* page 148). Deficiency of specific nutrients such as iron (*see* page 114) or iodine can also affect development.

▶ **Sensory deficits.** Vision and hearing problems affect many aspects of development.

▶ **Physical health.** This is important, both directly, and indirectly; for example, chronic upper respiratory symptoms not only predispose to hearing impairment, but also can cause disturbed sleep, which in turn can impair learning. Poor health may also lead to prolonged absences from school.

▶ **Stability of experiences and continuity of carers.** In infancy and childhood this is important because a variety of experiences can build resilience (*see* page 54) but too much change and uncertainty can be damaging.

Life course research

Early disadvantage is often compounded throughout life (*see* Figure 1.3). Poverty is associated with sub-optimal pregnancy outcomes. Children with a temperamental tendency to aggression are more likely to become aggressive adults if they grow up in poor, violent families and live in unattractive, violent neighbourhoods. Parents who have little support or interaction with other people may be more at risk of neglecting their children, with adverse effects on their children's learning, behaviour and brain development. Life chances are already reduced at school entry if children have fewer basic skills than their more fortunate peers. Early difficulties with language acquisition and behaviour are followed by conduct problems in school, educational failure, low earning capacity, increased criminality and failure to master reading and basic numeracy. Morbidity and mortality are increased compared with more fortunate families.

PREVENTIVE HEALTH SERVICES FOR YOUNG CHILDREN

Effective interventions to improve the health and lives of children depend on the expertise and commitment not only of the health professions but of many other agencies (e.g. social services, education, housing, and the voluntary organisations). In England, the creation of children's trusts represents an attempt to encourage these agencies to work together more effectively. General practitioners and primary care teams provide the majority of children's healthcare in the community. In the UK, the key professional responsible for the delivery of child health promotion programmes for the under-5s is the health visitor, though many other professionals are involved. Midwives make an important contribution in the first weeks of life, school nurses take over when the child starts school and general practice teams are involved throughout childhood.

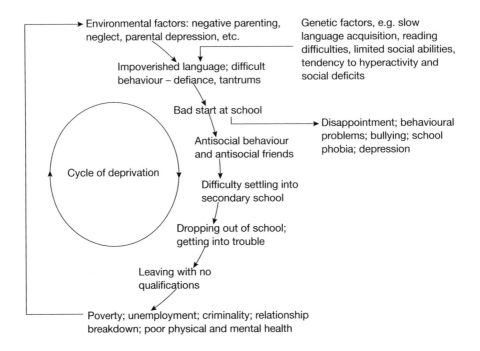

FIGURE 1.3 Cycle of deprivation.

The aims of preventive child health services, as set out at the beginning of this chapter, are relevant to all children and families. A *universal programme* – one that reaches every family – is essential, for three reasons:

▶ some services, such as immunisation and screening programmes, are necessary for every child irrespective of circumstances;
▶ it is only by providing a universal service that the individual and unique needs of each family can be assessed and agreed;
▶ if a service is universal, it is more readily accepted by parents, whereas they may resent or reject something perceived as special, needed only by parents with problems.

Families differ widely in how much help, advice and support they need and want. A confident prosperous couple with their third healthy child are likely to have very different needs from those of a single teenage first-time parent living in a high-rise flat (*see* Box 1.2 for further examples). Families with high levels of need are seldom easy to engage and they do not readily trust professionals or share concerns with them, so it is essential to build a long-term relationship; ideally, this relationship should start before the birth of the child.

Health professionals have to balance the importance of maintaining a universal service with the need to *target* their energies where they are likely to have the maximum benefit. Some form of targeting is adopted in most community child health services; for example, classifying clients into low, medium and high need groups.[5] More detailed scoring systems that aim to quantify the risk, vulnerability and needs of individual families have been devised but do not appear to be any better than professional judgment or to improve time allocation. This is not surprising, because vulnerability changes over time, families may not disclose all their circumstances, their situation may change (for instance the arrival of a new boyfriend with a history of violence can dramatically change the level of risk), and most importantly, because families differ in their resilience and their social support. Health professionals report that the most stressful situations arise in families where they perceive a substantial risk to the child, but this has not reached a level that triggers the active involvement of social services.

BOX 1.2 Extra support

The following are examples of situations where increased levels of professional support may be beneficial:

- parents with any of the three potent risk factors: domestic violence, substance abuse and parental mental illness, such as depression. These are problems that health professionals find exceptionally challenging;
- parents of limited intelligence and education;
- very young or unsupported parents, particularly with their first baby;
- death, serious illness or disability affecting any child in the family;
- families with multiple risk factors for child abuse or where abuse is known to have occurred;
- parents who are socially isolated due to personality factors, psychiatric problems, chronic illness, or linguistic and cultural barriers;
- families living in extreme poverty or temporary accommodation, or under threat of eviction, repossession or redundancy;
- high-achieving parents with extremely high personal standards for their children and for themselves as parents.

There can never be a simple formula to measure these complex social issues. Deprivation indices can be calculated for each case load or locality and these enable managers to allocate more staff and adequate expert support (e.g. specialist nurses – *see* Box 1.5) for the more challenging and demanding areas, but once they have agreed their overall policy objectives, the front-line staff must take responsibility for prioritising work with individual families.[6]

CHANGING CHILDREN'S LIFE CHANCES

We cannot alter the child's genes, but the way the child is brought up can, to some extent, be modified. Good parenting and good educational experiences can compensate to a considerable extent for other disadvantages. In the UK, recent research on child development is influencing parents' attitudes and public policy in several important ways.[7] Well-informed parents have become enthusiastic – and sometimes overly anxious – about the need to give their offspring optimal opportunities for early learning. Politicians and educators have acknowledged the benefits of early support and intervention for young children, especially those starting with any kind of disadvantage, and have initiated programmes such as Sure Start (*see* Box 1.3). The protection of young children has taken on a new urgency as we learn just how serious and common is the damage caused by abuse and neglect. Interest in postnatal depression has also grown as its impact on young children becomes clearer. These topics have, in turn, focused attention on parents' quality of life and what affects it. In Chapters 2, 3 and 5, we discuss how parents can be supported and helped, and the particular issues faced by parents in a variety of difficult circumstances.

In complex cases, professionals can be involved in managing a whole host of difficulties affecting a particular child. Brief interventions focused on single problems are unlikely to protect the child against cumulative negative factors that persist all through childhood and into adult life. In order to avoid overwhelming or de-motivating the family, it is important to select the interventions that are most likely to be effective. A long-term view may help, in which urgent problems are managed immediately while others are deferred to the next visit or the next year, for example. There is particular value in improving parenting skills as the benefits continue for years and include other children as well. Therefore, most value is achieved by targeting families with their first child. Helping unemployed parents to obtain work and thereby reduce their reliance on benefits and increase their self-esteem is part of government policy and was one of the Sure Start objectives.

BOX 1.3 The aims and objectives of Sure Start

Sure Start was launched in 1998 as a major government programme in the UK, with the aim of '... working with parents and children to promote the physical, intellectual, social and emotional development of children – particularly those who are disadvantaged – to make sure they are ready to thrive when they get to school'.[8] It built on early intervention research, mainly from the USA, research on nursery education and ideas about community development and ownership. Each scheme was locally based and typically served 500–1000 children. Sure Start multi-agency partnership schemes, costing over £1bn in total, were planned in 500 deprived areas between 1999 and 2004, and intended to reach one-third of children under 5 years who lived in poverty.[9] The programme is now integrated with the Children's Centres.

Objective 1: Improving social and emotional development:

- an increase in the proportion of babies and young children aged 0–5 with normal levels of personal, social and emotional development for their age by promoting greater parental understanding of and engagement in children's development, supporting early years and childcare providers in early identification of difficulties and increasing the contribution that out of school provision makes to older children's development as citizens;
- reduce inequalities between the level of development achieved by children in the 20% most disadvantaged areas and the rest of England;
- improve educational support for children who are looked after and increase the stability of their lives.

Objective 2: Improving health:

- a reduction in the proportion of mothers who continue to smoke during pregnancy;
- improve awareness of healthy living amongst children and their service providers and, in particular, in disadvantaged areas, by helping parents to support their

---

children's healthy development before and after birth;

- ensure information and guidance on breastfeeding, nutrition, hygiene and safety is available to all families with young children in the Sure Start local programme and Children's Centre areas;
- halt the rise in obesity; enhance the take-up of sporting opportunities;
- reduce the number of children aged 0–4 living in Sure Start local programme and Children's Centre areas admitted to hospital as an emergency with gastro-enteritis, a lower respiratory infection or a severe injury.

Objective 3: Improving learning:

- an increase in the proportion of children having normal levels of communication, language and literacy at the end of the foundation stage and an increase in the proportion of young children with satisfactory speech and language development at age 2 years;
- increase the use of libraries by families with young children;
- increase the proportion of children who have their needs identified in line with Early Years Action and Early Years Action Plus of the Special Educational Needs Code of Practice (*see* page 348) and who have either a group or individual action plan in place;
- improve levels of school attendance and reduce school absences.

Objective 4: Strengthening families and communities:

- A reduction in the proportion of young children (aged 0–4) living in households where no one is working;
- Increase access to and quality of childcare.

The impact of the programme is discussed on page 11.

BOX 1.4 Characteristics of successful early intervention programmes
- Clearly specified aims.
- Precise guidance, based on a theoretical framework backed by research evidence, as far as possible, as to what should be provided by the professional undertaking the intervention.
- A quality maintenance system that ensures staff are following this guidance. The term 'programme fidelity' is used to denote the importance of adhering to a structure that has been shown to work in tightly managed research and demonstration projects, when the programme is rolled out on a wider scale.
- A well-informed programme leader who understand the aims and supports the staff.
- Well-trained and highly motivated staff.
- A high intensity of intervention and, in most cases, a prolonged programme lasting months or even years.
- Caseload size that allows staff to provide this level of intervention.
- A targeted approach with a focus on the mothers at highest risk – typically young, poor, single and with limited social and psychological resources.

Which interventions work?

Some interventions in preventive child health have specific objectives and are of proven effectiveness; for example, immunisation, some screening procedures, the Nurse-Family Partnership (*see* Box 1.5), parent education in managing behaviour problems, some injury reduction programmes and the 'Reduce the Risk' advice to minimise the risk of sudden infant death syndrome.

Programmes like Sure Start have broader and more ambitious aims and objectives (Box 1.3 and Box 1.4). They seek to ensure that 'children are ready to benefit from their education when they go to school' and ultimately to bring about a wide-ranging improvement in their development and life course. Being ready to benefit from school is an important goal, though one not easy to define.[10] All such programmes are expensive in terms of finance and skilled staff and so it is important to ask – which ones are effective and what distinguishes the ones that work from the ones that don't?

The main features of the most successful programmes seem to be consistent in a wide variety of settings, both in home visiting and in centre-based programmes. When these principles are not followed, quality suffers and the benefits are at best modest. Box 1.4 summarises details of research findings from the UK and USA; Box 1.5 outlines some of the programmes that have been evaluated and are said to be effective.[11–18]

Parenting education

Several programmes focus on training parents to better understand their children's emotions and behaviour. Examples of programmes that have been shown to be effective include:

▶ PIPPIN (Parents In Partnership – Parent Infant Network), a UK-based project to prepare parents for parenthood during pregnancy;
▶ Triple-P, which originated in Australia. It is available for all parents and more intensive approaches are offered for parents having problems with their children;
▶ Incredible Years, which is a behavioural programme for children aged 1–16 years, developed in the USA by Webster-Stratton;
▶ Mellow Parenting, which is a flexible and less tightly defined programme of support for parents.

Evaluation of such programmes suggests that their effectiveness depends on a clearly structured curriculum, active parent participation (including practising ideas and approaches that are unfamiliar) and recognition of practical difficulties, such as working hours, transport and childcare during sessions.[19]

Injury prevention programmes

These are important because accidents and unintentional injuries are the leading cause of death in childhood in the UK and a major cause of morbidity and disability.[20] Young children are more likely to suffer burns, scalds and poisoning; older children are more at risk of fractures and head injuries. Boys are more at risk than girls and there is a relationship between adverse social circumstances and injury risk.

Some single-issue interventions have been shown to be useful; for example, safe packaging of poisons, fitting safety devices to the windows of high-rise apartment blocks, and reducing the temperature of the domestic hot water supply. Environmental changes, such as safer playgrounds and traffic calming schemes, are important in reducing injuries outside the home. Basic training for parents in first aid has obvious attractions and may raise awareness of potential hazards. Health visitors' advice and parent education on a range of hazards, combined with guidance on obtaining and using safety equipment, is effective, but education alone has little impact. Both professionals and parents should use the excellent information available on the web site of the Child Accident Prevention Trust.[21] (*See* Chapters 10–13 for age-related risks.)

BOX 1.5 Examples of effective early intervention programmes

The High/Scope study of the Perry Preschool in Ypsilanti, Michigan, USA, involved a daily 2.5-hour classroom session for 3- to 4-year-old children on weekday mornings and a 1.5-hour home visit to each mother and child on weekday afternoons, for 30 weeks per year. There was one teacher for every six children. When compared with controls, the intervention children had higher IQ scores at the end of this pre-school programme, but this effect disappeared after a few years; however, they had higher school achievement, and in adult life they earned more money and committed fewer crimes.

The American *Head Start* programme began in 1965 and aims to improve the outcomes for poor children. *Early Head Start* provides a variety of services including home visits and centre-based childcare and education to low income families with pregnant women, infants and toddlers. Programmes vary widely in quality, but small to moderate benefits in education and health measures are reported. Benefits were not found among families with multiple risk factors and some such families had worse outcomes than expected.

First Parent Health Visitor Scheme (FPHVS) is for first-time mothers from deprived areas who are offered a programme of regular home visits by a specially trained health visitor who aims to help, support, and advise the mother during the first phase of parenting. It emphasises empowerment, using written materials and cartoons. Families are visited at home antenatally (in the third trimester), at the statutory primary birth visit, at three weeks postnatally, and then every 5 weeks until the infant is 8 months old. Some families continue until 2 years of age. A randomised trial did not show any significant benefits over conventional health visiting.

Dublin Community Mothers' Programme uses volunteer experienced local mothers who advise and support new parents with monthly visits during the first year. Participating mothers appeared to do better on a variety of measures than those receiving only conventional visiting by a nurse.

Nurse-Family Partnership programme was developed by Olds in the USA. This is a high-quality, high-intensity home visiting programme delivered by nurses to high-risk mothers. Key features include a robust theoretical base, detailed guidelines, regular supervision, detailed monitoring of delivery and small case loads (typically the average case load for each visitor was around 20–25 families – barely one-tenth of the typical case load for a UK health visitor). The parents receive up to 13 visits during pregnancy and 47 during the first 2 years of the child's life. Significant long-term benefits have been shown for these mothers and children. Results were less satisfactory when the programme was delivered by non-professional staff.

Sure Start evaluation shows wide variation in local programme content, quality and coverage. Some improvements in a range of measures were found in Sure Start communities and could be related to the quality of the local programme, but so far the impact seems to be modest in relation to the investment made. (*See* discussion on 'hard to reach' families, page 13.)

Research on day care for children under 3 years old suggests that:

- for most children, high quality day care has little effect on language or intellectual development; with high levels of group day care, there may be a modest increase in antisocial behaviour;
- quality day care can be beneficial for children in poor circumstances;
- disadvantaged children are more likely to experience low quality day care. A combination of family disadvantage and low quality care may have negative effects on all aspects of development (*see* page 55).

Research on pre-school education for children over 3 years old shows that:

- pre-school educational experience enhances all-round development;
- duration of attendance and an earlier start are related to better intellectual development;
- some types of pre-school settings are more effective than others in promoting positive child outcomes;
- more effective settings combine education with care and have a high proportion of teachers trained in early child development and therefore promote stronger intellectual benefits;
- a pre-school curriculum that benefits all children (but particularly those from disadvantaged backgrounds) includes an effective intentional curriculum that involves active engagement with children; develops nurturing and emotionally supportive relationships with early childhood staff; integrates childcare and education; responds to cultural diversity; fosters social, emotional and regulatory skills; promotes early literacy and math skills;
- the quality of the home learning environment is more significant for intellectual and social development than parental occupation or qualification.

The inverse care law: 'hard to reach' families

Most parents will access medical care when they think their child is ill, and child health professionals often assume that parents will also welcome advice and support about preventive care and health promotion, but this is not always so. Even well-funded Sure Start local programmes with a substantial investment in their community found that many families were 'hard to reach'. There are many reasons for this (*see* Box 1.6).

The greatest difficulty faced by health professionals in seeking to provide a service for all parents is encapsulated in the inverse care law. This states that people who have the greatest need are those least able to access and make use of healthcare services. Competent 'middle class' families seek out any available expertise when they have any concerns and expect competent and detailed assessment. Professionals respond readily to such requests because meetings are easier to arrange, communication is more straightforward, and advice more likely to be acted on. In addition, professionals often empathise more when they identify with the clients.

Health professionals commonly believe that they know all the children in their 'patch' and are in touch with all or most families. This optimism is probably misplaced. In the first few months of life, screening and immunisation programmes achieve high uptake, but thereafter the coverage of routine health checks decreases as the children age and are generally lower in deprived areas (*see* Figure 1.4). In one deprived area, a comparison of health authority databases, health visitor lists, GP age-sex registers and Sure Start enrolment lists suggested that one-third or more of families were not engaged in any way with preventive and health promotion services.

BOX 1.6 Why do health professionals have difficulty in reaching some families?

Factors in the families:

- high mobility of young families (multiple changes of address);
- parents overwhelmed by problems (debt, poverty, bad housing, difficult neighbours);
- changes of address concealed to escape debts or a violent partner;
- parents returning to work, leaving their baby with a minder;
- lifestyles that don't fit within the hours of the professional working week;
- parents working long or unsocial hours; they are too exhausted to contemplate any additional activities with their children or to meet health professionals unless the child is ill;
- transport to children's facilities is expensive for those on low incomes;
- low level of trust in, or respect for, the health professionals they know;
- previous conflicts with health professionals (arguments about smoking or weaning);
- perception of professionals as intrusive, unsympathetic, authoritarian and out of touch;
- feelings of inadequacy about entering the territory of middle class health professionals;
- phobia of social encounters at children's clinics or health centres;
- fear of exposing poverty, poor quality childcare, abuse or domestic violence to 'prying eyes' of professionals;
- embarrassment over poor reading ability;
- parental mental illness, domestic violence or substance abuse;
- not seeing any need for professional advice about their children.

Factors in the professionals:

- ethnic, cultural and linguistic barriers (in both families and professionals);
- shortages of well-trained staff;
- professional ambivalence about how to allocate their time and how many 'no-access' visits to make before giving up;
- professional fear of being too intrusive or of uncovering problems that have no solution;
- inaccurate record systems (data entry errors, parents changing their or their baby's name);
- professional inertia, reluctance to change ways of working (greater throughput can be achieved with well-organised families).

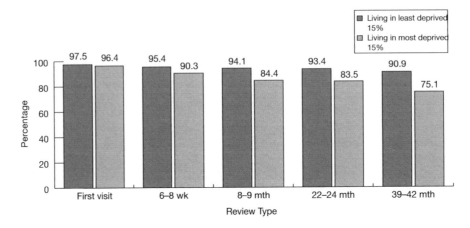

FIGURE 1.4 Histogram showing coverage in relation to age and social class from 0–5 years. In spite of a policy of regular universal reviews, the coverage declined at each successive health check, and declined more steeply for the more deprived social classes. (Courtesy of Simon Fraser, Information Services Division, Scotland; data based on Health Board reports for children born in 1999, to the Child Health Surveillance Programme.)

Intervention programmes, such as those listed in Box 1.5, can be effective for children in poor but functional families who have sufficient personal resources to make use of whatever is on offer; however, the poorest and most deprived families often do not benefit and may even be worse off in areas with active pre-school programmes.[22] Possible explanations for this finding are, first, that they are overwhelmed by services that make demands on them and are unable to respond; and second, that the more capable families make good use of available services, leaving fewer resources for the less competent. The net result is that pre-school programmes can actually widen the gap between the better off and worse off families.[23] Not all interventions are wholly positive.

The Family-Nurse Partnership programme in England aims to reach those parents who are difficult to engage and who are at increased risk of having problems in managing their children.[24] The programme is modelled on, and closely follows, the Nurse-Family Partnership in the USA (page 11).

Groups

Some mothers find support groups unpleasantly stressful. Provision of professional help, from outside a mother's normal social network, can lead her to spend less time with her network, and the normal supportive role of the network can be impaired. Parent training interventions can make parents feel incompetent, and a bad experience with one professional can make a family and their friends disengage from services for years.

INDIVIDUALS AND COMMUNITIES: SOCIAL EXCLUSION, SOCIAL CAPITAL AND COMMUNITY DEVELOPMENT

When the basic essentials of life are insecure, it is extremely difficult to be a good parent (*see* Figure 1.5). All the parents' energy is focused on coping with one day

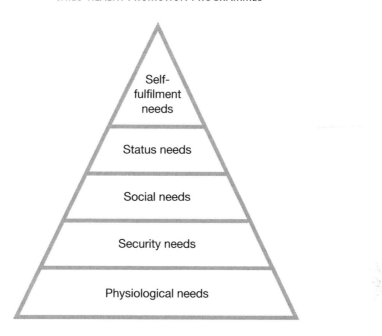

FIGURE 1.5 Maslow's 'Hierarchy of Needs'. People have to meet the essential needs of life before they can address issues such as mutual support, planning their futures or contributing to their community or society.

at a time. One way to improve the lives of children is to make it easier to be a good parent. Being a good parent is more straightforward for those who have an adequate income and a home in a supportive community. Poverty, unemployment, disorganised services in run-down housing estates with high unemployment, shifting population, poor schools, inadequate public transport, vandalism, burglary, violent crime, etc., all affect children both directly and through the negative impact on their parents. The term 'social exclusion' is used in the UK to describe the situation of people living in such circumstances.* It can be defined as the inability of our society to keep all groups and individuals within reach of what we expect as a society and the tendency to push vulnerable and difficult individuals into the least popular places.

Poverty creates chronic stress for parents trying to keep their children safe, well-fed, and properly educated. Poor people experience more adverse life events, and have fewer resources to deal with them. The term 'food insecurity'[25] describes the anxieties of those who cannot be sure that they have enough money to buy food. For many people the cost of achieving recommended dietary intakes is probably unachievable on the national minimum wage. Food insecurity includes running out of food, running out of money to buy food, skipping meals, experiences of going hungry and buying cheaper, less healthy foods because of financial constraints. In one London study, 20% of subjects were classified as suffering food insecurity.

---

* Social exclusion was originally a French concept, referring to the difficulties of disabled people in participating fully in society. In the UK, it includes the disability caused by poverty and disadvantaged circumstances. *See* Cabinet Office. *Reaching Out: An Action Plan on Social Exclusion.* London: HM Government; 2006.

Food-insecure families buy the cheapest available foods, which are often high in carbohydrate and fat, and as a result are more likely to become overweight or obese (*see* page 122). Breakfast clubs have been introduced in many schools as a response to the inadequate diets and family problems experienced by many children and these have several benefits, including improved attendance at school.[26]

Social capital

Material resources are a necessary, but not sufficient, requirement for improving the situation of parents living in poverty. The term 'social capital' describes the intangible wealth that results from mutual trust, good neighbourliness, friendships, relationships, organisations, activities and so on, within a community. 'It is the glue that holds a community together.'[27] High social capital in a community is said to have an influence on health and well-being, independent of any measures of material wealth. Conversely, communities that have little or no social capital are perceived as undesirable and stressful places to live. Neighbourhoods and community relationships are an important influence on how people feel about themselves and their lives, but social capital is a complicated concept; for instance, neighbourhoods with high social cohesion can also be intolerant of individuals who are 'different'. The term 'community' itself means different things to different people. For children, it may refer primarily to their school.

Increasing social capital and developing community resources may have beneficial effects on health – at least, for the majority of residents (but *see* note on 'Head Start' in Box 1.5). The experience gained in a community development project initiated by two health visitors is summarised in Box 1.7. There is no single formula for success, since every community is different and measuring changes reliably is difficult.[28]

Housing

Cold, damp housing in unsavoury and unsafe neighbourhoods is a common complaint of parents, and health professionals are often asked to assist with applications for re-housing or home improvements. This was an important issue in the Beacon project described in Box 1.7. The impact on specific aspects of ill health (e.g. asthma) is unclear, but poor housing in childhood adversely affects health in later life; re-housing reduces use of medical services and the frequency of mental health problems.[29] In strict scientific terms these relationships are complicated; for example, poor health may be the *cause* of reduced income, which in turn may lead to poor housing; but no-one really doubts the importance of good living conditions in bringing up children. If one approaches housing officers in the local authority as fellow professionals, most will be very willing to help, within the constraints of what is available, and to advise on local policies.

BOX 1.7 A community development project

The context
In 1995, the Beacon and Old Hill estate (pop. 6000) in the council ward of Penwerris, Falmouth, Cornwall, was a 'no go area' for the police; drug dealing, crime and vandalism were spiralling out of control, and the community had become disconnected from the statutory agencies. Mothers were fighting mothers on school premises, breaking bones, and children as young as four were stoning each other. Of 23 child protection registrations

---

in the council district of Carrick, 19 lived on the estate. More than 30% of households were living in poverty; there was a high unemployment rate; more than 50% of the 1500 homes were without central heating; and the illness rate was 18% above the national average. People living there described feeling 'hopeless' and talked of a lack of community spirit.

Initiating change
Two health visitors, deeply concerned by the escalating decline and unable to cope with increasing demands of their case load, decided that individual health promotion would have limited impact in such a setting. They recognised that community involvement would be key to changing the situation.

What was done?
From their intimate knowledge of this estate, the health visitors identified 20 tenants who they considered had the necessary attributes to engage their peers. They were invited to work in *joint* partnership with the HVs and statutory agencies that had yet to be engaged. Of the 20 people, 5 agreed to participate and they proved to be key to the engagement of the whole estate. They produced a hand delivered newsletter, knocked on every door of 1008 homes and invited all households to attend a 'listening' meeting. Residents established that the main problems affecting their health were crime, poor housing, and unemployment, together with the historical failure of the statutory agencies to address these issues.

The Beacon Community Regeneration Partnership was set up with people from the community as well as from police, education, health and the council. Health visitors worked with lead residents in identifying training needs, submitting grant applications (resulting in self-generated funding) and forming and maintaining a constituted committee. Visible quick wins were identified; dog fouling was an important issue and the council agreed to provide more dog waste bins.

The outcomes
By 2000:

- community activities for all age groups were introduced, including a new skateboard park;
- the overall crime rate fell by 50%;
- affordable central heating and external cladding were installed in over 90% of the properties;
- child protection registrations fell by 42%;
- postnatal depression fell by 70%;
- the educational attainment of 10- to 11-year-old boys rose by 100%;
- the unemployment rate was down 71%;
- breastfeeding rates were increased by 20%;
- a strong sense of community spirit was reported.

Why did it work?
It worked because:

- facilitative leadership from the outset was by health visitors known and trusted by the community;

- self-selection of key residents by HVs was made from a position of reciprocal trust and respect;
- the enablement of a lead role was for residents rather than professionals (the community retained ownership of the process);
- the partnerships were based on what the community wanted to change, *not* around money that was available;
- the partnerships were not forced (at first the police refused to come onto the estate!) but a community policeman began to attend and still attends all the meetings;
- project management skills were drawn from the community;
- it was ensured that every meeting had more people from the community than from agencies, to preserve the community voice and provide a critical mass of residents;
- every win was celebrated (photographs and success stories were widely disseminated).

From Durie R, Wyatt K. and Stuteley H. Community Regeneration and Complexity. In: Kernick, D. editor: *Complexity and Healthcare Organisation: A view from the street.* Oxford: Radcliffe Publishing; 2004. Reproduced with the permission of the copyright holder.

Benefits

Some parents find it difficult to negotiate the complexities of obtaining all the benefits to which they are entitled. The Citizens Advice Bureau[30] is a UK organisation that gives independent advice to clients on matters such as welfare and benefit entitlements, housing problems, debt management, legal advice, consumer rights and public services and utilities. It tackles poverty by enabling people to improve their financial circumstances and avail themselves of their rights. In a few areas, locating a bureau in a primary care setting has been found to be very useful for young families. A positive well-informed attitude among health professionals facilitates the use of the service.

CHILD HEALTH PROGRAMMES: PRACTICAL ISSUES

A service that is friendly, welcoming, culturally sensitive, employs local people, is easily accessible at convenient times and allows drop-in visits as well as fixed appointments is likely to be more popular with parents. Working parents welcome flexibility of appointment times and some families may only be able obtain non-urgent care by taking time off work unless services take account of local needs and lifestyles. Feedback from parents shows that a telephone answering service and a prompt response to telephone requests for advice are essential.

Community nursing teams, which have geographically defined responsibilities, are more likely to be aware of arriving and departing families, but on the other hand access to the general practitioner's records is often more difficult if staff are not directly associated with one general practice. This may become more difficult if changes in health service structures weaken the links of health visitors with GPs. Access to and regular updating of population and general practice registers are crucial so that all staff know who and where the children are and can identify children who have not received basic services. This is an important issue with hard to reach families.

Policy development at local level

Service plans for child health promotion should follow national recommendations (*see* page 196). Local guidelines for child health services are essential to meet the particular needs of children and families in the area. They should define the recommended pathways of referral for the more common clinical problems identified in everyday practice. Multi-disciplinary input is vital and shared training and study days are desirable, so that consistent advice is given by all staff (health visitors, doctors, midwives, practice nurses and receptionists, school nurses and nursery and playgroup leaders).

Unqualified staff – para-professionals – are also employed in many areas. Professionals are not essential in every situation, but those carrying out a task must have the necessary competencies to do so. Lay workers with specific expertise, for example in breastfeeding support, can be a particularly valuable resource. The needs of some families can be met by non-qualified staff that live in the community they serve, so they are familiar with its lifestyle and its problems. These staff usually need initial and ongoing training, which must be funded. Most can manage only small case-loads and need professional support to cope with stressful problems, particularly if they themselves are subject to similar life stresses. Some families may be reluctant to disclose personal problems to people they know locally. Complex long-term early intervention and support programmes seem to be less effective if provided by non-qualified staff when compared to professionals.

Premises

Community services can be provided in a wide variety of settings. Safe access, including facilities for the disabled, and car parking, are essential. If general practice premises are used, there should be set times when healthy children are not in contact with patients who are unwell and waiting to see a doctor. Timing is important as many mothers will have older children at school or playschool. A few robust, safe and interesting toys help to create a child-friendly atmosphere. Space to park pushchairs and prams is important. If health education material is displayed, it needs to be kept clean and up to date. A few clinics have invited the local Citizens Advice Bureau to provide a service and this has been welcomed by parents.

Essential equipment includes scales suitable for weighing babies, toddlers and older children, a height-measuring device, a mat for measuring length in babies (*see* page 134) and a tape-measure for measuring head circumference. Hearing and vision testing equipment should not be purchased unless recommended by local policy and those who are going to use them must be specifically trained to do so.

Toys and books are essential. If a standardised testing kit for eliciting developmental skills is used, items from the kit must be kept for that purpose and a separate set should be used to secure the child's attention and cooperation.

PARENT-HELD RECORDS: THE PERSONAL CHILD HEALTH RECORD

The introduction of parent-held records was welcomed by parents and professionals. National agreement has been reached on the format and core content of a Personal

Child Health Record (PCHR); this has been endorsed by the Department of Health and is widely available, though there are often local variations in layout and content. There should be a page prominently displayed at the front of the PCHR, setting out key facts about the record and the information in it (*see* Box 1.8).[31]

BOX 1.8 The Personal Child Health Record (PCHR)

The PCHR is the property of the parent as is the information in it. To be used to its full potential, all professionals and carers involved with a child should recognise this and should use the record at every opportunity. The following information sets out these principles.

This record is the main record of your child's health, growth and development and therefore we ask you to keep it in a safe place. The record is to be used jointly by you and others caring for your child. **Bring this book with you whenever you visit:**

- the child health clinic
- your health visitor
- your family doctor
- a hospital emergency or outpatients department
- a therapist (e.g. speech and language therapist)
- the dentist
- the school nurse
- any other health appointment.

You may like to show it to other carers of your child such as:

- childminder
- playgroup leader
- nursery school teacher
- primary school teacher
- and anyone else who cares for your child.

How we handle information

We wish to make sure that your child has the opportunity to have his/her immunisations and health checks when they are due. We also want to be able to plan and provide any other services your child needs. Therefore, we enter some of your child's details from this record on to our computer system. We treat this information as strictly confidential and only release it to:

- yourself as parent(s)
- your child's healthcare professionals, who work directly with your family.

This information may be used anonymously so that we can plan services for all children.

We will not normally release any information that could be linked to your child to any other person or organisation without seeking your permission first. However, it is sometimes necessary to use this sort of information for audit purposes and public health reasons, such as monitoring the effectiveness and safety of vaccines. We are subject to the terms of the Data Protection Act 1998 in respect of personal data held by us. **You have the right under the Act to ask to see details of the information held regarding your child.**

Experience to date is that parents, particularly first time and teenage mothers, welcome this system. Parents are less likely to lose the record than are the professionals. Additional health education material is sometimes included although it does not replace the Department of Health book, *Birth to Five*, which contains most of the information that parents need.

The PCHR has *potential* advantages:

▶ It makes the information about the child's health and development easily accessible to the parents, who are the people who need it most. Thus it is a useful vehicle for health education, particularly specific advice relevant to their child's immediate needs.

▶ It accompanies the child to hospital appointments and school; it goes with him when he changes doctors or moves to another district and simplifies communication between professionals, both for routine and emergency or out-of-hours care.

▶ It reduces the existing duplication of records between health visitors, GPs and other health services, although it is still essential to negotiate how the information held by the general practice and the community nursing team can best be shared.

▶ It encourages openness between professionals and parents. Parents expect to be kept informed of any professional concerns about their child and resent any secrecy. The NHS Plan specifies that parents should have copies of important letters about their child – indeed, for some years this has been the policy in many child development centres and paediatric units. Nevertheless, there are occasions when a confidential file may need to be maintained; for example, where a possibility of child neglect or abuse is being considered (Chapter 4 – Safeguarding and promoting the welfare of children. *See* page 58).

PCHRs have been found to be less used by more disadvantaged families and those where the child has been in hospital. Since parents are more likely to take the record seriously if it is used by health professionals, it is important that GPs, health visitors and school nurses record the opinions, advice and information given to parents in the PCHR. It should therefore be used by all healthcare professionals in both routine and emergency situations and, preferably, used as the main record – yet it must also be accessible to parents. These sometimes conflicting requirements present practical difficulties, which may only be fully resolved when web-based electronic records become widely available.

HOW DO YOU KNOW IF YOU ARE MAKING A DIFFERENCE?

Many of the aims of community child health teams are long-term and the desired outcomes depend on many other factors that are outside the control of health professionals. This makes it difficult for staff to assess the impact of their efforts, but to some extent this can be addressed by specifying short-term goals as proxy measures for the long-term aims. Goals need to be SMART: Specific, Measurable, Achievable, Realistic and Timely. Data collection should, as far as possible, follow agreed national guidelines, both for reasons of economy in software development and managing computerised databases, and to facilitate comparisons between teams and districts. The following are examples of aims and self-audit questions that might be agreed by primary care teams; however, an audit of any one of these is time consuming unless the team maintains and can access a well-designed information system.

Coverage and engagement. This is crucial (*see* page 13). Does the team know all the children for whom they are responsible? What checks are in place to ensure that details are available of children moving in or out of the locality? How many children are there in the locality whose families are not in touch or not using any preventive healthcare or pre-school services? How many no-access visits and other unsuccessful contacts are attempted and what is done to ascertain the reasons? Do children receive screening tests and immunisations at the recommended times? How do parents perceive the service? How many children, who were referred for assessment by specialist services (e.g. speech and language therapy, audiology, physiotherapy, etc.), took up their appointments and completed whatever investigations and interventions were recommended by the specialist(s)?

Immunisation uptake. Even in the face of media scares and negative publicity, immunisation rates are very dependent on good organisation and professional commitment (*see* page 153).

Newborn screening uptake. The uptake of the newborn 'blood spot' test should approach 100%. Rates for the hearing screen may not be quite as high, but follow-up of those not having this screen must be carefully monitored (*see* page 181).

Other screening tests. Uptakes for specified screening visits and procedures should be monitored. By definition, a screening test is considered to be sufficiently robust and important that it should be offered to every child.

Breastfeeding rates and duration. It is important to monitor intention to breast-feed, initiation and duration (*see* page 97).

Public Service Agreement targets for Sure Start. These are subject to change as Sure Start programmes become incorporated into children's centres; however, the original objectives are likely always to be relevant. The desired outcomes of pre-school services include enhanced language development, fewer behaviour problems and reductions in child abuse and in obesity – but these are very difficult to measure except in a formal research programme.

Smoking cessation. Even a modest reduction in the number of parents who smoke pays dividends for children (*see* page 30).

Dental status. Dental health is not only important in its own right (*see* page 122), but is probably a good proxy measure of the impact of dietary advice in general.

Safety equipment. If there is a loan scheme for home or car safety equipment, how well is it used and by whom?

Critical incident reviews. Examples of incidents that might usefully be reviewed include episodes of child abuse, avoidable injuries, cases of unexplained infant death and sudden infant death syndrome. Late diagnoses of major disabling conditions, such as cerebral palsy or severe hearing loss, and delays in identifying undescended testes or congenital heart disease, might be studied as well. It may also be useful to review how much worry and unproductive investigations are generated by over-diagnosis and over-referral.

REFERENCES

1 www.everychildmatters.gov.uk
2 Shonkoff JP, Phillips DA, editors. *Neurons to Neighbourhoods: The Science of Early Child Development.* Washington, DC: National Academy Press; 2000. Available at: www.nap.edu/openbook.php?isbn=0309069882 (accessed 13 November 2008).
3 Blair M, Hall D. From health surveillance to health promotion: the changing focus in preventive children's services. *Arch Dis Child.* 2006; **91**: 730–5.
4 Caspi A, Sugden K, Moffat TE, *et al.* Influence of life stress on depression: moderation by a polymorphism in the 5-HTT gene. *Science.* 2003; **301**: 386–9.
5 Crofts DJ, Bowns IR, Williams TS, *et al.* Hitting the target: equitable distribution of health visitors across case loads. *J Publ Health Med.* 2000; **22**: 295–301. *See also* Appleton JV. Establishing the validity and reliability of clinical practice guidelines used to identify families requiring increased health visitor support. *Public Health.* 1997; **111**: 107–13.
6 Pollock JI, Horrocks S, Emond AM, *et al.* Health and social factors for health visitor case load weighting: reliability, accuracy and current and potential use. *Health Soc Care Comm.* 2002; **10**(2): 82–90.
7 Hallam A. *The Effectiveness of Interventions to Address Health Inequalities in The Early Years: a review of relevant literature.* 2008. Available at: www.scotland.gov.uk/socialresearch (accessed 15 November 2008).
8 Glass N. Sure Start: the development of an early intervention programme for young children in the United Kingdom. *Child Soc.* 1999; **13**: 257–64.
9 Sure Start. Available at: www.surestart.gov.uk (accessed 16 November 2008). *See* also Evaluation Data. Available at: www.ness.bbk.ac.uk (accessed 16 November 2008). *See* also Melhuish E, Belsky J, Leyland AH, *et al.* Effects of fully-established Sure Start Local Programmes on 3-year-old children and their families living in England: a quasi-experimental observational study. *Lancet.* 2008; **372**: 1641–8. For Sure Start Children's Centres, *see* www.surestart.gov.uk/surestartservices/settings/surestartchildrenscentres
10 *Rethinking School Readiness.* 2008. Available at: www.rch.org.au/ccch/policybriefs.cfm (accessed 15 November 2008).
11 *The High/Scope Perry Preschool Study Through Age 40.* Available at: www.highscope.org/Research/PerryProject/PerryAge40SumWeb.pdf (accessed 15 November 2008).
12 US Department of Health and Human Services, Administration for Children and Families. *Head Start Impact Study: First Year Findings.* Washington, DC: US Department of Health and Human Services, Administration for Children and Families; 2005 (May).
13 Ludwig J, Miller DL. Does Head Start improve children's life chances? Evidence from a regression discontinuity design. *Working Paper 11702.* Available at: www.nber.org/papers/w11702 (accessed 15 November 2008).
14 Emond A, Pollock J, Deave T, *et al.* An evaluation of the first Parent Health Visitor Scheme. *Arch Dis Child.* 2002; **86**(3): 150–7.
15 Johnson Z, Molloy B, Scallan E, *et al.* Community mothers' programme: seven-year follow-up of a randomized controlled trial of non-professional intervention in parenting. *J Public Health Med.* 2000; **22**(3): 337–42.
16 Olds DL, Hill PL, O'Brien R. Taking preventive intervention to scale: the nurse-family partnership. *Cogn Behav Pract.* 2003; **10**: 278–90.
17 Belsky J, Melhuish E, Barnes J, *et al.* National Evaluation of Sure Start Research Team. Effects of Sure Start local programmes on children and families: early findings from a quasi-experimental cross sectional study abstract. *BMJ.* 2006; **332**(7556): 1476–82.
18 Sylva K, Pugh G. Transforming the early years in England. *Oxford Rev Educ.* 2005; **31**(1): 11–27. *See also Rethinking School Readiness* Policy brief No 10 2008. Available at: www.rch.org.au/ccch/policybriefs.cfm (accessed 17 November 2008).
19 Scott S. Parent training programmes. In: Rutter M, Taylor E, editors. *Child and Adolescent Psychiatry.* London: Wiley Blackwell; 2005.

20 Kendrick D, Barlow J, Hampshire A, *et al.* Parenting interventions for the prevention of unintentional injuries in childhood. *Cochrane Database Syst Rev.* 2007; Oct 17; **4**: CD 006020. *See* also Towner E, Dowswell T, Errington G, *et al. Injuries in children aged 0–14 years and inequalities.* London: Health Development Agency; 2005.

21 www.capt.org.uk

22 Belsky, *et al.*, op. cit.

23 Ceci SJ, Papierno PB. The rhetoric and reality of gap closing. *Am Psychol.* 2005; **60**: 149–60.

24 www.everychildmatters.gov.uk/parents/healthledsupport/

25 Tingay RS, Tan CJ, Tan NC-W, *et al.* Food insecurity and low income in an English inner city. *J Public Health Med.* 2003; **25**: 156–9.

26 Shemilt I, Harvey I, Shepstone L, *et al.* A national evaluation of school breakfast clubs: evidence from a cluster randomized controlled trial and an observational analysis. *Child Care Hlth Dev.* 2004; **30**: 413–27.

27 Putnam R. *Bowling Alone.* New York: Simon & Schuster; 2001.

28 Durie R, Wyatt K, Stuteley H. Community regeneration and complexity. In: Kernick D, editor. *Complexity and Healthcare Organisation: a view from the street.* Oxford: Radcliffe Publishing; 2004. More details and research issues arising from this work are available at: www.healthcomplexity.net (accessed 17 November 2008).

29 Shaw M. Housing and public health. *Annu Rev Public Health.* 2004; **25**: 397–418. *See* also Thomson H, Petticrew M, Morrison D. Health effects of housing improvement: systematic review of intervention studies. *BMJ.* 2001; **323**: 187–90. *See* also Thomson H, Morrison D, Petticrew M. The health impacts of housing-led regeneration: a prospective controlled study. *J Epidemiol Community Health.* 2007; **61**: 211–14.

30 Reading R, Steel S, Reynolds S. Citizens advice in primary care for families with young children. *Child: Care, Health and Development.* 2002; **28**: 39–45. *See* also web site of the National Association of Citizens Advice Bureau www.citizensadvice.org.uk (accessed 18 December 2008).

31 Walton S, Bedford H, Dezateux C, *et al.* Use of personal child health records in the UK: findings from the Millennium Cohort Study. *BMJ.* 2006; **332**: 269–70. *See* also Walton S, Bedford H. Parents' use and views of the national standard Personal Child Health Record: a survey in two primary care trusts. *Child Care Health Dev.* 2007; **33**(6): 744–8.

CHAPTER 2

Communication and consultation

CHAPTER CONTENTS

A consultation may be parent- or professional-initiated, and it is often easier to consider them separately, as we have done here. Many of the principles apply to both and this chapter should be read with that in mind. Box 2.1 summarises some general points about giving advice.

A MENTAL CHECKLIST

Every consultation and contact, whatever its reason, offers the opportunity to take stock of how the child is doing. Parents expect and welcome this because they often see it as one of the main reasons for providing a universal children's health-promoting service. It is worth developing the habit of an instant 'checklist' with every child you see. With practice, this can be done in a matter of seconds. Ask yourself:

- Does this child look well?
- If not, does he show signs of acute or of chronic illness?
- Does he look physically normal? Are there any unusual physical features?
- Is he within the range of expected height and weight for his age?
- Is his development within the normal range; that is, is he doing what one would expect for his age?
- Does he show signs of any unhappiness, anxiety or distress beyond what might be expected for the situation?
- Is his relationship with, and response to, the parent appropriate for his age and the situation?
- Is he suitably dressed for the weather and generally well cared for?
- Does the parent look well (physically and emotionally)?

THE PARENT-INITIATED CONSULTATION

The consultation is at the heart of any child health professional's practice. The most familiar type of consultation is where the parent requests advice because of a perceived problem with their child or their circumstances. The relationship is clearly defined – the 'client' seeks out the professional and initiates the process; the professional tries to resolve the problem within the limits of their ability and available knowledge (*see* Box 2.2).

Problem solving

This is most likely to be successful when it is a shared enterprise. You listen to the problem and offer a suggestion as to what might be a sensible course of action, based on your knowledge and experience. You are prepared to discuss and modify your advice if it proves ineffective or unacceptable. You review the outcome jointly with the parent at follow-up. This is the usual model when advising about emotional, behavioural and developmental problems. When applied to parents, it effectively turns the parent into a co-therapist who carries out therapeutic intervention and observes results, which they report back to you.

Advocacy

Professionals are also sometimes asked to act as advocates for parents. Problems with housing, benefits and educational assessment procedures are three common issues (*see* Chapters 1 and 15). Although these often seem to be beyond the expertise and role of health staff, a willingness to offer guidance and facilitate access to whatever help is available may be a pre-requisite to, or at least a big help in, building a closer relationship with the parents. It is often tempting to avoid issues for which no service or solution is available, but if the professional response is seen as negative or unhelpful in an area that is uppermost in parents' minds, it will be very difficult to address more sensitive or intimate topics.

BOX 2.1 General principles to be followed when giving advice

- Advice should be seen to be **logical, relevant, and sensitive**. This means that you have to be seen to acquaint yourself with the problem by taking a history, conducting a physical or developmental assessment where relevant, and, if possible, witnessing the problematical behaviour for yourself.
- Advice should also be relevant to the **stage in the child's life**. For example, developmental concepts like 'turn-taking' behaviour, or the process of language acquisition, are interesting to parents if explained in simple terms and demonstrated at the relevant stage in the child's development.
- **Be practical.** The parents have to be able to carry out your advice. Also be **specific.** Avoid vacuous exhortations such as 'Be more consistent'. If you cannot think how to be specific, ask the parent: 'Suppose I said you ought to be more consistent. How would you put that into practice in real life?'
- **Demonstrate** ways of dealing with behavioural and developmental problems, rather than just describing them. Role-playing can be useful and fun. Where necessary, find other parents, nursery nurses or playgroup leaders who can help the parent to learn how to play with and teach a young child.
- Rather than giving advice to stop doing something give **positive advice** to do

---

something different instead. This means saying 'Go out of the room when you feel like shouting at him', rather than 'Stop shouting at him'.

- **Ensure you are understood.** Use specific examples that you have gathered from your experience (or, better still, specific problems on the parent's mind) to illustrate your points. Check the parent understands what you have said ('Do you know what I mean?', 'Can you tell me what you think I've just said?', etc.).
- **Limit the amount** of advice given at any one session. If it is complex, **write it down** and give it to the parents, checking that they can read your writing. Record your suggestions in the Personal Child Health Record (PCHR) (*see* page 20).
- **Try to understand parents' doubts** about the advice given and the reasons for non-compliance.
- **Use a range of devices** to develop an understanding with parents: for example, illustrate that their child's problem is a common developmental stage by giving an example from your experience of another similar child; invite parents to keep a diary as a way of gaining insight into when and why problems occur; use a screening test as an instrument to explain why you think a child has or hasn't got a problem (*see* page 177); follow up hunches ('I get the feeling that you . . .') and cues given by parents ('You said just now that . . . and I was wondering if you meant . . .'). This calls for a respectful curiosity about people's lives and why they make the decisions they do.
- **Time your advice** and don't overwhelm parents with demands that they cannot handle. In particular, balance the undoubted importance of helping parents to stop smoking with the stress they may be under at a particular time.
- **Reassurance is not always reassuring!** Parents who have some concern about their child may be quite prepared to accept that (a) their GP does not know whether there is a problem or not; and (b) that the best course of action is to wait and see. They do *not* like to be told that there is nothing wrong or that they are worrying without reason, when they can see themselves that their child has some symptom, sign or anomaly that is not observed in other children of the same age. It *is* reassuring for them to know that their worries are being taken seriously.
- **Don't give unnecessary advice.** It reduces the parents' self-confidence.
- **Praise what they are doing** whenever possible; it is much better than simply advising them to do it.
- **Find out whether your advice is contrary to the way** their parents or other people in their culture do things. If it is, you need to explain why your spoken suggestion is more reliable than a method they have actually seen working.
- **Use peer groups.** Many young or disadvantaged parents relate more easily to peers in similar social circumstances than to health professionals, who are inevitably more middle class in their orientation. Organisations like Newpin enable parents to share experiences and provide mutual support, which may promote better child rearing and reduce the risks of neglect and abuse.

Social support

People with worries or problems often refer to a relative, colleague or friend as being 'supportive', yet support is a difficult concept to define, study and measure, particularly when it is provided by professionals. Some people value a supportive relationship with a professional on a long-term basis; whereas for others this is only helpful during periods of exceptional stress. There is a risk of creating undue dependency on the professional and in order to avoid this it may be more profitable in the long run to help the parent(s) build supportive networks among other parents, friends or relatives. For some people, this can be very difficult and they may need help to establish any peer support or friendships.

BOX 2.2 Good practice in consultation

- Listen to the parents' story in their own words and avoid interrupting if possible (on average, doctors interrupt their patients' account in less than 30 seconds!).
- Initial questions should be broad and open.
- Use focused and closed questions to get specific information or exclude possibilities.
- If the parent asks a question while you're talking, stop and answer it straight away.
- Invite clarification if something is not clear. If the parent looks puzzled, or frowns, or looks away, find out why before going on.
- A 'genogram' is useful. Map out who is who in the family and how they are related. This can be used to clarify awkward points, like uncertainty over who is the father of the child or whether there are tensions between family members.
- Use the ICE check: *Ideas* about what they think is wrong; *Concerns* about what the future might hold or what might be going to happen next; *Expectations* as to what they hope to get from the consultation and what solutions might be acceptable.
- For behavioural problems and other unexplained episodic behaviour: use the ABC check: *Antecedents* – what happens before the episode; *Behaviour* – what is observed; *Consequences* – what happens afterwards (*see* page 273).
- With young children, talk to the parents first and then to the child; use closed questions initially and don't pressurise the child to talk. Depending on age, you can ask about who lives at home, about school and about friends.
- Use a final check to ensure nothing has been missed: 'Is there anything else you want to mention?'
- If you need more information, don't be afraid to say so: you can ask the parents to keep a diary (*see* page 312); say that you want to speak with nursery or playgroup leaders; discuss the case with a colleague. The parents will probably look up on the internet any terms you use; there is no reason why you shouldn't do the same!

THE PROFESSIONAL-INITIATED CONSULTATION: HEALTH PROMOTION

Health promotion has several inter-related dimensions (*see* Chapter 1). Here we are mainly concerned with one-to-one health promotion with parents of young children. This often involves more complicated relationships than in parent-initiated consultations. A large proportion of preventive healthcare and health promotion for young children is initiated by professionals and this changes the nature of the relationship between professional and parent.

What do parents expect?

Most new parents are grateful for basic information and advice about basic baby care, immunisation, feeding, etc., but they do not necessarily welcome what they fear may become a more intrusive or authoritarian relationship. Health visitors are still perceived by some parents as hygiene inspectors or as child abuse police.

What are professionals aiming to do?

Child health promotion programmes have many different aims and objectives (*see* Chapter 1). Some of these are defined by policy-makers and managers rather than by the individual practitioner, who may not share them or may consider that they are not relevant to the immediate needs of the parent with whom they are working. Professionals may be more interested in small but important changes in the lives of individuals.

Access

You cannot begin to create a relationship in which health promotion can be undertaken until you obtain access. This has two aspects. The first is physical access: you need an opportunity to meet the parent(s), preferably by entry to their own territory at home, but alternatively in a clinic or other premises. In order to achieve that, the first step is to 'market' the service on offer. You need to present the service as something you and your colleagues are proud of. Such a service would have continuity from pregnancy through delivery and infancy; it would be delivered by smart, confident professionals, who respect the views and worries of parents; it would have warm welcoming premises. The organisation of clinics and services would take account of the lifestyles of local people.

Establishing contact with parents is not enough on its own; you also need 'mental access'. Many parents will accept that their child will be seen for routine procedures by healthcare staff and they may share their anxieties about material needs and practical problems, but this is no guarantee that they will permit access to their more private personal concerns and worries. Most people will only share such private information with a professional who has earned their trust and respect and who is capable of sensitive observation and empathic questioning. Unless such a relationship is achieved, it will be possible only to deliver the basic routines of care, such as immunisation or weighing; little health promotion will take place.

Often the parents who could benefit most from pre-school support and intervention for their child have the greatest difficulty in making use of such services. This is known as the 'inverse care' law. Interviews with parents who have been 'hard to reach' reveal a number of obstacles and concerns that are relevant to the ways professionals practise (*see* page 13).

Modes and styles

One-to-one work with a parent involves switching between several different modes. Perhaps the simplest is a **linear hierarchy**. This is where you are the expert, telling the parent quite firmly and clearly what to do; there is a well-recognised practice; and you are quite clear what should be done. Advising on how to manage febrile convulsions, or explaining immunisation or screening programmes, are common examples. You may also need to adopt this style when dealing with concerns about child protection or with a parent who is not coping.

Analyses of tape-recorded encounters between community nurses or health visitors and their clients have shown that many staff tend to follow this hierarchical approach in a large part of their work, giving advice, which, though important, is often unasked for and gets in the way of hearing about the parents' immediate concerns. Some health professionals are more comfortable with this authoritative style of communicating than with any other. This tendency is reinforced by the pressure on them to follow an agenda of tasks and questions set for them by policy-makers.

The example of smoking

All health professionals and most parents know that smoking is bad for parents and for their children, but advising parents to give up smoking, though justified, is rarely successful.[1] Helping parents to quit requires a variety of approaches, combining clarity of information with an understanding of the individual's motivation and the extent of their dependence on smoking (*see* Box 2.3).

BOX 2.3 What every health professional should know about smoking

- Cigarette smoking is the single biggest avoidable cause of death and disability in developed countries. Of the people that smoke, half will die prematurely, losing an average 8 years of life. Smokers aged under 50 have a more than five-fold increase in risk of heart attack. For smokers who quit before age 35, survival is about the same as that for non-smokers. Poor people are more likely to smoke and much less likely to quit than the affluent.
- Smoking in pregnancy is associated with increased rates of fetal and perinatal death, reduced birth weight for gestational age, and behavioural problems, such as attention deficit disorder.
- Mothers' self-reporting to professionals of how much they smoke is unreliable.
- Exposure to cigarette smoke increases the infant's risk of cot death (*see* page 30), chest infections, otitis media and meningitis. Parents or visitors do not significantly reduce the child's exposure by smoking outside. Passive smoking in cars is also damaging to children.
- Nicotine is a more addictive substance than cocaine or heroin. Nicotine is a stimulant, but tolerance soon develops. The effect is the same as that produced by other drugs of misuse (such as amphetamines and cocaine). Cigarette smoking is a manifestation of nicotine addiction. Smokers regulate the way they puff and inhale to achieve their desired nicotine dose, which is why 'cutting down' or using low tar cigarettes has little benefit.
- Absorption of cigarette smoke from the lung sends a dose of nicotine that reaches the brain within 10–16 seconds. Smokers need regular cigarettes to maintain nicotine concentrations. Overnight, the blood levels drop to close to those of non-smokers.
- Withdrawal symptoms make it hard to quit: irritability, restlessness, feeling miserable, impaired concentration, and increased appetite. They begin within hours of the last cigarette and are at their worst in the first week, resolving over 3–4 weeks. Hunger can persist for longer.
- All health professionals should ask smokers, 'How do you feel about your smoking?' and give simple brief advice routinely to all smokers. Most pregnant women know they ought to stop smoking, so asking about smoking and their partner's smoking is unlikely to cause offence.
- It is important to assess motivation to quit, and the degree of dependence on cigarettes, indicated by the number smoked per day and how early the first cigarette is smoked after waking.
- Smoking cessation services may offer interventions through groups or individually.

The combination of behavioural support and either nicotine replacement therapy or bupropion is more effective than either alone.

- Nicotine replacement therapy can be used in pregnancy and during breastfeeding. It is suggested that short-acting formulations should be used. Bupropion is not recommended as there is no safety evidence.
- Health professionals who smoke are very poor role models for their patients/clients!
- Undue pressure on clients to stop smoking is counter-productive; motivational interviewing approaches are more likely to work (*see* below).

Partnership: the 'empowerment' model

Most health promotion consultations will contain an element of giving expert advice and information, but the aim of health promotion is not merely to educate but also, when appropriate, to shape and change parent behaviour. This cannot be done simply by telling them to do or not do certain things.[2] It is necessary to establish, with the parent(s), what their needs are and to develop an understanding with them that change can be achieved and may be worthwhile. The relationship should be established on equal terms, rather than with the professional in the dominant role. The aim is to enable the parent to develop as an individual and to increase their confidence and abilities in child rearing, so they can make appropriate decisions and take action about their own and their children's health.

Partnerships are dependent on mutual trust and respect. Hilton Davis[*] suggests that there are four key qualities needed to achieve this:

- **unconditional positive regard**[†] – valuing parents as people, and assuming competence and strength, not weakness and incapacity; assuming that parents *are* genuinely trying and have good intentions;
- **genuineness** – attempting to be yourself, honestly and openly, not hiding behind a professional façade;
- **empathy** – understanding the viewpoint of the person you are talking to;
- **humility** – allowing the person seeking help to play the lead role.

Staff who seek to develop these qualities are more likely to be perceived as useful and helpful, although the result will often be increased emotional demands made by parents and the sharing of often complicated and apparently insoluble life problems. Professionals may need to 'de-brief' with experienced colleagues to avoid being overwhelmed by the troubles of their clients.

One practical implication of partnership working is that decisions such as where and when to meet a parent or when to terminate a professional–parent relationship should be agreed between the parties, and not made solely by the professional. Casual termination of supportive relationships, and frequent changes of health professional with no hand-over and loss of continuity, are insulting to the parent and devalue the staff and the service.

---

* Hilton Davis is Professor of Child Health Psychology, London.

† A term derived from the work of Carl Rogers (1902–87) – a leading American psychologist and psychotherapist.

Motivational interviewing

This is a cognitive-behavioural approach that aims to help individuals identify and change behaviours likely to adversely affect their health.[3] The technique originated in addiction therapy, but now has wide application in many fields, including health promotion. It emphasises five principles (which overlap with those set out in the previous paragraphs):

1 expressing empathy;
2 avoiding argument (don't encourage the individual to rehearse all the arguments for not changing their behaviour);
3 supporting self-efficacy (help individuals to re-frame negative thoughts in a positive way);
4 rolling with resistance (instead of arguing, try to gently challenge the underlying thought processes that need to change);
5 developing discrepancy (defining the difference between where the individual is now and where they want to be so they can generate their own achievable goals).

Staff who have learned and applied motivational interviewing skills report a considerable improvement in their ability to work with clients, while clients confirm that the approach results in a better working relationship with the professionals.

Stages of change

The 'stages of change' model is a way of describing how individuals approach health issues like giving up smoking.[3] It recognises that some people have not seriously thought about whether they should stop; some know they should, but have not made any serious effort to do so; and some are ready to make the attempt. It is easier to provide a service for those in the latter group, but health professionals need to adopt different approaches for those who have not reached that stage.

Providing information

Parents want information in many different situations. The PCHR and the publication *Birth to Five*[4] may be sufficient for many parents, but more is needed if the child has any medical or developmental disorder. Parents may want:

▶ general information about health, illness and disability in general, entitlements and local services, and specific information relevant to their child's problem;
▶ information about voluntary groups and how to find the most relevant one;
▶ details of schemes that provide parents the opportunity of meeting others facing similar problems;
▶ guidance on how to assess the reliability of information (e.g. rejecting out-of-date books or web sites, checking the credentials of those who advise voluntary groups, and being aware of the wide range of severity even within specific conditions) (*see* Box 2.4).

BOX 2.4 Medical information on the internet – guidelines for parents

Families with a child who has a disability or health condition often use the internet to search for information and support.

Be careful when looking on the internet

- You may come across information which is upsetting to read – most information about conditions includes a spectrum of how someone might be affected including the most severe cases.
- If the professionals involved in your child's care seem unsure of the underlying condition it can be tempting to do your own research. Many conditions share features and you may come across something that sounds just like your child. Be wary of this. You risk going down the wrong route entirely.
- Always go back to the health professionals and ask them to relate the information you have found to your child.

Assessing the quality of information

Expert information on conditions, including rare disorders, can be found from verifiable sources such as universities, government libraries or hospitals and the information is often posted on their web sites. Information from other sources should give details of date of writing and authorship. Key points to remember:

- Conditions affect children in very different ways. Information on the internet about symptoms or treatment may or may not be relevant to your child
- Look for evidence of who wrote the medical information – names and qualifications of professionals for example
- Web sites can be set up by anybody. Look for contact details and registered charity numbers to help you decide if the web site belongs to a respected organisation – or a commercial one that may have biased information to sell a treatment or product
- Information on the internet can be out of date or even factually incorrect
- Discuss medical information found on the internet with a health professional
- Some information on the internet is very academic and specialized; some is sensational and extreme
- Information from outside the UK might not be relevant in this country.

Extracts from guidance produced by 'Contact a Family' and the Information Management Research Institute (IMRI) – *see* www.judgehealth.org.uk.

Reproduced by kind permission of 'Contact a Family' © 2008, registered charity number 284912 (209–211 City Road, London. EC1V 1JN). 'Contact a Family' provides support, advice and information for families with disabled children, no matter what their condition or disability. Further information including links to a wide range of reliable data sources can be found at: www.cafamily.org.uk/medicalinformation/additionalmedicalinformation/medicalinformaitioninternet.html.

Parents prefer to decide for themselves whether and when to access information, meet other parents or join voluntary groups. Providing guidance about sources of information and support reduces parents' stress by giving them more control over their lives and makes them less dependent on professionals (*see* page 344 for further discussion).

WORKING WITH FATHERS

Most of the research on working with parents of young children focuses on mothers, but fathers' needs are important too.[5] There is a risk that community health professionals (who are mainly female) can inadvertently exclude fathers and even make them feel superfluous (*see* Box 2.5).

BOX 2.5 Where do fathers fit in?

What the research tells us
The research informs us that:

- fathers are generally thrilled with the arrival of their infant(s);
- they show intense involvement with their newborn child and worry as much as mothers about the baby's welfare, separations, etc;
- as with mothers, fathers' sensitive care-giving is linked to secure attachment;
- young infants can show strong attachment to more than one person; the preferred person when distressed is often the mother rather than the father in the early months of life, but this preference diminishes markedly by the second year;
- fathers see their role in various ways: 'just being there', support, discipline, being involved, being responsible;
- fathers' play tends to be more physical and more exciting than that of mothers;
- fathers can play as valuable a role as mothers in children's language acquisition and early literacy;
- they are less inclined to engage in joint book-reading unless encouraged, but it may be important for boys to have a male role model emphasising the importance and benefits of reading;
- fathers' 'fund of knowledge' often differs from that of mothers; for example, they may be able to transfer mechanical and tool-handling skills, enthusiasm for physical fitness and coordination, or computing and technological expertise.

The effect of professional attitudes
Below are some examples of the effect of professional attitudes:

- many services are planned and delivered 'for mothers and children', thus marginalising fathers;
- there is a culture of anxiety about men's involvement with young children and about aggression and violence, which can make men feel unwelcome in many early years services and premises;
- extreme feminist views of men and male roles can exacerbate this negative influence;
- early years services are overwhelmingly used and provided by women;
- premises are seldom decorated and furnished with any masculine influence or décor.

What can be done to strengthen fathers' role and increase involvement?
Here are some examples:

- centres and services need a policy about engaging men; developing and publicising a policy in itself is helpful;
- address correspondence and plan services for 'parents' not just mothers;
- be aware that many men have literacy problems themselves and are very embarrassed about this;
- remember changing lifework patterns for men and women; adapt times of services accordingly;
- involve men in core issues relevant to aims of service, not just fringe activities;
- a staff gender and ethnicity mix is very helpful in making men feel more welcome;
- be open about current negative attitudes on 'men as monsters', paedophiles, etc.;
- provide fathers with information on child development at different ages, for both girls and boys;
- identify the abilities, interests and needs of fathers and incorporate or address these issues;
- listen to and learn from fathers and let them know their opinions are valued;
- offer classes in life skills training including parenting, relationships, and leadership;
- promote tolerance by encouraging cultural diversity and acknowledging the roles of mothers;
- provide peer support, e.g. by matching new fathers with current participants;
- create an atmosphere where men as well as women are expected to be involved; e.g. bulletin boards showing photographs or posters that include men.

Some of this material is derived from the 'Engaging Fathers' research programme, Family Action Centre, University of Newcastle, Australia and is reproduced with the permission of Richard Fletcher.[5]

READABILITY

If you prepare written information for parents or use literature provided by other organisations, consider how many of your patients will be able to understand it. Readability is increased by (a) short words, short sentences and short paragraphs; (b) a high human interest factor, which is achieved by the use of personal pronouns, incomplete sentences (e.g. 'What next? well . . .), and references to experiences of individuals and groups; and (c) a large clear font, with well spaced text, and subheadings if the information provided is lengthy.

A significant proportion of the population is illiterate, or nearly so, and many people with severe reading problems will go to great lengths to conceal the fact, particularly from professionals. A sympathetic question such as 'Did you or anyone in the family have problems with reading at school?' may be useful. Adult literacy classes are widely available, but it takes courage to admit one's difficulties and enrol.

It is crucial to have information translated into the right language; such translations can sometimes be obtained from other professions or other geographical areas. This is very important with information about children, as in some families only the father reads English and may not pass on all the information to his partner.

CULTURE, LANGUAGE AND INTERPRETERS

Families who have limited English proficiency (LEP) can sometimes find a health professional who speaks their language, but often staff need the services of an interpreter. In some situations, the use of a family member to translate may be unavoidable, but this is often unsatisfactory. It is unfair to give children the responsibility of interpreting to their parents. If the father is the only family member who speaks English, there is a risk of misunderstandings with other family members when complex health information has to be shared. It is vital to ensure that the mother and other key family members are fully informed. Wherever possible, use a trained interpreter, link worker or health advocate. Professional interpreters are trained to a high standard and are expected to abide by an ethical code of conduct. Health professionals need to learn how to make the best use of an interpreter. Box 2.5 summarises key points about the use of interpreters.

Professional interpreters can play any one of four roles:

1 **Message converter.** Interpreters listen, observe body language, and convert the meaning of all messages from one language to another without unnecessary additions, deletions, or changes in meaning.
2 **Message clarifier.** Interpreters are alert for possible words or concepts that might lead to misunderstanding and identify and assist in clarifying possible sources of confusion for the patient, provider, or interpreter.
3 **Cultural clarifier.** Interpreters are alert to cultural words or concepts that might lead to misunderstanding and act to identify and assist the parties to clarify culturally-specific ideas.
4 **Patient advocate.** In this role, interpreters also actively support the patient or parent; they can explain how the NHS functions, explain screening tests, etc.

Deafness

The word 'Deaf' with a capital 'D' may be used to refer to people whose first or preferred means of communication is by signing. The term 'Deaf' can, in addition, denote a sub-group of those with profound hearing impairment who have a (sometimes militant) pride in their culture and traditions. In the UK, 'signing' means BSL – British Sign Language. BSL is recognised in the UK as a language in its own right. There are many other sign languages around the world. The term 'deaf' with a lower case 'd' refers to all people with a significant hearing impairment, including those who are or have become hard of hearing, as well as the Deaf community.

For many hearing impaired people, the use of health services is as difficult as for a hearing person who has limited ability in the use of English. BSL is not just a manual representation of spoken English, it has its own word order and grammar, and facial expressions and mouth patterns play an important part. While some Deaf people can read and write standard English fluently, it should not be assumed that communication problems can be solved simply by writing out everything one wants to convey. Parents who rely on BSL often avoid contact with health professionals because of communication problems and many have difficulties with instructions about treatments and medicines. In general, communication with a Deaf parent about their own health or that of their child needs an interpreter and the same principles apply as for any other interpreter.

BOX 2.6 Using interpreters

Before the consultation
Things the healthcare professional should do:

- Plan ahead – consider when you might need an interpreter; consider not only the English proficiency of the parent but the complexity of the information you want to convey or discuss.
- Allocate enough time as the consultation will take much longer when using an interpreter.
- Brief the interpreter on what kind of information will be discussed.
- Ethnic communities are often small and tightly knit, so introduce the interpreter and enquire before beginning whether the patient and the person interpreting know each other.
- If possible, plan for a face-to-face interpreter rather than using a telephone service, but for some languages a telephone service may be the only option (use the internet for up-to-date service details; enter 'telephone interpreting NHS' into Google; for BSL interpreters, enter 'sign language interpreters').
- Remember that it is not only planned visits that may need an interpreter, but conveying results, appointments, etc., by post or phone; and those with LEP cannot phone for information or to change appointments.
- Be aware that some people may be too proud to admit that they need an interpreter.
- Put a reminder sticker on the notes of families who may need an interpreter.

The wishes of the client/parent must be taken into consideration:

- Check with the parent about the use of an interpreter – who would they trust?
- Make sure you have the correct language (not always obvious) and don't make assumptions about their preferences for which language they are most comfortable with.
- For healthcare issues, most families prefer a professional interpreter from their own country and culture.
- Some may prefer an interpreter from a different background to ensure absolute privacy, while others may prefer a friend or relative.

The skills and duties of the interpreter:

- Some basic knowledge of how the NHS and other relevant services work.
- Accurate consecutive and simultaneous language translation.
- Avoiding showing religious, racial, political or sexual prejudice.
- Honesty about linguistic and specialist competence.
- Complete impartiality irrespective of their own religious, cultural or political beliefs.
- A duty of complete confidentiality.

The consultation or interview
Things the healthcare professional should do:

- Plan the seating arrangements and consider the lighting; try to avoid having bright lights or windows behind the professional or interpreter. Sit facing the parent and child and address questions and comments to them (trained interpreters can sit beside the health professional and slightly behind, but if untrained they should be beside him/her, but within line of vision).

- Ask the interpreter to translate everything that is said; if what the parents say is much longer than what the interpreter says to you, ask him/her to translate word-by-word.
- Listen to the parent, smile and nod encouragingly even if you don't understand.
- Some English words and concepts cannot easily be translated and vice versa – be patient.
- A trained interpreter will not try to translate word for word, but will try to convey what the parent meant.
- You may need to define or discuss terms like stress, depression, pain.
- Check with the person interpreting to see if they understand any technical term, and ask how they translated it.
- Be aware that diagrams and sketches to explain medical concepts can present problems for many people from other cultures.
- Written information or instructions must also be clarified through the interpreter.

SUMMARY

Communication and consultation are core skills for health professionals and particularly for those who are involved with community services and health promotion. Self-monitoring, feedback from colleagues and service users, and reflection on lessons learned are important so that one can go on improving throughout a professional career.

REFERENCES

1 Stanton HJ, Martin J, Henningfield JE. The impact of smoking on the family. *Cur Paediatr.* 2005; **15**: 590–8. *See* also Britton J, editor. *ABC of Smoking Cessation.* Oxford: Blackwell Publishing; 2004. (The articles in this book are also available on the BMJ web site – www.bmj.com)
2 Davis H, Spurr P. Parent counselling: an evaluation of a community child mental health service. *J Child Psychol Psychiatry.* 1998; **39**(3): 365–76. *See* also Baggens C. What they talk about: conversations between child health centre nurses and parents *J Advanced Nursing*, 2001; **36**(5): 659–7.
3 Rollnick S, Mason P, Butler C. *Health behaviour change: a guide for practitioners.* Oxford: Churchill Livingstone; 1999.
4 Department of Health. *Birth to Five.* 2007. Available at: www.dh.gov.uk/en/Publications andstatistics/Publications/PublicationsPolicyAndGuidance/DH_074924 (accessed 18 December 2008).
5 www.newcastle.edu.au/centre/fac/efp/index.html (accessed 18 December 2008). *See* also Sarkadi A, Kristianson R, Oberklaid F, *et al.* Fathers' involvement and children's developmental outcomes: a systematic review of longitudinal studies. *Acta Pædiatrica.* 2008; **97**: 153–8.

CHAPTER 3

Mental health, temperament and behaviour

This chapter considers how parents and children interact, the influences of parental mental health and the child's temperament and the ways in which relationships can go wrong. It is important to take into account the family background and circumstances, and the history of the pregnancy, when considering anxieties about a child's health, development or behaviour. Understanding how all these factors interact can help to avoid emotional and behavioural problems in the child, promote optimal development and reduce the risk of abuse or neglect.

PREGNANCY: A TIME OF MENTAL PREPARATION

Pregnancy is the ideal time for professionals to forge a sound working relationship with the prospective parents. However, in UK practice it is usually the midwife who relates closely to the family during pregnancy; as a result, the health visitor only gets to know them after the baby is born and this may make it more difficult for the health visitor to build up the level of trust needed to work with parents in difficult circumstances (*see* page 13).

Pregnancy is an opportunity for the parent(s) to consider how they will respond when there is a new member of the family and how they will cope with the inevitable changes in their lifestyle. If their relationship is under strain or breaks down, this phase of preparation may be disrupted. Either or both partners may be ambivalent about the pregnancy; some may have bad memories of their own childhood; the pregnancy may have been planned to salvage a failing relationship, or to replace a stillborn baby or a child who died; or it may follow a series of distressing miscarriages. Young, poor and unsupported mothers need special attention (*see* page 11).

Another increasingly common situation is where a successful high-achieving couple defer pregnancy until their mid-30s because of career and financial considerations. Difficulties in conceiving may heighten their anxieties. These couples often have very high expectations of their medical advisers and when the child is born they may be very worried about health, development and making decisions on issues such as immunisation.

The role of antenatal classes

Antenatal classes, whether held by hospitals, health clinics, the National Childbirth Trust (NCT; originally called the *Natural* Childbirth Trust), or privately, offer education about pregnancy, delivery and parent-craft. The latter includes preparation for parenthood; the change from competent business or professional person to nervous inexperienced carer of a small, demanding and apparently fragile infant is a challenging role-transition for first-time mothers. Intentionally or unintentionally the classes provide a peer group for new mothers, during pregnancy and afterwards. This can provide companionship and support for women who would otherwise be socially isolated. Postnatal classes and postnatal support groups (run by most branches of the NCT) offer the same possibility. A peer group can prove a valuable source of informal advice on problems, concerns and feelings related to childbirth and infant care. To some extent it can replace the support offered by an extended family and this may help diminish the risk of depression. Child health clinics can extend this function and this point should be considered when planning services.

MATERNAL BONDING

Introduction

Early studies in the 1970s suggested that the first hours and days after birth were crucial to the developing relationship between mother and baby. Separations in this period might interfere with the new mother's feelings towards her baby so that she might never achieve a loving closeness to the baby and might subsequently abuse him.

The situation became confused by the practices advocated by Leboyer* and his disciples.[1] Birth was seen as a potential source of psychological trauma for the baby, the effects of which might persist throughout life. Therefore, babies should be delivered in silence or to music, possibly underwater, and should be placed on the mother's belly as soon as possible in order to minimise the trauma of separation and emergence from the amniotic environment. The beneficial result of all this was to humanise obstetric and neonatal care. Unfortunately, there were adverse effects too. Novice mothers began to panic that they would not 'bond' to their babies. Some hospitals insisted on placing newborn babies to the breast or belly 'to help the bonding' even when both mother and baby were exhausted, or in the face of a squeamish mother's protestations that she would prefer her naked baby wrapped up in order to hold him. Ordinary pain relief during labour became suspect because of fears that the baby's responsiveness to the mother would be diminished.

---

* Frederick Leboyer (born 1918) – a French obstetrician.

These anxieties are largely unfounded. *The facts are*:

▶ The original studies on the adverse effects of neonatal separation have been repeated with better methodology and the original findings have *not* been confirmed.

▶ Most mothers whose babies are removed into incubators or are otherwise separated from them shortly after birth find that they develop normal feelings of love towards their babies.

▶ Some perfectly normal mothers do not feel anything special towards their new baby for several hours or even days, but this does not usually matter. By the time several weeks have passed virtually all have discovered that they love their babies. The few exceptions to this are usually under obvious stress, have developed post-partum depression, or had negative feelings about the baby throughout the pregnancy.

▶ If there is a link between a failure of the mother to feel love towards her new baby and a subsequent risk of child abuse, this is extremely weak and only seems to apply when other stresses, such as marital breakdown or eviction from housing, occur.

▶ There is no obvious link between maternal 'bonding' and the development of attachments by the baby later on in the first year of life (*see* page 46).

▶ Ambivalence about the pregnancy (unwanted child, etc.) may only be fully evident at or after the birth and may be transferred to the baby. Whether this is dependent upon events in the first few days after childbirth is unclear.

▶ Some premature babies are insufficiently physically attractive to elicit feelings of love towards them as easily as a term baby might. The same is true for babies with physical handicaps. They may initially repel (facial deformity) or may be unlikely to live long, in which case the parents may intentionally withhold affection to avoid bereavement should the baby not survive.

▶ Some babies are too exhausted following birth to be very responsive to their mothers, which may alarm the mother who perceives it as her fault.

It is doubtful whether any process in human development is so mechanical as to be switched on or off by different handling practices within a critical period of a few days. Life is more complicated than that and people more adaptable. However, a mother's self-confidence can be undermined, for example, by neonatal separations (which are largely avoidable) or unwarranted hysteria about possible 'bonding' failure.

Action

A mother who seems not to have any loving feelings towards her new baby is more worrying if she does not complain about the fact. One who is concerned that she has not 'bonded' will probably be all right. Probably, the most helpful thing to do is to undress the baby and carry out a neonatal physical examination, commenting on the baby's skills in looking, hearing, reaching, sucking and showing alarm. It is comparatively easy to show how the baby responds preferentially to the mother, looking towards her voice, gazing at her face, settling in her arms. The demonstration is essentially that the baby prefers his mother to the doctor and is a little person who can discriminate between and value different people.

While doing this, some careful questioning of the mother as to her perceptions of the baby may reveal anxieties or ambivalence, which are blocking ordinary affection. Asking about sleeping and feeding will give some idea of handling and the extent of maternal exhaustion. Is the baby's father pulling his weight and what are his attitudes? Could this mother be depressed or overwhelmed with childcare? In most instances, the health visitor will be the appropriate professional to support the mother, reassure her, discuss ways of increasing support and monitor the development of her feelings towards the baby. A mother with a serious post-partum depression will need referral to a general psychiatrist (*see* page 44).

TEMPERAMENT

Temperament and personality influence the relationship between parent and child. Some parents, for example, may be very proud of a lusty, angry baby with a fierce temper, while others see this as an undesirable characteristic and would prefer a placid, peaceful infant.

There are inherited determinants of a child's style of behaviour, which are usually referred to as 'temperament' and are not the result of his upbringing. Controversy continues as to which variables are best selected in order to describe and classify temperament, and there is some uncertainty as to how great is the contribution of inheritance.

An influential project (the New York Longitudinal Study[2]) proposed nine particular variables:

▶ activity level
▶ regularity of biological functions (sleep, hunger, etc.)
▶ approach or withdrawal to novelty
▶ adaptability to altered situations
▶ threshold of responsiveness
▶ intensity of emotional reaction
▶ quality of general mood
▶ distractibility
▶ attention span or persistence

This is not a list to be learned, but an indication of what types of descriptive variables are used. Other studies have differed by introducing other variables, such as fastidiousness, sociability or impulsiveness.

Temperament can change over time according to the child's experiences and may be particularly prone to change in the first year of life. Parental actions may intensify or ameliorate certain temperamental traits. However, it is crucial to realise that temperament itself can shape parents' reactions. The child plays an active part in shaping his environment, which can then, in turn, shape him.

A highly active child may irritate his parents who react irritably and negatively, with the effect that his general mood is soured. Of course, the opposite may be true: a quiet, reflective, introverted child may be a disappointment to an extrovert energetic father. It follows from the above that a 'goodness of fit' concept is important: the match between parents' expectations and personalities and their child's temperament. A poor fit leads to distress and even psychiatric disorder.

In the New York Longitudinal Study, three particular patterns of temperament emerged which, taken together, accounted for about two-thirds of the children involved:

Easy:

▶ regular biological rhythm
▶ positive approaches to novel situations
▶ rapid positive adaptability to change
▶ predominantly sunny mood
▶ mild intensity of emotional reactions

Slow to warm up:

▶ negative
▶ withdrawing responses to novel situations
▶ slow adaptability

Difficult:

▶ irregular negative
▶ withdrawing responses to novel situations
▶ slow to adapt to change
▶ predominantly negative mood (whines, grumbles, feels cheated)
▶ intense emotional reactions

The children with difficult temperaments (about 10% of the sample) showed an increased risk of developing behavioural disorders later in childhood. From a theoretical point of view, the importance of the concept is that it emphasises the interactive nature of social and emotional development. The child is an active element and contributes to the quality of those interpersonal interactions, which help shape his development.

From a clinical point of view, the principal implication is that some parents will need to be told that their child's difficult behaviour is not their fault and has not been caused by upbringing. It is the way he is and they need to devise ways of responding to it which are patient and positive. In other words, they must learn to respond to him as an individual in his own right and not to blame themselves for his difficult style. Nor should they become angry with him or themselves because of their failure to produce much change in him; change will be incremental and slow.

MATERNAL DEPRESSION

This is a common problem and the following should be considered:[3]

▶ Within 2 weeks of giving birth about two-thirds of all women experience instability of mood with ready weepiness. This maternity blues or baby blues is innocent and passes within hours or days.
▶ Rarely, an acute puerperal psychosis develops, but if it does, it is nearly always in the first 2 weeks post-partum. Early signs can include confusion, over-activity or disturbed behaviour. The woman becomes severely disturbed, usually with a mixture of affective and schizophrenic features and a degree of

disorientation. There may be a past history of psychosis or bipolar disorder in the mother or in a close relative. Response to treatment is good, as is prognosis, but because of the implications for child safety this is a psychiatric emergency requiring urgent assessment and admission to hospital.

‣ Mothers with babies and young children may be easily upset and emotionally labile. They may suffer feelings of helplessness when a difficult baby and lack of parenting expertise combine to put pressure on their coping ability and confidence. Mothers seldom get any feedback as to whether they are 'good' mothers. Depression is common and there are probably many other contributing factors, including:
— loss of previous social contact and support (friends, job, etc.);
— continuing reduced social contact because of baby's demands;
— general exhaustion and lack of sleep;
— partner spending more time away from home in evenings;
— friction with partner, in-laws and parents;
— ambivalence about becoming a mother;
— ill or abnormal child, previous loss or bereavement (stillbirth, miscarriage, infant death);
— unrealistic expectations of infant responsiveness;
— being unable to breastfeed;
— the resurfacing of problems from childhood.

Postnatal depression does not differ from depression occurring at other times in the parent's life and is not necessarily more common in the first few months after childbirth, but it is particularly important at this time for two reasons: first, mothers expect to feel happy and fulfilled at this time and feel profound guilt and disappointment that they do not; secondly, prolonged periods of maternal depression can have adverse effects on the child's development. Infants try to elicit interaction with their main caregivers[4] (page 52 and page 202) and may become upset or withdrawn if the adult is unable to respond appropriately because of depression. Many depressed mothers are both irritable and inert and these factors may contribute to the child becoming aggressive, under-stimulated, uncontrolled and/or cross.

There are dangers in regarding all depressed new mothers as having 'postnatal depression'. Those with a past history of mental illness or substance abuse and those who are victims of domestic violence are at serious risk of harming themselves and/or their babies, or being harmed themselves. The Confidential Enquiry into Maternal Deaths[5] showed that, when grouped together, such situations now cause more maternal deaths than obstetric disasters. If a mother is seriously depressed, not looking after herself or her baby properly, or even having thoughts of harming one of them, her GP should be consulted urgently as psychiatric referral may be needed.

Identification

In many districts it is usual to 'screen' mothers for depression, usually using the Edinburgh Postnatal Depression Scale.[*] However, it does not satisfy the criteria for a good screening tool and the National Screening Committee recommends that it

---

[*] An alternative, recently recommended by NICE, is a three-question screen, though its validity for postnatal depression is unproven.

should not be used in this way but 'it may serve as a check list, as part of a mood assessment for postnatal mothers . . . alongside professional judgement and a clinical interview'.[6] It can be useful as a trigger or focal point to open up a discussion about how a mother is feeling, but it should not just be handed to parents to complete or use in isolation. Some women find checklists unhelpful and even insulting. They may deliberately conceal their true feelings when completing them, because admitting to depression makes them feel guilty, or they do not identify their feelings as depression, or they may have no confidence in their health visitor or doctor and fear that the baby might be taken away. Sensitive questioning about how a mother is feeling and coping, good listening and awareness of danger signs, such as slow monotonous speech and lack of eye contact, are likely to be more effective ways of recognising women who need help and the smaller number who are at serious risk (*see* Box 3.1).

BOX 3.1 Examples of questions that can be useful in assessing a new mother's mood

It is important to show that you are really interested in the answers and care about the person, so this takes time. These questions should be asked one-to-one, in a private place, without rush. They should not be read off a form.

- How have you *been*?
- Are you alright in yourself?
- I guess things have been tough recently (followed by a smile and a pause).
- Do things seem pretty impossible at the moment?
- Are you coping OK?
- What help are you getting?
- How is your baby?
- How is the (breast)feeding going?
- How much sleep are you getting?
- What did you have for breakfast this morning?

Questions about self-harm can start rather vague then become more focused if needed (the last questions aren't necessary if there's no sign of depression and no worrying answers to the first questions in this list):

- Are you thinking this is all pretty unbearable?
- Do you sometimes think life might not be worth living?
- Are you thinking that might be true for your baby too?
- Do you think you might do something about it?
- Do you think you might harm yourself, or your baby?
- Do you have any plans to do that?

Management

After identifying and referring those mothers at serious risk who may need urgent psychiatric referral, the *management* is, in the first place, two-pronged:

- to attempt to correct situational factors which are thought to be causal;
- to minimise stress on the mother.

There is no single formula, but the following are common manoeuvres:

- Individual support from a health visitor or social worker (practical advice is often better received than counselling).
- Help with taking the baby out: friends, relatives or day nursery.
- Assistance with building a social network (if a self-help group such as Newpin is available locally, this may be helpful).
- Psychological or 'talking' therapies may be useful. Anti-depressant drugs are commonly prescribed but their role is poorly evaluated. They are thought most likely to succeed when biological functions (sleep, appetite and weight) are disturbed. There are no grounds for preferring any one over another, but the modern derivatives of the tricyclics or SSRIs are usually favoured. If effective, they should be taken for 6 months.

Prevention

Maternal depression may sometimes be prevented before it starts, in socially isolated women, by developing relationships with home visitors during pregnancy. This is more useful than simply providing information and resources. The benefit is greatest for mothers suffering from multiple risk factors.

Fathers

There is a natural tendency for staff, particularly health visitors, to focus on mothers. Much less is known about depression in fathers. Fathers who lose their jobs are more likely to be explosive, rejecting, and punitive. The children of depressed fathers, particularly their sons, have an increased risk of emotional and behavioural problems. Men may feel excluded from childcare and if they do not have a stable relationship with the mother they may have difficulty with access even to see their child, yet many really want to be involved and be good fathers. A child's good relationship with the father can reduce the developmental risks (to attachment, emotion regulation, cognition, and behavioural modelling) associated with having a depressed mother (*see* also Box 2.5).

ATTACHMENT AND AFFECTIONAL BONDING

Attachment theory states that the clinging behaviour that young children display towards their parents and close carers is normal and biologically determined, has particular characteristics, and is especially important in psychosocial development.[7] Selective clinging to one (or a few) person(s) is understood as evidence of an individual's first close personal relationship and the experience of that relationship will influence the quality of subsequent close relationships throughout life.

Attachment behaviour refers to what you actually see: the clinging, or conversely, the separation anxiety shown by the child at separation from his or her attachment figure.

Small babies accept separation from parents with apparent equanimity. At an average age of about 6–7 months they start to show signs (i.e. attachment behaviours) which indicate that they are becoming psychologically attached to another person, usually their mother. In most cases it is one particular individual (occasionally two, simultaneously) in the first instance. This person is singled out from others by the baby as being especially significant and important. She or he does not have to be related by blood and certainly does not have to be the biological mother. There is little or no relationship with events during the neonatal period.

The attachment figure is usually someone who has had a lot to do with the baby in terms of play and comforting; feeding is not the crucial element and breast or bottle-feeding is simply irrelevant. Even harsh physical treatment or 'battering' is compatible with the development of an attachment to the abuser; as long as the carer has involved themselves in intense, physically close social interactions with the infant, it may be sufficient. The amount of time spent together each day is not crucial, provided that it lasts for many months and is physically close. Working parents are quite able to elicit attachments from their infants so long as they do things with them at some time during the average day.

In practice, the first attachment figure is nearly always the baby's mother (or attachment is formed equally with mother and father). For the sake of simplicity the term mother is used here.

Normal attachment behaviours comprise:

- crying when mother leaves the room and calling for her;
- crawling or toddling after her;
- clinging hard when anxious, fearful, tired or in pain;
- hugging, climbing onto her lap, talking and playing more in her company;
- using her as a secure base from which to explore.

All attachments are intensified by anxiety, tiredness and illness. These are evidence of normal psychosocial development in toddlers between about 6 months and 3 years. These are quite compatible with secure attachment formation and can be detected during medical consultations. They may be less obviously selective when the baby or small child has been reared in a larger or extended family. They abate gradually after the age of about 3 or 4 years.

At the same time as the appearance of attachment behaviour (average age is 6 months), there is usually the development of stranger anxiety, a wariness towards and shyness of strange people, which promotes clinging to the attachment figure in their presence. This can also be noted during ordinary medical consultations and is likewise a normal developmental feature, quite compatible with the formation of a secure attachment. The mother's presence calms the child; her absence (or threatened absence) precipitates separation anxiety. This is normal, but can interfere with settling at night. Some children find that they can deal with it by having a cuddly toy, known as a comfort object or transitional object, such as a blanket or teddy bear. These are useful devices and do not usually need to be discouraged, even though parents sometimes disapprove of them. Their existence does not indicate insecurity.

Usually, a child gradually learns to tolerate separations, so that separation anxiety wanes over the pre-school years, although it will still appear at times of distress and pain in young schoolchildren. The rate at which this happens depends on three variables:

- the temperament (personality) of the child;
- the way in which the mother handles the child;
- what experiences the child has of actual or threatened separations.

Adequate resolution of separation anxiety is promoted by the mother being sensitively responsive to the child's needs and providing a sense of security. It follows that if a mother responds to clinging by pushing the child away brusquely, if she uses threats of abandonment as coercions, or if her health and constancy are threatened in the child's eyes, then the child continues to feel insecure and anxious. The resolution of separation anxiety and observable attachment behaviour goes hand in hand with the development of faith that the mother will always return after separation; in other words, a relationship has developed that can persist in the temporary absence of the mother. It is usually thought that this depends upon the child having formed an internal mental representation of his mother; an idea and an image. The term bonding was originally used to describe this process and it was held that the development by the child of affectional bonds allowed the proximity-seeking attachment behaviour to subside. Unfortunately, the term 'bonding' has more recently also been used to describe the warm feelings a mother may have towards her newborn baby as explained on page 40.

The development of secure affectional bonds in early childhood makes it much more likely that an attitude of trust and optimism in personal relationships will persist in later life. Conversely, a failure to develop affectional bonds may result in a lack of what is often called basic trust, with resulting shallowness, suspicion and selfishness in future relationships. Although the acquisition of affectional bonds means that the child no longer has to maintain proximity to his or her mother, if she dies or otherwise disappears, grief ensues. Most children form one initial attachment, but others follow. The usual sequence is for mother to be the first, father to follow some months later, and then other figures, such as grandparents or siblings. It is often assumed that each successive attachment is rather weaker than the previous one. Nevertheless, some children form two or more attachments simultaneously, especially in families where childcare is shared between a number of adults. In such families, separation anxiety is less evident because the departure of the child's mother merely means that the care of the child is likely to be in the hands of another attachment figure. The child still feels secure even though the person changes.

The process of attachment formation and the establishment of affectional bonds usually takes place between age 6 months and 3–4 years. After that time it is more difficult to form deep attachments and bonds to parental figures, though not impossible; many late adoptions, even in adolescence, are successful from that point of view. The whole process is echoed in late adolescence and adult life by falling in love, which is sometimes called pair bonding. In turn, this is followed by the development of deep affection for one's own children.

Abnormalities of attachment formation

In experimental settings it is possible to define several patterns of attachment behaviours: secure, avoidant, ambivalent and disorganised; however, there is no reliable link between the behaviours you observe and the underlying attachment type or disorder. For example, some children who have been constantly with their mother (as is common in some cultures) can be very stressed by separation, quite misleadingly giving the impression of 'insecure attachment'. The measurement and assessment of attachment is difficult and there are no simple reliable methods suitable for routine primary care settings.[8]

Absent or attenuated attachments

Attachment behaviours may fail to develop adequately. The child may appear endearingly friendly to the examining doctor, but closer questioning or longer acquaintance reveals that he or she does not discriminate between familiar and unfamiliar adults in terms of seeking comfort and affection. Although appearing intimate (sitting on your lap, offering kisses) the relationship is superficial and easily broken by separation without any separation anxiety. There are several possible reasons for this:

▶ prolonged institutional rearing, for example in poor quality orphanages;
▶ depressed, emotionally cold or rejecting parents;
▶ learning disability;
▶ autism.

In such cases, referral to a child psychiatrist is sensible. In the case of prolonged neglectful orphanage care, the long-term outcome is often poor with a general difficulty forming and sustaining close relationships, a difficulty learning social rules and a propensity in adult life to aggressive, promiscuous, or feckless behaviour. This is essentially what used to be called maternal deprivation. Adoption often results in considerable catch-up but some of these characteristics may persist (*see* page 79).

Avoidant attachment

There is no indiscriminate attachment behaviour; the child has formed a selective attachment. Clinging and separation anxiety are muted; the child separates from his mother reasonably easily and plays by himself in her absence. On her return he is indifferent to her presence or even actively avoids her greeting. On other occasions he is likely to behave aggressively towards her, although not all the time. The clinical task is differentiating between avoidant attachment from what can look like secure self-sufficient behaviour. Simply asking the mother whether she feels emotionally close to her child is the easiest test. Secure children have gone through a phase of clinging and subsequently share emotions and experiences readily with their mother without demanding reassurance or excessive attention. Avoidant children have always kept their mothers at a distance and seem to strive for emotional self-sufficiency prematurely.

In some instances this pattern reflects elements in the *child's* personality; he dislikes cuddles and intimacies even though the parents are loving and affectionate. He wriggles off laps and dislikes kisses. Such a pattern has a good prognosis so long as the parents can accept their child's individuality. There is no strong link with aggressive behaviour.

In other instances the pattern arises on account of harshness, coldness or rejection on the part of the *parent*. This is evident when mother and child are seen together and it is this configuration that is associated with a tendency for the child to behave aggressively to his mother in other settings. This has a poor prognosis for future antisocial behaviour. The situation can be improved if the parent can be persuaded to act in a more sensitive, affectionate and child-centred way, but this is not easy. In theory, professional counselling is indicated, but such parents will not readily accept it and continue to berate their child.

Insecure attachment

The child is chronically clingy and obviously ambivalent to the mother, being actively cross with her following the briefest separations. The origins of this usually lie in an unfortunate mix of the child's temperament and mother's state of mind or personality. A depressed and irritable mother, for instance, may be short-tempered with a querulous child and her rejecting attitude promotes further clinging by the child. A mother with an immature personality may find herself unable to separate out her needs from the child's and turns to the child for caring or gratification in a way that makes the child anxious and clingy. However, some insecure infants have been exceptionally anxious and irritable throughout their lives and have perfectly satisfactory mothers; it is wrong to *always* blame the child's mother for causing an insecure attachment.

It has generally been held that insecure attachments are often followed by emotional disorder in childhood, particularly school refusal, and it is appropriate to refer insecure children to a child psychiatrist if the problem has not resolved by the age of 5.

Recovery from early deprivation: a sensitive period?

Severely neglected children, such as those reared in understaffed orphanages or by abusive parents, may display 'disorganised' responses to their caregivers. In these, the child acts somewhat unpredictably with his carer, as if not knowing whether to seek closeness with her or not. Orphanage rearing and severely deprived institutional care may result in severe deficits in emotional, physical and cognitive development, which are related to the time spent in care. Similarly, disastrous effects can occur in infants who have repeatedly had severely disrupted relationships with caregivers. When children enter adoption or long-term fostering they can still form attachments, even after a number of years in care, but these may sometimes be insecure and there may be persisting deficits in social interactions. Good outcomes require extra sensitivity on the part of the new carers. Long-term fostering produces better outcomes than residential group homes, but early adoption is the preferred option, because the child's security and self-worth are promoted by the adoptive parents' long-term commitment.

There seems to be a relatively sensitive period for the effects of poor quality rearing of the type that does not allow for the development of adequate attachments. For instance, an institutional upbringing during the first few months of life only, or admission to an institution in middle childhood after an adequate home life in the early years are not associated with the above problems. As a rough guide it would appear that the years between ages 1 and 4 are the crucial ones, although there is wide variation and many adoptions later than age 4 can work well. *See* page 80.

EMOTIONAL AND SOCIAL DEVELOPMENT: CLUES TO LATER MENTAL HEALTH

Theory of mind

A theory of mind is the ability to recognise that other people have minds that hold information, desires, beliefs and fears and that these, in turn, determine and explain their behaviour (*see* Box 3.2). This ability is crucial in the development of empathy and relationships, within the family and with peer groups.

BOX 3.2 Theory of mind

- From about 2 months onwards, infants enjoy 'conversations' with adults. They become the focus of each other's attention and take turns in exchanges of looks, mouth movements and noises; this is called 'joint attention'.
- At around 9 months, objects such as toys or pets become the focus of these conversations. Adults use these opportunities to teach the infant the names of the objects that attract their interest, which is an important contribution to language acquisition.
- During the second and third years of life children begin to understand that other people have intentions or preferences.
- By the age of 4 years, most children are able to reflect on other people's different perceptions of the world but it takes several more years before they fully understand conversational subtleties like lies or jokes that rely on working out what other people know or think.
- Theory of mind is related to the quality of empathy, the ability to recognise the emotions and concerns of other people. Therefore, it is a valuable part of developing social skills and friendships and makes it less likely that disputes will be resolved by violence (but some children use their insights into other children's emotions to bully them by exploiting vulnerable points).
- Children with autism spectrum disorders (and many with learning disability) typically can be shown to have a weak or absent theory of mind.

Friends and peer relationships

Early peer relationships (Box 3.3) are important to a child's self-esteem, to his reaching his full potential and also for the development of the children around him. Children vary widely in the number of friends they have and in the way they interact with them, which can vary from week to week. The pattern of relationships at school can be quite different from those in the home neighbourhood.

BOX 3.3 Milestones for playing with other children

- 2–6 months: interested in other infants.
- 6–9 months: smiling and babbling at other babies.
- 9–12 months: copying each other.
- 12–24 months: simple interactions ('you do it'); turn-taking. Toddlers play more warmly with children they play with often. Such relationships can be viewed as rudimentary friendships and toddlers can become upset at loss of friends.
- 2–3 years: simple role-play.
- 3–4 years: children rapidly set up complicated role-play games, and negotiate decisions about what should happen next. They learn to control aggression, deal with conflict and seek resolution.

Some aggression directed at peers is normal. This peaks at age 2–3 years. Moderate aggression has a good side: it is more common in the most outgoing children, who are more actively trying to initiate social play; indeed, submissive or withdrawn children are more likely to be rejected by peers. When conflict arises in a game, unfamiliar children tend to give up; friends are much more likely to compromise and continue to play. While moderate, and occasionally severe, aggression and conflict should be seen as normal, frequent severe aggression with peers is a cause for concern (*see* page 326).

Fostering emotional and social development

The newborn infant's day can be divided into 'states'. He spends much of the day either asleep or awake and restless or crying, but there are short periods when he is calm and wakeful. In this state, the phenomenon of 'turn-taking behaviour' can be observed. This is a social activity that normally involves both vision and hearing. The infant looks intently at the parent and this gaze is returned. When the parent makes sounds to the baby, he stills and listens. When the sounds stop, the baby vocalises and increases his bodily movements. If these do not elicit a response from the parent, for example if the parent is depressed or distracted, the baby may look bewildered, become distressed or withdraw from further attempts at social engagement.

Important tasks for every infant are to develop social competence and the ability to regulate his emotions. Subsequently he must develop more sophisticated skills, such as attention, planning, and the ability to delay gratification, which will help him control his environment, including other people, and himself.

By the middle of the second year, toddlers make active efforts to avoid or ignore emotionally arousing situations, engage in encouraging or reassuring self-talk, change or substitute goals that have been frustrated and acquire other quite sophisticated behaviour strategies for managing emotions. This is easier if their parents manage the emotional tone of family life, provide demonstrations of acceptable behaviour and offer reliable comfort when the child is overwhelmed. They need to monitor, correct, reward and gradually let go, entrusting tasks to children so they feel proud, trusted and confident to tackle the next task. In this way, parents provide 'scaffolding' and supportive challenges to help their children's emotional development, much as they do with language development. Children who are not nurtured in this way are more likely to develop problems in managing their emotions and may show a variety of emotional problems in adulthood.

Effortful control is the ability to stop doing something that one wants to do, or is already primed to do. The game of 'Simon Says' tests this ability, as do waiting in queues, taking turns, and following instructions. Children who are better at effortful control are also better on measures of conscience and moral behaviour, they are criticised less, find it easier to make friends and are less likely to have behavioural, school, relationship, and occupational problems in later life. It is closely related to flexibility in shifting between different tasks, or between different ways of thinking, or of changing one's mind; this helps in making friends, solving conflicts, and generally achieving social goals. On the other hand, inflexibility, or behavioural rigidity, can become a significant behavioural problem.

Encouraging learning

Families and cultures differ in the emphasis they place on academic success, sports, personal contentment, or reading versus arithmetic. Cultures differ in practices relating to sleeping, feeding, discipline, self-discipline, crying, parental roles, and gender differences in the children, often with different expectations for boys and girls. For example, Japanese mothers tend to use soft sounds to describe toys, and to encourage warm feelings toward the toys; American mothers are much more likely to tell a child the toy's name and to speak *with* their children; some African and Central American mothers use a lot of commands. There is no evidence that any of these approaches is best, although they may well play a role in shaping a child's interactional style, and even his way of thinking. Not surprisingly, families can feel extremely threatened when outside 'experts' who are not familiar with cultural differences seem to be undermining or questioning their efforts to bring up their children 'properly'.

There are several things parents can do to encourage their child's cognitive and cultural development:

▶ provide generous, reliable and responsive emotional warmth, creating a climate in which the parent's values and standards are likely to be accepted and adopted by the young child;
▶ give the child rich exposure to language (having books in the house, showing them in use and reading to them, having constructive conversations with their children, encouraging interactions with other children and carers, going to the library, playing games involving quantities);
▶ go on educational outings;
▶ seek out the best quality childcare they can afford;
▶ encourage exploration (as opposed to 'overprotective' parenting).

Children learn new information and skills best when they are within their '*zone of proximal development*', which means being set challenges that are fairly difficult, but achievable, with or without assistance. This can be described as 'scaffolding'. The parent connects to what a child already knows, but leaves gaps for him to fill in himself. For example, children will acquire language fastest if the parental speech they hear is well matched to their comprehension; that is, it is directed to them, and is not too simple or too complicated. Babytalk – parents using 'baby' words and grammar – is not encouraged.

Adults can also contribute to children's *social development* by playing with them, sharing meals and by arranging for them to visit and play with peers. Parents of more popular children are likely to use explanations to encourage compliance, to be warm, and to discuss feelings. Conversely, children are likely to acquire poorer social skills if their parents view social skills as unchangeable characteristics of a child, or 'not my job'. Children are more likely to be aggressive if their parents are rejecting, inconsistent, overindulgent, or uninvolved. Parent training that addresses these factors can improve outcomes for children.

Infants who are very anxious and inhibited sometimes retain these characteristics for many years. They can be cautious about new experiences or objects, but over-cautiousness in social situations tends to be their most disabling characteristic as they grow older. Sometimes over-protectiveness by parents contributes to the persistence of this 'social reticence'.

Quite different is the child who relishes new experiences, is exuberant and generally in the centre of things socially. This is generally only a problem if the child is disinhibited, so he breaks rules and annoys everyone.

Avoiding and managing conflicts

Minor conflicts often arise between children and their siblings and carers, concerning everyday matters, such as sweets and tidying up. Children will learn and copy the way their carers handle such disagreements. The child learns that, one way or another, conflict must be resolved. What happens after a conflict can be even more important than the conflict itself, providing learning for the child and, for the carer, opportunities to discover what works with a particular child. Children as young as 2 or 3 years can learn several strategies to deal with disagreement, such as 'I'll do it later', 'I won't because. . .', 'I'll do part of it', 'Well can I have just a little?' and pretending they didn't hear. They learn these manoeuvres by copying what they hear carers and peers doing. Once this has been achieved, the next step is for the child to learn which areas are likely to be negotiable, and how best to phrase his disagreement.

As the child grows older, parents use more explanations, complicated bargaining, and indirect guidance. They have to decide when to push the child to cooperate; when to offer choices; when to give up; when to accept the child's suggestions and when to say no. Children who feel that they have some control over what they are doing are much more likely to be cooperative.

Children pick up their parents' ways of interacting. The ideal, at least in Western society, is seen as generous parental affection, clear and consistent boundaries, low levels of emotional upset, and de-emphasis of threats and criticism. Parents can also encourage moral behaviour, both by modelling it themselves and by pointing out opportunities when the child could help someone else. Escalating battles of will, on the other hand, teach children a way of behaving that can lead to major social dysfunction later.

Routines of everyday life (such as bedtime, mealtimes and so on) are important to help parents feel life is not out of control and make it easier to obtain children's cooperation. Routines are reassuring for children and help them become accustomed to doing shared activities.

Stress, emotional development and resilience

Life will always contain stressful events and children must learn to handle a degree of stress appropriate to their age and stage of development. Complete protection from stress is neither possible nor desirable. Long-term stress coupled with the inability of carers to help a child regulate his anxiety levels (as may occur when there is prolonged marital conflict, violence or extreme situations, such as war) is much more likely to be damaging than infrequent stressful events. There may be effects on stress hormone levels and changes in brain structure that are detectable on scanning.

Physical abuse makes children more aggressive and more likely to attribute hostile intent to other people. It is associated with difficulties in emotional and behavioural regulation, an increased risk of depression in childhood and an increased risk of mental illness as adults. The impact of abuse on a particular child depends on its severity, duration, associated threats, emotional support from a carer, general risk factors (e.g. learning disability and additional stressors), general protective factors (e.g. a resilient temperament and a long-lasting close supportive relationship with an adult) and genetic factors (*see* page 4). Children as young as 4 years, and perhaps younger, can experience post-traumatic stress disorder (PTSD) in a way comparable to adults, although the symptoms may be less clear-cut.

Resilience is the ability to cope with, and respond constructively to, stressful events, misfortunes and adverse circumstances. Factors that increase a child's resilience include innate temperamental characteristics, normal or advanced language and social development, attractive physical appearance and having at least one adult (not necessarily a relative) who has a close, personal, long-term relationship with the child.

How much do young children remember?

Children can seldom articulate early childhood memories and it is difficult to know how much they remember, but the answer is probably very little (so-called childhood amnesia). By about 20 months of age children can begin to say something about recent events, if they are in the same or similar situation. By about 3 years they can recount events of several months ago, but may focus on different aspects on different occasions, giving the wrong impression that they are being inconsistent or unreliable. Events that have occurred on many occasions, particularly if stressful or unusual, become incorporated into a script or schema that describes a typical episode rather than a specific one. Limitations of language are also important in determining how much a young child can convey of what has happened (*see* page 291). Therefore, interviewing young children does require considerable skill, especially when the stakes are high as, for example, in suspected child abuse cases.[9]

Gender identity

Gender identity is the perception of one's own gender. It is the result of interaction between genetic and prenatal influences, endocrine function and psychosocial and environmental experiences (*see* Box 3.4).

BOX 3.4 Gender identity

Children will display the following aspects of gender identity:

- By the end of the first year, infants are able to discriminate between the sexes and some also show sex related toy preferences.
- Between 2 and 3 years of age children can correctly label themselves and others as boys or girls.
- By the age of 3 years, there is a clear preference for the roles of boy or girl. At this age, children seem to use cues like clothing or hair to make these judgments, and are less aware of genital differences.
- Five-year-olds have learned that gender stays constant and they are interested in the differences between male and female.

IMPACT OF DAY CARE

With the increased emphasis on getting poor and unemployed people into work, and the pressures on professional women to return to work as soon as possible after childbirth, staff are likely to be asked for advice about day care for the parents' young child. In 1999, 53% of British mothers with a child younger than 5 years of age were employed, and 49% of children under 1 year of age had a mother working. Childminding allows the mother to work, which can have financial and emotional benefits for the whole family; however, low incomes and high costs of day care may mean relatively little increase in disposable income.

Many children are cared for when parents are at work by grandparents or other relatives. Children develop attachments to people who provide physical or emotional care with some continuity (probably at least a few months) and who have an emotional investment in them. Secure attachments to childminders may lead to improved social skills, both in children who have a secure attachment at home and probably even more so in children who do not. Such attachments do not become as important as the attachment to the mother, even in children who are spending most of their waking hours in childcare. During the first 2 years of life, child-minders need to be consistent, warm and long-term if the child is to progress as he would with the biological parents. A corollary of this is that during periods when parents are having severe difficulties (e.g. due to mental illness) childminders can usefully support and nurture the child's development.

For many people, childcare provision in groups, for example day nurseries, is an unavoidable part of modern life. High quality day care can produce benefits for cognitive, language and social development, particularly for disadvantaged children. Children are likely to be more positive and cooperative if they remain with the same peers long-term. Poor childcare produces either no benefit or negative effects – this is a controversial issue because some researchers have found that early extensive continuous care by someone other than the mother leads to less harmonious patterns of parent/child interaction and higher levels of non-compliance and aggression in later childhood.[10] The effect is usually modest in size and is mainly seen in vulnerable children who are in low quality day care, but is important in terms of public policy since so many children are cared for in such settings. Infections, particularly middle ear disease, are more common in children attending day care.

REFERENCES

1 Leboyer F. *Birth Without Violence*. Rochester: Inner Traditions Bear and Company; 2002.
2 Chess S, Thomas A. *Temperament: Theory and Practice*. Abingdon: Routledge; 1996.
3 Musters C, McDonald E, Jones I. Management of postnatal depression. *BMJ*. 2008; **337**: 399–403.
4 Murray L, Andrews L. *The Social Baby: Understanding Babies' Communication from Birth*. Richmond, UK: The Children's Project; 2005 See also Poobalan AS, Aucott L, Ross L, *et al.* Effects of treating postnatal depression on mother–infant interaction and child development: Systematic review. *Br J Psychiatry*. 2007; **191**: 378–86.
5 *Why mothers die: 2000–2002 report*. London: CEMACH; 2002. Available at: www. cemach.org.uk/Publications/Saving-Mothers-Lives-Report-2000-2002.aspx (accessed 18 December 2008).
6 www.nsc.nhs.uk/ The guidance of the National Screening Committee was clarified at: www. amicus-cphva.org/pdf/prbepds1.pdf (accessed 18 December 2008). *See* also Shakespeare J, Blake F, Garcia J. A qualitative study of the acceptability of routine screening of post-natal women using the Edinburgh Postnatal Depression Scale. *Br J Gen Pract*. 2003; **53**: 614–19.
7 Grossmann KE, Grossmann K, Waters E. *Attachment from Infancy to Adulthood: The Major Longitudinal Studies*. New York: Guilford Press; 2006.
8 O'Connor TG, Byrne JG. Attachment measures for research and practice. *Child Adolesc Mental Health*. 2007; **12**(4): 187–92.

9 Jones DPH. *Interviewing the Sexually Abused Child: investigation of suspected abuse.* 4th ed. London: Royal College of Psychiatrists; 1992.

10 Belsky J. Developmental risks (still) associated with early child care. *J Child Psychol Psychiatry.* 2001; **42**(7): 845–59. *See* also HM Government. *Choice for Parents, the best start for children: a ten year strategy for childcare.* 2004. Available at: www.hm-treasury.gov.uk (accessed 19 December 2008). *See* also Melhuish E. 2004. *Literature Review of the Impact of Early Years Childcare Provision on Young Children (paper in support of the National Audit Office Report (HC 268 2003–04).* 2004. Available at: www.nao.org.uk/system_pages/search. aspx (accessed 19 December 2008).

CHAPTER 4

Safeguarding and promoting the welfare of children

TERMINOLOGY

The term 'safeguarding' is a concept that has evolved from a concern about children and young people in public care, to include the protection from harm of all children and young people and to cover all agencies working with children and their families. It reflects a shift from a narrow focus on diagnosis and management of child abuse to a broader concept that includes prevention and early intervention. The definitions of this and related terms are as follows:

Safeguarding and promoting the welfare of children means protecting children from abuse and neglect *and* helping children and young people get the most from life. It is defined in *Working Together to Safeguard Children* as:

▶ protecting children from maltreatment;
▶ preventing impairment of children's health or development;
▶ ensuring that children are growing up in circumstances consistent with the provision of safe and effective care.

These aspects of safeguarding and promoting welfare contribute to the five outcomes for improving the well-being of children set out in Section 10(2) of the Children Act 2004, namely:

- physical and mental health and emotional well-being;
- protection from harm and neglect;
- education, training and recreation;
- making a positive contribution to society;
- social and economic well-being.

Child protection: everything that is done to protect a child or young person from significant harm.

Significant harm: where a child or young person is being badly treated or where they have been stopped from growing and developing well. This can happen in a family as well as in an institution (e.g. school, children's home, prison or the army).

Children in need: children and young people who need extra help and/or services in order to be well and healthy. This includes disabled children.

PREVENTION

Prevention of child abuse is an important goal. It has three components: (i) primary prevention of child abuse by support and guidance at the individual level, and by community-wide initiatives (page 16); (ii) secondary prevention by early identification and intervention where a child may already have been abused; and (iii) tertiary prevention, which means ensuring safety and providing treatment for abused children and adults and, in some cases, for the abuser as well.

BOX 4.1 The Children Act – Sections 47 and 17

Threshold for Section 47 of the Children Act 2004 (Child at Significant Risk, also called 'Child Protection Enquiries'):[1]
Where a local authority
a   are informed that a child who lives, or is found, in their area;
   i is the subject of an emergency protection order; or
   ii is in police protection; or
b   have reasonable cause to suspect that a child who lives, or is found, in their area is suffering, or is likely to suffer, significant harm

the authority shall make, or cause to be made, such enquiries as they consider necessary to enable them to decide whether they should take any action to safeguard or promote the child's welfare.

Threshold for Section 17 (Child in Need):[2]
For the purposes of this Part a child shall be taken to be in need if
a   he is unlikely to achieve or maintain, or to have the opportunity of achieving or maintaining, a reasonable standard of health or development without the provision for him of services by a local authority under this Part;
b   his health or development is likely to be significantly impaired, or further impaired, without the provision for him of such services; or
c   he is disabled.

In order to safeguard children and young people, all agencies working with children, young people and their families are required to 'take all reasonable measures to ensure that the risks of harm to children's welfare are minimised'; and where there are concerns about children and young people's welfare, all agencies must 'take all appropriate actions to address those concerns, working to agreed local policies and procedures in full partnership with other local agencies'. Sections 17 and 47 of the Children Act 2004 specify these definitions and duties in more detail (*see* Box 4.1).

CHILD PROTECTION

Worries about child abuse are a major cause of stress to primary care staff. Doctors worry about 'missing' the diagnosis, making 'false accusations', wrecking their relationship with the adults in the family and being the subject of complaints. Community nursing staff have the same worries and often complain that they are supporting many families who are at risk of abusing their children and who they feel should be the responsibility of social services. Many of these families are hostile to any professional intervention and some have a reputation for verbal aggression and physical violence, which can make child protection work unpleasant, hazardous and worrying.

Although the focus of this book is on the pre-school age group, it is important to remember that abuse of young children may come to light, or be prevented, by appropriate prompt review of the whole family when an older child or teenager discloses that they have been abused. This may happen in various ways. Sometimes they present directly to a professional or by a call to Childline, but the abuse may only be disclosed in response to sympathetic interviewing; for example after episodes of repeated running away from home, reluctance to return home after school, intentional overdose or self-harm or diagnosis of pregnancy or a sexually transmitted disease.

Defining child abuse

Incidents of cruelty or mistreatment probably occur briefly in most families; but the term *child abuse* is reserved for when it is sufficiently extreme or persistent to be damaging. It implies that a child has been treated in a way that is unacceptable when judged against current standards for the care and protection of children. These standards evolve over time as social expectations change and people from different cultures learn from each other.

It is important to avoid the trap of accepting 'cultural differences' as an excuse for findings unequivocally indicative of abuse.[3] For example, female genital mutilation, ritual beatings and 'exorcism' are unacceptable no matter what the cultural rationale might be. There is a trap at the other end of the spectrum too, in that some perfectly safe practices can seem damaging to those unfamiliar with them, and so can be wrongly labelled as abusive; for example, wearing beads around the waist can lead to minor bruises or abrasions. In the middle of the spectrum, some unexplained and baffling findings may be due to unfamiliar child rearing practices that need to be treated with respect and call for education; for example, the use of enemas for inner cleansing.

CATEGORIES OF ABUSE

There are **four main categories** of child abuse:

▶ physical abuse
▶ sexual abuse
▶ emotional abuse
▶ neglect

Many children suffer several forms of abuse. Emotional abuse often accompanies the other three forms.

Physical abuse

This is also often known as non-accidental injury (NAI) and is defined as 'Any non-accidental physical injury to a child which results in tissue injury'. Rates are difficult to determine, but the National Society for the Prevention of Cruelty to Children (NSPCC) estimates that 1–2 children die as a direct result of abuse each week in the UK. The severity of the injury does not necessarily correlate with the underlying psychopathology. For example, cigarette burns will heal, albeit with a small scar, but suggest deliberate, considered, sadistic abuse; whereas a subdural haemorrhage, which may be associated with permanent brain damage, may be due to a caring but stressed parent losing control for a few moments.

Clues in the history that suggest a non-accidental cause of an injury include unexplained delay between injury and presentation to medical services, a vague, inconsistent, varying account of how injury occurred, and an explanation that is incompatible with the child's developmental status or with the actual findings on examination. Parents sometimes respond to questions in an irritable or touchy way. Box 4.2 summarises pre-disposing factors and key features of abuse and Box 4.3 reviews the interpretation of bruises.[4]

There are continuing debates about some aspects of physical abuse; in particular, how 'shaken baby syndrome' relates to subdural bleeding and a suggestion that some infants may have unusually fragile bones without necessarily having a recognised disorder such as brittle bone disease (osteogenesis imperfecta).[5] Such issues are sometimes raised by parents, but are essentially a matter for specialist advice.

BOX 4.2 Predisposing factors and physical findings in child abuse

The following apply in particular to physical abuse, but also to abuse in general:
Predisposing factors in the family:

● socially isolated family or single unsupported parent;
● materially disadvantaged with little privacy for individual members;
● young parent(s);
● male co-habitee who is not father of child;
● lack of child-centred attitudes;
● unreasonably ambitious or perfectionist expectations of child;
● parents were abused themselves in childhood;
● habitually violent household;
● chaotic, multi-problem family;
● alcohol or substance misuse or other mental illness in a parent.

Predisposing factors in the child:

- biologically unrelated to potentially abusing adult;
- unacceptable (wrong gender, malformed, handicapped);
- children with severe communication impairment (hearing loss, language disorders, learning disability, etc.);
- unwanted;
- difficult temperament or perennially crying (*see* page 214).

Precipitants:

- physical or mental illness in child or parent;
- social disaster, such as eviction from home, loss of job, etc.;
- marital or child/parent dispute.

Examination for additional physical features:

- head or eye injury (black eye, detached retina, subdural haematoma, skull fracture in a non-ambulant child);
- long bone or rib fracture in a child under 2 years old;
- burns with unusual outlines resulting from being held against hot object;
- burns to buttocks, groin, or in glove-and-stocking distribution from part immersion in hot water;
- deep circular cigarette burns;
- weals or abrasions with unusual configurations (e.g. crescentic, as inflicted by beating with loop flex);
- bite marks (do not make judgments as to whether they were made by an adult or a child);
- finger and thumb grip marks or bruises especially on cheeks, ears, upper arms or back (from child being held and shaken);
- injured lip and/or torn frenulum from ramming bottle or spoon into mouth, or forcing lips against teeth;
- serious injuries of different ages.

BOX 4.3 Bruises and skin lesions

How old is the bruise? The only reliable rule is that a bruise that is going yellow is more than 18 hours old. Do not be drawn into saying more than this as you cannot tell.

Non-abusive bruises:

- bruising in non-independently mobile babies is very uncommon;
- 17% of infants who are starting to mobilise have bruises;
- at least half of walking children have bruises;
- the majority of schoolchildren have bruises;
- the bruises that are small, usually <10–15 mm, often have an explanation, are sustained over bony prominences, and found on the front of the body (knees and shins, forehead);
- bruises on the buttocks, forearm, face, abdomen or hip, upper arm, posterior leg,

or foot are uncommon, though bruises on the lower back are occasionally seen in very mobile young children. Accidental bruises on the hands or ears are very rare;

- many children acquire a few scattered bruises, which cannot always be instantly explained.

Abusive bruises:

- any part of the body is vulnerable and bruises are away from bony prominences; the most common site is head and neck (particularly face) followed by the buttocks, trunk, and arms;
- bruises are large, commonly multiple, and occur in clusters; for example, due to finger tip pressure on the face while forcibly feeding the child, around the chest when the child is shaken or on the thighs in children who have been sexually abused;
- bruises are often associated with other injury types;
- some bruises carry the imprint of the implement used.

Bleeding disorders:
Bruises that occur in improbable sites such as the axilla, or are palpable, or are developing very rapidly, may be due to disease. Consider bleeding disorders and leukaemia. A blood count and the standard basic clotting tests do not exclude all types of bleeding problem. Such investigations should be overseen by a paediatrician with access to the advice of a haematologist.

Other skin lesions:

- old chickenpox scars, vaccine scars (especially BCG), and insect bites that have been secondarily infected and then healed, can all produce marks that can be mistaken for healed cigarette burns;
- localised rashes, due to medications or other substances, can be misdiagnosed as marks from an implement;
- bite marks are often difficult to interpret but are one of the few injuries that may identify the abuser (don't try to judge who or what made them – leave it to the experts)!

Child sexual abuse (CSA)

This is 'the involvement of dependent, developmentally immature children and adolescents in sexual activities that they do not fully comprehend, are unable to give informed consent to, and that violate the social taboos of family roles'. This includes a variety of acts: exposure, fondling, sexual intercourse and rape. Victims are more commonly girls and can be any age. Most sexual abuse of young children is perpetrated by family members or people known to the family; stranger abuse is less common. It is often assumed that abuse by someone outside the family has no implications for the family and therefore does not call for a child protection conference, but it may be linked to intra-familial problems (*see* Box 4.4).[6]

BOX 4.4 Child sexual abuse

Predisposing factors in intra-familial child sexual abuse include:

- mother who was herself sexually abused in childhood;
- poor marital sexual relationship;
- opportunity for perpetrator to abuse.

Examination – points to consider:

- examination is often normal or there are only non-specific findings;
- abnormalities of the hymen may be significant but can be difficult to interpret;
- consider the need to check for sexually transmitted organisms in vagina or throat and sexually transmitted disease;
- look for bruising or laceration to vulva or anus, enlarged vaginal opening;
- non-specific findings that *may* be significant include vaginitis and recurrent dysuria.

The prevalence of all forms of sexual abuse, including exposure to pornography and verbal sexual overtures, is difficult to assess. Differences in definition, sampling and data collection result in estimates that range from 3% to 36% for females and from 3% to 29% for males. The experience of confidential phone help-lines like Childline, and research interviews with adults, suggest that many episodes of sexual abuse in childhood are never revealed to anyone. Adults' knowledge of Childline, and school-based programmes, which teach children to say 'No' to sexual advances, are thought to make a contribution towards the prevention of sexual abuse.

Child sexual abuse is often chronic and secret, presenting after it has been happening for years. Its origins may have been very early in childhood even though the child only discloses what is happening later on. In pre-school children, abuse may present in several ways:

▶ The child may say that s/he has been abused. This should be taken seriously. A spontaneous, detailed, consistent account with an accompanying display of emotion is likely to be valid.
▶ More often, suspicion arises because of something ambiguous that the child (or another child) has said and this can be very difficult to interpret (*see* page 55).
▶ The child may say that they do not like a particular adult or do not want to be alone with them.
▶ Perineal soreness, discharge, dysuria or anal problems are usually not due to abuse, but the possibility must be considered.
▶ Sexualised behaviour may worry parents or staff though it may be picked up from peers or television.
▶ An older sibling may disclose abuse, leading to a review of the whole family.

Sexual and sexualised behaviour
Sexual behaviour
This means any behaviour that involves touching, exploring one's own body and that of others, sexual language, masturbation and games or interactions that can have sexual connotations. What is seen as 'normal' behaviour in one culture or generation

can be regarded as a problem by another. The sexual behaviour of children is likely to be affected by the attitudes and openness of their parents. Many children discover that sexuality is surrounded by value judgments, prejudices and emotions and may think that sexuality is secret.

Children learn at an early age that sexuality is private and is not something that one performs in front of an audience. When socialisation has been disrupted for some reason, children may not set boundaries for themselves and their bodies and protect their personal privacy to the same extent. Commercial and media pressures often seem to encourage provocative and sexual behaviours in children who are not yet able to fully understand their significance.[7]

Sexualised behaviour

This refers to sexual behaviour in a child which is not appropriate for the child's age and stage of development, is recurring, takes over other activities and becomes a central aspect of the child's everyday life, involves the child attempting to involve other children (or adults) in sexual activities and to which the children and/or adults surrounding the child react with concern. It is important to be aware of the range of normal sexual behaviours before labelling a particular pattern as sexualised, because of the inevitable assumption of exposure to inappropriate sexual activity (*see* Box 4.5).[7]

BOX 4.5 Normal sexual behaviours in children

Normal children:

- are curious about their bodies and can take part in sexual investigations of their own body and in games with other children;
- vary in their interest in sexuality;
- play 'peeking games', often in conjunction with visits to the toilet, motivated by curiosity about each other's sexual organs (this is common around the age of 3 years);
- enjoy bodily contact in the form of hugs, sitting on the knee of staff and holding hands; these are common (if not discouraged by staff policies);
- are observed to masturbate (about 1 child in 20) but as a frequent or daily event this is rare;
- participate in sex play which is spontaneous, good-humoured and mutual in nature;
- may use provocative sexual language, but usually either in anger or imitating a TV/ game character; not intending for sexual content to be taken factually.

Normal children rarely:

- use provocative sexual language in which the sexual content is intended to be explicit and taken literally;
- exhibit behaviour that appears to imitate adult sexuality; e.g. attempted intercourse or imitation of sex with another child or dolls/soft toys;
- attempt to insert objects in the child's own anus or vagina or the anus or vagina of another child or oral-genital contact;
- demand that others take part in specific sexual activities;
- engage in repeated problematic sexual interaction with other children characterised by force, threats, dominance, violence and aggression.

Emotional abuse

This includes all *relationships* (rather than merely actions and inactions) that significantly damage a child's development, socially, emotionally, or cognitively. The relationships are characterised by pervasive, harmful, non-physical interactions. These are categorised in more detail in Box 4.6. The boundary between ordinary parental anger and abuse is not rigid, but is transgressed if it is so severe, frequent, or unpredictable that the child learns maladaptive behaviours or attitudes as a consequence.

The severity of emotional abuse is measured by the *effects on the child*. This is crucial because treatment that would be damaging to one child may not be to another of a different age, temperament, or culture, or a child protected by strong relationships with other family members. When there are other difficulties affecting the child as well, clinical judgment is needed to work out whether the unusual parental behaviour is likely to have had a significant effect.

Beyond these broad statements already given, it is difficult to generalise about such a varied topic as emotional abuse. Emotionally abused children tend to be either extremely compliant or aggressively defiant rather than anything intermediate, but it is important not to assume that the child who clings to the parent and seeks comfort, or who has an apparently good relationship with the parent, cannot have been abused (*see* section on Attachment – page 46).

In other cases, parents may describe a child as always difficult and reveal grotesque disciplinary practices that they appear to believe are necessary in order to control such a wayward child. Descriptive terms such as 'he's evil' may be used. The child may be handled roughly by the parents, with little or no eye-to-eye contact or comfort when distressed. Some forms of emotional abuse can occur without any intention of hurting the child; for instance, in mothers who, through depression or incapacity, cannot make their children attend school.

Perpetrators of emotional abuse and emotional neglect rarely try to conceal the abuse (fabricated illness is an exception). The hurdle is not disclosure but professional willingness to recognise and deal with the issue. Box 4.6 illustrates the range of behaviours included in the category of emotional abuse.

BOX 4.6 Emotional abuse

There are various categories of ill-treatment within emotional abuse:[8]

- Parental emotional unavailability, unresponsiveness, and neglect towards the child (this is usually due to parental mental illness, substance abuse, or overwhelming work commitments).

- Negative attributions and misattributions to the child:
    - hostility;
    - harsh non-physical punishments (e.g. prolonged isolation, refusing to speak to the child, exposure to feared stimuli, threats of severe violence);
    - denigration, mocking, or taunting;
    - attributing inherent badness to the child;
    - rejection.

- Developmentally inappropriate or inconsistent interactions with the child:
  - expectation of the child beyond or below her/his developmental capabilities;
  - exposure to confusing or traumatic events and interactions (including domestic violence, incorrect accusations of motivations such as persecution);
  - inducing guilt or terror, or fear of abandonment, to promote compliance;
  - overprotection.

- Failure to recognise or acknowledge the child's individuality and psychological boundary:
  - using the child for the fulfilment of the parents' psychological needs (e.g. in one parent's conflict with the other; in a parent's delusional system; or in fabricated or induced illness; or fulfilling the carer's unfulfilled ambitions);
  - inability to distinguish between the child's reality and the adult's beliefs and wishes.

- Failure to promote the child's socialisation within the child's context:
  - actively corrupting mis-socialisation (e.g. promoting drug misuse);
  - failure to promote the child's social adaptation (including isolation);
  - failure to provide adequate cognitive simulation and opportunities for learning.

Neglect

Neglect occurs when a parent fails to provide conditions or measures required for a child to develop physically, emotionally and socially, or when they fail to protect the child from avoidable suffering. Neglect with or without concomitant emotional abuse can cause growth failure, short stature and limited intellectual development, as well as leading to avoidable and treatable physical disorders, such as skin infections due to poor hygiene.

Home alone

A common concern is young children being left alone in the house. If urgent action is needed, social services contact the police to gain entry and, if necessary, an appropriate Order (Box 4.9) can be obtained pending further review. When children are left alone or have accidents, the question arises as to whether the parents' care of the child was acceptable. Professionals may be asked for their opinion on these issues. There is little evidence on such questions and a wide range of professional opinion (*see* Table 4.1).

Non-organic failure to thrive

The term 'failure to thrive' is sometimes used to denote a pattern of weight gain in infancy that appears to fall below 'normal'. It implies a judgment that the growth pattern is abnormal due to incompetent or neglectful parenting. There may also be developmental delay. (*See* page 137 for further discussion.)

Fabricated and induced illness

This was previously known as Munchausen's Syndrome by Proxy and as Meadows' Syndrome. It includes deliberate airway obstruction or suffocation, poisoning by drugs, salt, etc., the invention of non-existent symptoms such as fits, and the deliberate creation of physical findings, such as blood in the urine. Diagnosis is difficult; suspicion usually arises from inconsistencies between the history, parental behaviour and observed findings. The underlying psychopathology is complicated, probably variable and poorly understood. Expert multi-disciplinary assessment is essential when fabricated induced illness is suspected.*

TABLE 4.1 Results of a survey of more than 200 professionals on their views about the age at which children could safely undertake a variety of activities compared with best evidence or best available opinion.

Activity	Best estimate from literature (years)	Range of answers given by most respondents (age in years)
Eat peanuts safely	5	2–8
Bath without adult present	6	3–12
Go to the shops (crossing a road)	9	5–11
Cycle in the street	10	5–17
Be left alone in the house	10	7–17
Play in playground without adult	9	3–14
Climb a tree	No evidence found	4–10
Make a cup of tea	No evidence found	6–12
Play with other children on housing estate	No evidence found	3–14
Use matches	No evidence found	6–14
Play near water with no adult nearby	No evidence found	5–16

Source: Derived from Tomlinson and Sainsbury[9] (*Child Care Health Dev.* 2004; **30**(4): 301–5) with the permission of John Wiley and Sons and the authors.

CHILD PROTECTION SITUATIONS IN COMMUNITY AND PRIMARY CARE

Fractures, other serious injuries and unequivocal signs of sexual abuse or assault are likely to result in direct referral to A&E departments rather than to primary care staff and there should be a well-rehearsed response to such situations.† Community staff working with young children are likely to be faced with less dramatic, but often more difficult problems, for example:

▶ concern that a family with multiple problems is having difficulty coping with their child(ren);

---

* *See* Department for Children, Schools and Families. *Safeguarding Children in whom illness is fabricated or induced.* London; DCSF; 2008.

† *See* Woodman J, Pitt M, Wentz R, *et al.* Performance of screening tests for child physical abuse in accident and emergency departments. *Health Technol Assessment.* 2008; **12**(33).

- observation by staff of emotionally abusive behaviours (*see* page 66);
- worries about a family whose situation or lifestyle put a child at risk (e.g. heavy alcohol consumption, drug misuse, mental illness or learning disability (*see* page 93 for more discussion);
- unexplained bruises noted by childcare staff at playgroup or nursery or by a GP or health visitor while examining or weighing a young child;
- ill-defined symptoms that could be due to abuse but usually aren't, such as dysuria or a sore perineum in a little girl;
- concerns about possible sexual abuse based on something a child has said or done.

General principles

Every Trust that involves children will have a *named* doctor and nurse for child protection. Not only are they responsible for policy and training, but they can offer clinical advice to professionals. Each Primary Care Trust (PCT) has a *designated* doctor and nurse who are responsible for overseeing child protection matters in all the Trusts from whom the PCT commissions services.

The best interests of the child are paramount. Unless you think a child is in immediate danger of serious harm, you rarely need to act without first consulting colleagues, so do not panic, you are not alone! Make sure you have the contact details of your designated and named nurse and doctor available and get their advice.

Child protection cases are seldom straightforward and often the best course of action is to refer the child and family to the paediatrician responsible for child protection. There are a few key things to keep in mind, which you may find helpful:

- Make sure you are up to date with local policy. Keep local child protection guidelines to hand, along with details of how to contact the local Social Services Department – both in office hours and at other times.
- Take any allegation seriously – especially by a child.
- Always consider the child protection implications of adult illness. Reviews of child abuse tragedies often find that major health problems of a parent were well known to health professionals, but no-one had thought about the risks to the child(ren).
- Parents who have found themselves involved in child protection issues, whatever the circumstances, say that they appreciate being listened to, treated with respect and value, with honesty and in a non-judgmental way by professionals.
- For primary care staff, there may be an apparent conflict between your worries about the child and your concerns about your long-term relationship with the whole family. In child protection issues, if you feel that your duty of confidentiality to the parents (or other adults involved) conflicts with your duty to protect the child, you owe a duty of care only to the child.[10] Sometimes it may help to remind the family of this.
- There is generally no need for primary care staff to get into detailed discussions about what happened or to find out who was responsible. Once you have decided that you need to refer the child, leave the rest to the paediatrician, the social worker and the Police Child Protection Team.
- Similarly, it is important not to conduct multiple in-depth interviews with young children or cross-examine them as this may produce confused and

unreliable evidence; but do not be afraid to simply ask the child what happened. Record the answer. Do not ask leading questions (e.g. 'Did X do this?').

▶ It is never good practice to use family members as interpreters, but this is particularly unwise in possible child protection cases. Misunderstandings are all but inevitable. This applies both to languages other than English and to people who use communication systems other than speech – for example, British Sign Language for the Deaf. Arrange for an interpreter to be present before embarking on interviews (*see* page 37).

▶ Record full and accurate details of the history and examination, including details of the person(s) from whom the history was obtained. Make sure you date, time and sign your notes. Do not jump to conclusions, but record why you are worried. The parents will have access to your notes and they may be used in legal proceedings.

▶ If you are asked to attend a child protection conference, your job is to present the facts. Important information must be shared. Remember that parents will often be present, so consult the chair in advance if there are things you do not want to say in front of the parents. Do not form pre-conceived ideas about the case, or the role or competence of professionals in other disciplines. No-one has a monopoly of wisdom and no single professional is likely to have a complete picture of a child's life or problems. Members of the primary care team such as the GP and health visitor may know the pre-school child and his family better than other professionals; whereas the school child is probably best known by his teachers.

▶ Attending child protection conferences is time consuming but vital if you have important information to share. If you really cannot go, write a report and try to speak to the social worker or chair of the conference on the phone beforehand.

MANAGEMENT OF A CASE OF SUSPECTED CHILD ABUSE

In every area there should be agreed guidelines on the management of child abuse and these should be kept to hand and consulted in every case. Whenever there is a significant suspicion of abuse the Social Services Department should be contacted as soon as any initial treatment has been carried out. The parents should be told of the immediate plans. Depending on the circumstances of the individual case and the strength of concern, it is usually best to share your concerns with the parents. Detailed notes of the examination and any discussions with the parents (and other professionals) should be made immediately. (*See* Box 4.7 for current guidance on sharing information and obtaining consent.) After discussion with the social worker, it may be helpful to arrange a planning meeting in order to share information and consider the best course of action.

If the possibility of abuse arises during a home visit or a consultation, the degree of continuing danger to the child should be assessed, remembering that even in long-term abusive situations the consultation may precipitate a crisis. You may have to make some decisions even before you contact Social Services.

BOX 4.7 Explanation and consent[11]

Matters to consider regarding explanation and consent:

- Explain to the parents at the outset what information will or could be shared, and why.
- Seek the agreement of the parents and, where appropriate, of the child, to the proposed course of action, except when to do so may put the child or others at risk of significant harm.
- The child's safety and welfare must be the overriding consideration.
- Respect the wishes of children or families who do not consent to share confidential information, unless there is need to override that lack of consent.
- Seek advice when in doubt.
- Ensure information is accurate, up-to-date, necessary for the purpose for which you are sharing it, shared only with those who need to see it, and shared securely.
- Always record the reasons for your decision; whether it is to share or not.

Points to consider regarding the sharing of information:

- Is there a legitimate purpose for you or your agency to share the information?
- Does the information enable a person to be identified?
- Is the information confidential?
- If so, do you have consent to share?
- Is there a statutory duty or court order to share the information?
- If consent is refused, or there are good reasons not to seek consent, is there a sufficient public interest to share information?
- If the decision is to share, are you sharing the right information in the right way?
- Have you properly recorded your decision?

Decide on the degree of urgency

The degree of urgency can depend on a number of factors:

- **The severity of the injury** and the need for immediate medical or surgical treatment. This must take priority.
- **The nature of the abuse.** Sexual abuse occurring within the past few days may require urgent examination to obtain forensic material and it may be important to obtain specimens from clothing or bedding before evidence is destroyed. Bite marks may also merit urgent assessment by a forensic dentist in order to obtain DNA specimens.
- **The informant**, if any. If a child makes an allegation of abuse, even if it happened a long time ago, it should be taken very seriously and it should be made obvious to the child that this is the case. If it appears, in the child's eyes, that nothing is happening, the allegation may be retracted and an opportunity lost. This is especially important in suspected sexual abuse.
- **The age of the child.** A young child may be in more imminent danger than a school child.

> ▶ **The abuser.** If the suspected abuser lives in the same house as the child, there will be concern as to whether or not the child can safely return home.
> ▶ **Family factors and attitudes.** Urgent decisive action may be needed if the family is hostile to any professional intervention or there is doubt about their cooperation.

Examination and assessment

Unless the well-being of a child is in immediate danger, it is rarely necessary to examine him without the consent of a parent or guardian. If a parent refuses to give consent, the child may still be examined if he is willing and mature enough to give consent. A child of sufficient understanding may refuse to be examined. A Court Order may be sought if necessary, but such a course of action should be undertaken only after careful thought and consultation.

Examination by more than one doctor

In the case of suspected sexual abuse, a physical examination should be carried out, but usually only after a detailed history (investigative interview*) has been taken. If there is an urgent need to collect forensic evidence or for treatment, this may take precedence over the interview. Young children should be interviewed by someone who has been specially trained to elicit information reliably and avoid leading questions. The interview may be video-recorded. The examination should be carried out by an approved doctor who may be a paediatrician, a specially trained forensic medical examiner or, occasionally, a gynaecologist. Ideally, two doctors conduct the examination at the same time; repeated examinations on different occasions often produce conflicting opinions. This is partly because subtle physical signs may not be interpreted in the same way by everyone and partly because they change over time. The use of a colposcope with recording facilities is becoming the norm when examining children who may have been sexually abused.

If emotional deprivation, non-organic failure to thrive or fabricated illness are under consideration, further specialist opinions will usually be necessary. When NAI is suspected, it may be helpful to have further clinical and radiological opinions when there is doubt as to the aetiology of the injuries.

Next steps
Removal of the child to a safe place

Rarely is it necessary to take a child away from its home (police officers, but not social workers, have a right of entry to a child's home). If it is necessary to urgently remove a child from its home, this should be arranged by a social worker. The Children Act 1989 makes provision for a child to be assessed medically, against his parent's wishes, but without being removed from them (*see* Tables 4.2 and 4.3).

Calling a child protection conference

An 'Initial Child Protection Conference' should be convened whenever there is concern that a child may be at continuing risk of significant harm. The purpose is for professionals to share information and to decide the most appropriate course

---

* Until recently, these interviews were often called 'disclosure interviews', but this term has now been discarded as it appears to be pre-judging the outcome of the interview. There may, in fact, be nothing to disclose.

of action in the child's best interests. Parents will almost always be invited for part of the conference, but professionals should be given an opportunity to share information and concerns in private.

Where the child is *not* considered to be at risk of significant harm, a 'Child In Need Plan' may need to be prepared, specifying the action to be taken to support the family in meeting the needs of the child. If it is agreed that the child *is* at continuing risk of significant harm, then the child becomes subject to a 'Child Protection Plan', which specifies what action is required to reduce the risk to the child. This is part of the Integrated Children's System.[12] Until April 2008 these children would have been on the Child Protection Register, but this has now been phased out; however, any child who would previously have been on the Register should still have a Child Protection Plan.

Planning

The plan for future management defines the responsibilities of the professionals and the parents; the aims and methods needed to achieve the specified objectives; and agreement on how and when progress is made will be reviewed. If there are continuing worries about the family, the primary healthcare team will have an important role in supporting and monitoring the family. Minutes of the case conference should always be sent to the GP. These are confidential and should be filed in a secure place. Many Social Services Departments circulate minutes to parents. If in doubt about what decision has been made in a particular case, the chairperson of the conference should be consulted.

The decisions made by the conference are based on the severity of the abuse, the risk of further abuse (which must be set against the risks of removing the child from his home) and the probability that the parents(s) are able to cooperate with and benefit from an intervention and support plan. In emotional abuse, a 'trial for change' is usually attempted before the child is separated from the perpetrator. If other forms of abuse are taking place, tackling those takes precedence. The child must be adequately protected before modification of underlying causes can begin.

When things go wrong

When a child dies or there is a serious incident that is of public interest or concern, a 'Part 8' review is undertaken. This is so called because it is based on Part 8 of the government guidance document, *Working Together* (1991). A study of Part 8 reviews revealed recurring problems:[13]

▶ Conferences focused more on whether or not to place the child on the Child Protection Register than on a practical intervention and support plan for the family. This criticism has also been made by parents when asked about their experience of child protection proceedings.
▶ There was failure to take full account of mental health problems in the parents.
▶ Optimism for progress and a good outcome was sustained in the face of recurring abusive incidents even while the family were being monitored.
▶ Frequent staff changes made continuity of support and assessment very difficult.
▶ There was a reluctance to take a firm line with parents about the changes they should make in how they managed their children and their lifestyle.

THE LEGAL FRAMEWORK FOR CHILD PROTECTION
Children's Rights and the UN Convention

The UN Convention on the Rights of the Child was adopted in 1989 and has been ratified by most countries, including the UK, and although it does not have the force of national law it is an influential document.[14] The Convention defines children as all human beings under the age of 18. Its guiding principles emphasise non-discrimination, the best interests of the child, opportunities for maximum survival and development, and the participation of children in decisions, particularly those that affect them personally.

The Human Rights Act 1998

This incorporates into UK law the European Convention on human rights. Article 8 requires respect for family life, allows intervention only where it is legally endorsed and to the extent necessary to protect the welfare of children. Childcare interventions under this legislation are limited and focused on family reunification.

The Children Act 1989

This Act brought together most of the legislation covering the care and protection of children in England and Wales. Great efforts were made to ensure that it was written in such a way as to be comprehensible to professionals other than lawyers. The types of Orders, and details of who can apply for them, are summarised in Box 4.8. The Act and associated guidance have a number of provisions relevant to health professionals; in particular, Sections 17 and 47 are used frequently and are, therefore, particularly important (Box 4.1).

The responsibilities of health professionals

Health professionals have a number of responsibilities:[15]

- to protect children and refer any concerns about child abuse to social services or police;
- to know who to contact in police, health, education and social services to express concerns about a child;
- to avoid doing anything that may jeopardise a police investigation;
- to keep meticulous records with due regard to confidentiality and record all concerns/discussions/decisions;
- to be aware of current guidance on accountability and confidentiality;
- to be aware of local child protection procedures and how and in what circumstances to contact the named and designated professionals;
- to have an understanding of the 'Framework for the Assessment of Children in Need and their Families';
- to receive training and clinical supervision in child protection.

BOX 4.8 The legal framework – the Children Act 1989

Protection, care and supervision of children – main legal provisions under Parts IV and V of the Children Act 1989

Order	Who can apply?	How long does it last?	Details and purpose
Child assessment order (section 43)	LA or NSPCC	7 days	Used where there is good cause to suspect that a child is suffering from significant harm but is not in immediate risk and the applicant believes that an assessment (medical, psychiatric or other) is required.
Emergency protection order (sections 44, 45)	Anyone, but usually LA or NSPCC	8 days, plus 7-day extension	Used if there is reasonable cause to believe that the child is likely to suffer significant harm if he is not moved to another place or if enquiries are frustrated by access to the child being unreasonably refused. Parents can challenge it after 72 hours if not present when the order was made.
Supervision order (sections 31, 35 and schedule 3)	LA or NSPCC	1 year	Child placed under supervision of SSD or a probation officer. It does not give the LA parental responsibility. The person with parental responsibility is the responsible person and the person in whose favour the order is made is the supervisor. ('Parental responsibility' means all the rights, duties, powers, responsibilities and authority which by law a parent of a child has in relation to the child and his property.)
Care order (sections 31–4)	LA or NSPCC	Until age 18 or the order is discharged	SSD obtains parental responsibility, which they share with the parents, but they have overriding power. They must plan and periodically review the child's future.
Interim supervision and care orders (section 38)	LA or NSPCC	8 weeks plus 4-week extensions as needed	Similar to full orders but more restricted.
Police Protection Order (section 46)	Police	72 hours	Allows the police to remove a child, keep him in safe accommodation and prevent his removal until satisfied about his safety. They must consult the child if practical, and notify parents and SSD. Parental responsibility is shared with SSD.

LA = Local authority; NSPCC = National Society for Prevention of Cruelty to Children; SSD = Social Services Department.

Orders with respect to children in family proceedings (section 8 orders) for child protection under Part II of the Children Act 1989

Order	Definition
Residence order	This specifies with whom the child is to live. It may be made when the child is in the care of SSD. It ends any care order and gives parental responsibility to the person with whom the child lives.
Contact order	This allows contact with person specified in the order and *requires* the person with whom the child lives to allow contact.
Prohibited steps	This order prevents parents or any other person from taking the steps stated in the order without first obtaining permission to the court.
Specific issue	This specifies how a specific issue is to be handled.
Family assistance (Section 16)	This enables the court to direct that SSD should provide assistance to a family involved in proceedings.

SSD = Social Services Department.

Rules of evidence

Hearsay evidence may be allowed in civil proceedings in connection with the upbringing, maintenance or welfare of the child. Children who are victims or witnesses of violent crime may give the main part of their evidence on video and will usually be cross-examined by a TV link to the courtroom.

Provision of accommodation to third party

Where it appears to a local authority that a child is in danger if a third party remains in the child's place of residence, the authority is empowered to provide assistance to the third party to seek alternative accommodation. The assistance could be in kind. This is designed to reduce the instances where the child has to be removed from his home.

Children Act 2004[16]

This Act introduced a number of new measures, including a Commissioner for Children (England), legislation to support development of child databases and information-sharing between agencies, and the establishment of Local Safeguarding Children Boards to replace Area Child Protection Committees.

Criminal Injuries Compensation Authority

The Authority can pay awards for physical damage or mental injury in cases of child abuse.[17] Adoptive parents, paediatricians, social workers and health visitors should investigate this when appropriate.

DOMESTIC VIOLENCE AND ABUSE – AND THE EFFECT ON CHILDREN

Domestic violence is defined as violence between current or former adult intimate partners.* It occurs in all social classes, all ethnic groups and cultures, all age groups,

---

* Some authors now prefer the term 'intimate partner abuse'.

and in disabled people as well as able-bodied. It may involve verbal abuse, accusation and innuendo, deprivation of freedom or of money, physical or sexual assault, threats and intimidation or attacks with deadly weapons. It accounts for one-quarter of all violent crime in the UK and, directly or indirectly, for a significant number of deaths.[18] Domestic violence and abuse are probably much more common than is currently recognised by professionals (Box 4.9). One in four women have suffered some form of domestic violence or abuse and on average a woman is assaulted by her partner 35 times before reporting it to police. The reported incidence of domestic abuse and violence by women against men is said to be one quarter to one half the incidence of abuse of women by men; in general, the abuse of men by women is less severe and of shorter duration.[19]

Children are often involved in domestic violence. Nearly 35 000 children per year pass through refuges for women victims of domestic violence in England and Wales; of these, 75% have witnessed violence, 10% have observed a sexual assault on their mother, and between one-quarter and three-quarters have been abused themselves. Hearing an assault take place can be as distressing for a child as witnessing one. They may be injured as an incidental consequence, or deliberately or while trying to protect one or other parent.

Children living in domestic violence refuges experience poor preventive health services. There are problems with inaccurate personal data, low uptake of immunisation, delayed development, mental health problems, delay in receiving appointments (often because mail is not delivered) and difficulty in follow-up. Mothers are reluctant for previous records to be obtained because of fears for their safety.

BOX 4.9 Domestic abuse and violence

When to suspect domestic violence:

- background factors include: marital separation, young children, financial pressures, drug and alcohol abuse, disability and ill health;
- professional women may be less likely to present to public agencies and to seek their own solutions, but violence occurs in all social classes;
- domestic violence often starts or intensifies during pregnancy and is associated with late booking, poor attendance and non-compliance, self-discharge against advice, unexpected fetal death, miscarriage, depression, suicide and alcohol and drug abuse;
- victims may attend their GP or A&E department with a variety of ill-defined complaints, unexplained or untreated injuries, self-harm or multiple psychosomatic complaints;
- other clues: unnecessary presence of the woman's partner at consultations, during which her partner answers questions on her behalf; direct or indirect evidence of jealousy, such as refusing to let a woman go out alone.

Don't be afraid to ask the person about domestic violence. It is not easy to enquire about it, but victims report that they would find it helpful to be asked even if at the time they deny any problems. By acknowledging that they know such things can happen, even in apparently stable relationships, professionals indicate that the subject is not taboo and that they are willing to listen and believe what they are told.

This makes it easier for the woman to seek help when she is ready to do so.

Exposure to domestic violence puts a child at risk and it is important not to ignore suspicions when there is evidence to justify them. Ways of opening up the subject include questions like:

▶ how are things at home?
▶ how do you get on with your husband/partner?
▶ are there any particular problems or worries at home?
▶ do you ever feel afraid of being attacked or assaulted?

If the child is old enough to express their concerns, they can be asked simple questions about life at home, what their father/mother's partner is like, whether people get cross at home, what happens and whether they worry about their mum.

What to do

There are a number of things a professional should do in the case of suspected domestic violence:[19]

▶ provide information or access to information about options (this means that you need a knowledge of local policies and facilities): i.e. displaying posters and leaflets about local and national sources of help regarding domestic violence;
▶ be sympathetic and supportive;
▶ do not make judgments about who is to blame or what provokes the violence;
▶ be cautious in offering unsolicited advice as to what the woman should do;
▶ consider with her the level of risk to her and the child(ren); if this is significant you may have to initiate the child protection process, even if the woman does not want you to; however, be aware that this may expose her (and sometimes you and your colleagues) to the risk of violence from the partner;
▶ remember that the best way to protect the child is to protect the non-abusing parent;
▶ if suspicion emerges during a visit to a GP, but the woman denies any problem, offer to arrange for her to see the health visitor, midwife or other member of the primary care team as appropriate;
▶ when in doubt as to what to do next, the named doctor or nurse for child protection, or the local domestic violence forum, may be able to offer advice and support.

If women search the internet for information on this issue on their home computer, they should be reminded that concealing which web sites they have visited is difficult even for experts.

LOOKED-AFTER CHILDREN

A 'looked-after child' is defined by the Children Act 1989 as a child in voluntary care of the local authority – 'accommodated' – or subject to a care order made by a Court to grant shared personal responsibility with the local authority – 'in care'.

The long-term outcomes for looked-after children are generally poor, for reasons set out on page 50. If children have been in care for 18 months they have an 80% chance of remaining in care for 4 years or more. The Local Authority is required to improve these outcomes for children in their care. The Quality Protects initiative (England) and the Children First initiative (Wales) aim to improve the welfare of looked-after children and a national performance-monitoring framework requires local authorities to report annually on 'life health chances' of children in their care.

The first health assessment of a pre-school child entering care needs to be thorough as these children usually have more physical and mental problems than other children. In addition, they may have missed out on medical care and routine checks; their parents may not have identified problems that would have been dealt with in other families; and their immunisations may be incomplete. Current regulations[*] require that a looked-after child should be assessed by a doctor (and undergo a physical examination when appropriate); a written report must be prepared and a plan for future healthcare must be made before or as soon as possible after a placement is made.

Looked-after children often lack advocates, such as parents or stable carers, to request assessment and treatment and ensure this is provided. The involvement of a specialist nurse for looked-after children leads to improvements in health assessments and health outcomes for such children.[20] The revised regulations allow more flexibility and the use of professional judgment with regard to follow-up health assessments. Some children will need much more monitoring than others. For instance, a child who has been taken into care and is having trouble with schoolwork may be depressed due to the family break-up as well as having a language disorder or hearing loss. Such cases probably should be managed by a paediatrician and/or child mental health team.

FOSTERING AND ADOPTION

Fostering has become increasingly important in recent years. Foster parents are often asked to care for children from very difficult circumstances. They may have disabilities, challenging behaviours or mental health problems. Foster parents need training and support to carry out this important task.[21]

Adoption is usually the best long-term solution for children who cannot return to their biological parents. Placement in a good children's home, or even with caring long-term foster parents, cannot provide the stability and security of adoption. Far fewer infants are in need of adoption in the UK than was the case in the past. Many of the older children who would benefit from adoption have had multiple placements and, in many cases, also have disabilities, health problems or difficult behaviour. This means that medical assessment for adoption is often more complicated and time-consuming than it used to be.[22]

The Adoption and Children Act 2002 updated the 1976 Act and aligned the adoption law with the provisions of the Children Act 1989, making the child's welfare the paramount consideration. It was fully implemented in 2005.[23] It places a duty on local authorities to provide an adoption support service; introduces an independent review mechanism for prospective adopters who feel they have been turned down unfairly; and widens the pool of potential adoptive parents, for example, by

---

[*] Amendment of the Arrangement of Placements for Children Regulations 1991: Health Assessments, Regulation 7. This replaces the earlier system, which required a twice-yearly examination for all children under five and an annual examination thereafter.

enabling unmarried couples to adopt jointly. The Adoption and Children Act 2006 regulates issues of contact with a child and inter-country adoption.

Health visitors and other primary care staff may need to offer advice and support to adoptive parents. Adoptive parents can be anxious about introducing the new member of their family to relatives and friends, particularly if the child has emotional or behavioural problems. They have often experienced lengthy assessment to determine whether they are eligible and fit to adopt, so may be wary of more in-depth professional contact and it is useful to begin by encouraging them and focusing on where they are doing well. Older children may exhibit difficult behaviour for many reasons; for example, they may have been abused; or they may be testing out the security of their new placement or grieving for lost foster carer attachments. Some of these children can be extremely difficult; for example, they may be angry, depressed, autistic, antisocial, drug-addicted, or even (rarely) psychotic.

It is natural to assume that parents will be thrilled with their new baby or child, particularly if they have had a long wait to adopt, but this is not always so. Parents may have worries about breastfeeding and bonding, feelings of disappointment over their infertility and loss of biological function, the stigma of adopting, worries and feelings about the child's history, origins and birth family, and concerns of when to start telling the child about his history. The adopted child is not the one they dreamed of originally, does not share their genes and brings with it no ancestral ties. The issue of links with the child's birth family may need to be addressed. Some adoptive parents report symptoms of postnatal depression indistinguishable from those of biological parents.[24]

International adoption presents some additional challenges. The parents must comply with the law on inter-country adoptions.[25] The child may have spent months or years in an orphanage where there is little emotional warmth or language stimulation. There is an increased risk of prenatal and postnatal growth impairment and a variety of health problems (*see* Box 4.10). One common worry of the adoptive parents is slow language acquisition. These children are not like other bilingual children who learn two languages either simultaneously from infancy, or sequentially; instead they have to abandon one half-learned language and start afresh.[26]

Adoption contact register

The legislation requires the Registrar General to maintain a register comprising adopted persons and relatives. The British Association for Adoption and Fostering (BAAF) took stewardship of the register in 2004.[27] An individual's name will only be entered on the register at their request. The Registrar General will then pass on to an adopted person (if at least 18 years old) who has registered with him, the name and address of any relative who has also registered. The address may be that of an intermediary. This should allow easier contact between adopted children and their natural relatives, but retains confidentiality where required.[*]

---

[*] Useful further information and links to key documents can be found at the web site of the BAAF: www.baaf.org.uk/info/lpp/adoption/index.shtml

> **BOX 4.10 Orphanage rearing and later adoption**
>
> - Children brought up in orphanages with inadequate stimulation have markedly delayed language development. They catch up well if they are placed in a more nurturing environment before the age of 6-7, but if placement is delayed much longer than that they are likely to have difficulty with subtler aspects of language, such as producing correct word endings, talking about emotions, or enthusiasm for talking; an example of a developmentally 'sensitive period'. However, other aspects of language have no such sensitive period; children can catch up when they are lagging in vocabulary and semantics.
> - Some children, after being removed from orphanages or neglectful institutions and then adopted, are left with permanent deficits in physical and cognitive development. These deficits are related to the duration spent in care, even after controlling for the possibility of congenital or nutritional effects.
> - Long-term fostering produces considerably better outcomes than modern residential group homes, at least for children who are at high genetic and early-childhood environmental risk.
> - When two or more children are adopted together from a deprived situation, they may have more difficulty catching up than children adopted separately. This is perhaps because of the complexity of the interaction with the parents (as seen in normal twin development), the effectively bilingual environment or the taxing of the adoptive family's emotional and financial resources.

THE COMMON ASSESSMENT FRAMEWORK

Early recognition of problems and their management is a major part of the government's strategy to shift the focus from dealing with the *consequences* of difficulties in children's lives to *prevention and early intervention*. The development of a Common Assessment Framework (CAF) aims to ensure that practices and services are determined by the needs of the child rather than by professional boundaries.* Children and families will receive a more 'joined up' and coordinated service, without multiple and overlapping assessments. It helps practitioners from a variety of agencies (health, education, social services, youth offending, etc.) to assess children's needs for additional services earlier and more effectively, develop a common understanding of those needs and agree a process for working together to meet them. This will avoid the need for families to repeat their story in a number of different, overlapping assessments.

The CAF is based on the Framework for Assessment of Children in Need and their Families, developed in 2000.[28] It has three main domains (*see* Figure 4.1). Where appropriate it links with other assessments such as those undertaken for Special Educational Needs or Connexions. It encourages staff from various agencies to think beyond their own immediate area of expertise and consider other aspects of the child's situation that might be helpful or relevant. The CAF consists of:

- a simple pre-assessment checklist to help practitioners identify children who would benefit from a common assessment. It can be used on its own or

---

* For more information, *see* www.everychildmatters.gov.uk/deliveringservices/caf/ and http://publications. everychildmatters.gov.uk/

complement the assessments of specialist staff, for example midwives or health visitors;

▶ a process of gathering and interpreting information about the the child, based on discussions with the child, their family and other professionals as appropriate;

▶ standard forms to record the findings and actions to follow.

ASSESSMENT FRAMEWORK

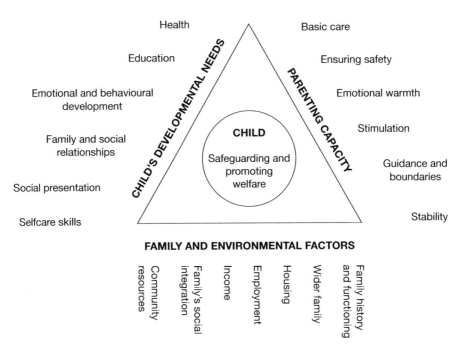

FIGURE 4.1 The Common Assessment Framework: assessment is undertaken along each of three dimensions.

The new role of 'Lead Professional' (LP) is an important part of the strategy. It is not a new job, but a way of delivering integrated support. The LP is a single point of contact for children, young people and their families; they coordinate services and reduce overlap and inconsistency. The LP is not responsible or accountable for other people's work. The LP should be the person best placed to work with a particular child and family.

COMMON SITUATIONS

We summarise in Box 4.11 and Box 4.12 suggested ways of responding to two common situations involving pre-school children in community or primary care settings.

BOX 4.11 Common situations – (1) unexplained bruising

BRUISES ARE FOUND when the child is taken to a health professional by a parent or when the child is in the care of someone else (playgroup leader, nursery staff, etc.).

- If the child has been presented to you by the parent, what reason do they give? Is the visit about the bruises or about something quite different?
- What explanation is given? Is it compatible with the shape, size and distribution of the bruises?
- Are these bruises normal? (*See* Box 4.3 for a summary of what is known about bruising in young children.)

If you are still concerned about possible abuse there are different approaches you can use:

- Be kind and sympathetic: whatever the truth of the matter, for most parents this is an awful situation.
- Express open concern for the bruises and say that you want someone else to look at them. For example, 'Mrs Jones, I am puzzled about these bruises [or other marks] and I am concerned about them. I would like the paediatrician to see them.'
- Don't lie to the parent; don't collude with the parent about, for example, being an 'easy bruiser', if you do not feel that is a viable explanation.
- If the parent is angry or hostile, you can say 'My job is to find out what is causing these bruises, not to blame anyone'. You can be certain that the bruises were non-accidental if they show the mark of an implement, and can then say, 'You can see that he has been hit with something, but it is not my job to find out who did it or why; that is a matter for the Police Child Protection Team.'
- If your concern is initiated by repeated episodes of unexplained suspicious bruising, you can say, 'We cannot let this go on; we have to look into it and find out why this is happening.'

BOX 4.12 Common situations – (2) anxiety about sexual abuse

A young child is brought to the doctor with SORENESS OF THE PERINEUM OR VAGINAL DISCHARGE or BLEEDING. Child abuse is not mentioned by the parent.

- Soreness, plus or minus itching and scanty vaginal discharge are very common in little girls, and are rarely due to child sexual abuse.
- Other causes are more likely: urinary infection, infantile masturbation, pinworms, soap powder or bubble bath reactions, lichen planus, non-venereal infections, or (in older children) the normal discharge that occurs as girls approach puberty.
- Predisposing factors include the low oestrogen levels and thin skin in pre-pubertal girls and poor hygiene.
- Severe itching, especially at night, is very suggestive of pinworms. The classic sellotape test is unreliable. A suggestive history may merit a trial of treatment (mebendazole 100 mg, repeated after 2 weeks; consider whether you need to treat the rest of the family).
- Culture may grow a group A streptococcus, *H. influenzae*, or a range of other

organisms. Antibiotics may be justified if there are leucocytes in the discharge and if there is a pure culture of one organism. Candidiasis is unusual in children no longer wearing nappies. Finding Trichomonas or genital warts in pre-pubertal girls is suspicious and gonococcus should be regarded as definite evidence of abuse.

- Unexplained vaginal bleeding before the normal age of puberty always merits specialist referral. There are many causes, including tumours, endocrine disorders and foreign bodies. Do not immediately assume it is due to sexual abuse; in the absence of other pointers it probably is not.

Nevertheless, the parents are likely to have thought about abuse; they will not mind being asked and may well expect questions like:

- Is it possible that someone might have interfered with the child – touching their private parts?
- Is there anything else you are concerned about or has he/she said anything to you to make you feel worried?

Depending on the age of the child, you need to convey the message that it is OK to talk. By asking the questions mentioned above, you may make it easier for the child to talk to the parent at a later stage.

REFERENCES

1 *Working Together to Safeguard Children.* Available at: www.doh.gov.uk/pub/docs/doh/safeguard.pdf (accessed 20 November 2008).
2 *Framework for the Assessment of Children in Need and Their Families.* Available at: www.doh.gov.uk/pub/docs/doh/frameassess.pdf (accessed 20 November 2008).
3 Koramoa J, Lynch MA, Kinnair DA. Continuum of child-rearing: responding to traditional practices. *Child Abuse Rev.* 2002; **11**: 415–21.
4 Maguire S, Mann MK, Sibert J, *et al.* Are there patterns of bruising in childhood which are diagnostic or suggestive of abuse? A systematic review. *Arch Dis Child.* 2005; **90**: 182–6.
5 Bishop N, Sprigg A, Dalton A. Unexplained fractures in infancy: looking for fragile bones. *Arch Dis Child.* 2007; **92**: 251–6. *See* also http://dontshake.ca/index.php
6 The Royal College of Paediatrics and Child Health. *Physical Signs of Child Sexual Abuse.* London: The Royal College of Paediatrics and Child Health; 2008.
7 Larsson I. *Child Sexuality and Sexual Behaviour.* Stockholm: Swedish National Board of Health and Welfare; 2000. Available at: www.sos.se/FULLTEXT/123/2001-123-20/2001-123-20.pdf (accessed 19 December 2008). *See* also Levin DE, Kilbourne J. *So Sexy So Soon: The New Sexualized Childhood and What Parents Can Do to Protect Their Kids.* New York: Ballantine; 2008.
8 Glaser D. Emotional abuse and neglect (psychological maltreatment): a conceptual framework. *Child Abuse Negl.* 2002; **26**: 697–714.
9 Tomlinson R, Sainsbury C. Childhood injury prevention advice: a survey of health professionals' responses to common scenarios. *Child Care Health Dev.* 2004; **30**(4): 301–5.
10 The Royal College of Paediatrics and Child Health. *Responsibilities of Doctors in Child Protection Cases with Regard to Confidentiality.* London: The Royal College of Paediatrics and Child Health; 2004.
11 Department for Education and Skills. *Every Child Matters: making it happen.* London: Department for Education and Skills; 2007.

12 www.everychildmatters.gov.uk/socialcare/integratedchildrenssystem/
13 Sanders R, Colton M, Roberts S. Child abuse fatalities and cases of extreme concern: lessons from reviews. *Child Abuse Negl.* 1999; **23**(3): 257–68.
14 www.unicef.org/crc/crc.htm *See* also *Lancet* feature on child protection – 3 December 2008: www.thelancet.com/journals/lancet/article/PIIS0140–6736(08)61709–2/abstract (accessed 7 January 2009).
15 The Royal College of Paediatrics and Child Health. *Child Protection Companion*. London: The Royal College of Paediatrics and Child Health; 2006.
16 www.opsi.gov.uk/acts/acts2004/20040031.htm
17 Sugarman N, David TJ. Criminal injuries compensation for abused children. *Arch Dis Child.* 2004; **89**: 300–2. *See* also www.cica.gov.uk.
18 Department of Health. *Domestic Violence: a resource manual for health workers*. London: Department of Health; 2000. *See* also www.doh.gov.uk/domestic.htm. *See* also Mullender A, Morley R. *Children Living with Domestic Violence*. London: Whiting and Birch; 1994. *See* also *Women's Aid Federation*. Available at: www.womensaid.org.uk (accessed 20 November 2008). *See* also www.domesticviolencedata.org.
19 www.dewar4research.org/DOCS/dvg-v3.pdf (accessed 19 December 2008).
20 Hill C, Wright V, Sampeys C, *et al.* The emerging role of the specialist nurse: promoting the health of looked-after children. *Adoption and Fostering.* 2002; **26**: 35–43. *See* also Newman T, Blackburn S. *Transitions in the Lives of Children and Young People: Resilience Factors*. Available at: www.scotland.gov.uk/library5/education/ic78–00.asp (accessed 19 December 2008).
21 National Children's Bureau. *Supporting and Training Foster Carers to Promote Health and Well-being*. London: National Children's Bureau; April 2007.
22 Mather M. Adoption: a forgotten paediatric specialty. *Arch Dis Child.* 1999; **81**: 492–5.
23 www.everychildmatters.gov.uk/socialcare/childrenincare/adoption/act2002/
24 Department for Education and Skills. *Practice Guidance on Assessing the Support Needs of Adoptive Families*. London: Department of Education and Skills; 2004.
25 *The Adoption (Intercountry Aspects) Act 1999*. London: Stationery Office; 1999. *See* also *Adoption Guidance – Adoption and Children Act 2002 annex C*. Available at: www.everychild matters.gov.uk/resources-and-practice/ig00032/ (accessed 20 December 2008).
26 Glennen S. Language development and delay in internationally adopted infants and toddlers: a review. *Am J Speech Lang Pathol.* 2002; **11**: 333–9.
27 www.adoptionregister.org.uk/
28 www.archive.official-documents.co.uk/document/doh/facn/fw-pf.htm (accessed 20 December 2008).

CHAPTER 5

Targeting services to specific needs

This chapter describes the needs of children in a variety of circumstances that affect the work of community health professionals. Irrespective of the particular problems that a family may face, there are some general principles that health professionals should try to apply.[1] Parents and children value certain characteristics in the people and services who support them through difficult times. These include reliability (keeping promises), respect, practical help, plus the ability to give support, take time to listen and respond and being able to take a holistic view of their lives (including their strengths) rather than just focusing on the problems. Continuity of professional care and regular use of the Personal Child Health Record are particularly important for families in difficult circumstances.

YOUNG CARERS

Many children unavoidably take on the role of carer to a parent who suffers from physical or mental illness or disability. Children growing up in these difficult circumstances often find it difficult to tell other people about their stress and the burden of care for the adult(s), and sometimes younger siblings, that they often feel they have to carry. Figures for young carers refer to children over 5 years old,[2] although some children under 5 years probably have some responsibility for care of a parent. Young carers like to have their efforts appreciated and they want some choice as to how much care they have to provide. These children often have reduced social and educational opportunities and should be offered support for themselves and for the adults in the family. In many areas, voluntary sector organisations make special provision for young carers.*

TEENAGE MOTHERS

The UK has a high rate of teenage pregnancies. Providing easy access to and knowledge of contraception or termination to teenagers is not the only answer to reduce this rate. Only a minority of teen pregnancies are planned; in many cases, contraception had not been used effectively or at all. Teen pregnancy in the 12- to 15-year age group is more likely to be unplanned and unexpected than pregnancy in older teenagers.

In previous generations, early marriage and motherhood was the norm. Teenage motherhood is now atypical since most women defer motherhood till their mid- or late-twenties. The well-recognised association between teenage motherhood and adverse child outcomes in the 21st century is due primarily to the social and educational background of these young women, rather than their age *per se*. Low social class, a history of being 'in care' and poor educational attainments associated with few career prospects are important factors in early motherhood; the same applies to young fathers, although they are usually several years older than the mother.

These young mothers share many of the characteristics of older single mothers growing up in social adversity, but they have specific difficulties as well. These include the incompatibility of motherhood with usual teenage lifestyles, interference with education and reduced opportunities for employment, which in turn may lead to low income and debt problems. Younger mothers are more likely to be depressed, to be less responsive to their children, and to use harsher discipline. Their children are more likely to have developmental and behavioural problems and are more likely to themselves become teenage parents.

In spite of these negative findings, many teenage mothers are keen to do the best for their children. They may be pleased when they fall pregnant, particularly if they see little prospect of academic success or of a satisfying career, which may make motherhood a desirable option. Although these young mothers may have limited knowledge of childcare, most will benefit from advice and support if offered in a flexible, respectful, and non-judgmental way.

The sharing of childcare responsibilities with other adults, such as the child's father or grandparents, may help the young mother to achieve more in school, and reduces the risk of maternal depression. The maternal grandmother can be particularly helpful for very young mothers, but only if she is supportive and gives the mother confidence. (Many young mothers have complicated and ambivalent relationships with their parents.)

Young fathers may initially be thrilled by the discovery that their partner is pregnant. Later, they may be overwhelmed by the responsibilities involved in fatherhood, but many are keen to be involved with the child in spite of the difficulties of continuing their education, finding employment and coping with the hostility of the mother's parents and of health and social work professionals (*see* also the Family-Nurse Partnership on page 11).

---

* For information on what's available in your area, *see* www.youngcarers.net/ or search for 'young carers' followed by the name of your area.

SINGLE PARENTS

Children of single parents tend to do less well, socially and educationally. One important factor contributing to this is poverty; others include lack of a male role model, time constraints reducing supervision and joint play, reduced emotional support, and reduced cognitive stimulation. Children of divorced and never-married parents have quite similar outcomes despite having quite different life experiences.

ASSISTED CONCEPTION AND MULTIPLE PREGNANCIES

Parents may worry about the health and development of babies conceived by assisted reproduction or conception. In general they can be assured that these babies do very well, but assisted conception is associated with less good outcomes for the pregnancy and the child than is the case with natural conception. Much of this may be related to the infertility that made the assisted conception necessary, rather than to the intervention itself. There is an increased risk of low birth weight and of short gestation, and a higher perinatal mortality rate. Assisted conception may result in a multiple pregnancy, which increases the risk of premature birth and its associated hazards, such as cerebral palsy.

Whether conceived naturally or by assisted conception, twins have an increased risk of various developmental problems when compared to singletons of the same weight and gestation. This is partly due to the additional burden of care so that parents have less time to devote to their babies, resulting in minor, but measurable, lags in language acquisition, for example. Parents of twins are likely to be more tired and less able to continue careers and employment. Of course, all of these issues apply even more to triplets and higher order births.

WORKING IN MULTI-CULTURAL COMMUNITIES

All parents want their children to be physically healthy and to become independent and self-supporting. Childrearing practices and attitudes differ *between* cultures, but social status and education can create just as many differences *within* cultures. Often the most marked differences are in gender roles, extended families, and views on discipline, religion and health.

Parents who move from societies in which the main concerns are physical health, nutrition and survival, sometimes find it hard to adapt to the very different pre-occupations and values of a rich Western country. Western cultures value and encourage autonomy, personal ambition and material success. African and Asian cultures are more likely to teach interdependence and responsibility to others, but their emphasis on courtesy, respect and conformity can cause conflict for children who, after school entry, are heavily influenced by their peers.

Parents arriving as refugees or asylum seekers in an unfamiliar country have to adapt quickly to a range of challenges. They may have experienced injury and stress in their home country, during the journey to a country of refuge and while finding respite and claiming asylum. They are often de-skilled both in employment opportunities and in childcare, as they cannot apply the strategies their own parents used, such as leaving children to play outside or sharing care with neighbours.

Discrimination in housing, racial harassment, bullying and poorly paid jobs affect both parents and children. However, young children are not intrinsically racist;

although they typically learn to recognise different races in the late pre-school years, race remains much less important than gender in guiding the choice of playmates. Racially-based behaviour usually only develops after school entry.

Families that have recently moved far from their homeland often go to great lengths to preserve what they remember of their traditional culture and sometimes seem very old-fashioned to relatives who are embedded in the rapidly evolving life-styles of their adopted society. As children in these families grow up, they pick and choose from the various cultures they meet. They may show quite different behaviour at home and school and value different aspects of the family's home culture at different ages. 'Generation gaps' and 'cultural gaps' rarely fit simple stereotypes.

Refugee children

More than half the world's displaced population are children. There is a high risk of psychological disturbance among these children, which may take various forms. The features of post-traumatic stress disorder (PTSD) may occur, but in young children various forms of behavioural and emotional disorder, sometimes with developmental regression, are more common than the classic features of PTSD. Physical illness may also need to be considered, depending on their home country; for example, anaemia, giardiasis, worms and other parasites, dental problems, thyroid deficiency, lead poisoning, hepatitis B, HIV and tuberculosis. Box 5.1 summarises points to be considered when working with refugees or asylum seeking families. (*See* page 80 for international adoption.)

BOX 5.1 Key mental health issues for refugees, asylum seekers and other immigrants

General:

- racism;
- language barriers;
- cultural beliefs and practices;
- poor public perception; stigma.

Social risk factors:

- poverty;
- unemployment;
- loneliness and isolation;
- homelessness and overcrowded housing;
- displacement and lack of belonging.

Health:

- mental and physical effects of deprivation, injury, bereavement and torture;
- high rates of anxiety and depression;
- lack of knowledge of services;
- shortage of interpreters and advocates;
- may need catch-up screening and immunisations.

Education:

- language barrier in school;
- language barrier at home: difficult for parents to support children's schoolwork;
- attributing all the child's difficulties to language barrier or trauma, hence contributing to delay in recognition of problems with hearing, cognition, or socialisation.

Institutional racism

This refers to practices and attitudes of organisations that discriminate, often unwittingly, against particular races or cultures. It does not imply that individual staff are racist. Specific actions may be needed to adapt to the needs of other cultures; for example, courses to aid understanding of particular cultures or religions and the appropriate use of interpreters. Indicators of successful multi-cultural provision may be obtained by monitoring service uptake in all local ethnic groups.

Practitioners working with a particular immigrant community can often give better service after studying their history and traditions. For example, disability is more common in Pakistani children because of consanguinity. This surprises many parents and it is vital that staff do not seem to be blaming parents for their child's disability. The provision of information by middle-class White professionals cannot be expected to change traditional practices, and local communities need to take on the responsibility of educating the younger generation.

PARENTS WITH MENTAL HEALTH PROBLEMS

A small number of parents have severe mental illness, such as bipolar affective disorder (manic depression) or schizophrenia, but alcoholism, personality disorder and most particularly anxiety and depression, are far more common. Children are affected in various ways: mental illness often results in reduced employment opportunities and poverty; the parent may be distant and unavailable emotionally to the child, resulting in behavioural and developmental difficulties; there may be an increased risk of parental discord or abuse.

It is important to assess the risks to the child. Some psychiatrists are reluctant to consider the child when dealing with adult patients who are also parents, but risk assessment and planning in collaboration with the general practitioner and/or Child and Adolescent Mental Health Services (CAMHS) are vital. Issues such as benefits, family support, medication, contraception, domestic violence and childcare should be considered.

DEAF PARENTS WITH A HEARING CHILD

The normally hearing child of deaf parents is in a unique situation. If the parents use sign language, they will usually want the child to learn this means of communication. Provided the child is also exposed to other normally speaking children and adults (it is suggested that 10 hours per week is sufficient), acquisition both of normal spoken English and of sign language presents little or no difficulty, and indeed, this bilingualism may be an advantage. However, there are many sensitivities among Deaf people (*see* page 36) and it is important to ascertain the parents' views and those of their relatives and peer group, and to avoid hasty conclusions as to what is best for the child.[3]

PARENTS WITH A LEARNING DISABILITY

Parents with a learning disability may have a number of problems. Some of these are related to the parents' difficulty in coping with the demands of everyday life and childcare, and their limitations in providing sufficient developmental opportunities for their child. Other problems may be related to the cause of the learning disability; for example, if this is a heritable disorder, the possibility must be considered that the child may have the same condition and may need the appropriate investigations.

The degree of the parents' learning disability needs to be assessed to ensure that adequate care and supervision of infants and children are provided and that appropriate support is available. This is most likely to be necessary in supporting their children's learning and in managing difficult behaviour in adolescence. Support by the extended family is ideal, but even this is unlikely to be sufficient if the child has special needs as well.

Parents that have mental health problems in addition to their learning difficulties may be quite able to deal with daily routines, but have much more difficulty during relatively brief episodes of severe illness.

TRAVELLER FAMILIES

The Caravan Sites Act 1968 defined Travellers as 'persons of nomadic habit, whatever their race or origin' but in 1989 the Commission for Racial Equality determined that Gypsies formed a distinct ethnic group. There are two main groups: new Travellers and traditional Travellers. The inclusive term 'Traveller' is acceptable to most. New Travellers are people from the settled community, who adopt a nomadic lifestyle. In the UK, traditional Travellers are a mix of English and Welsh Romanichal (or Romany) Gypsies, Irish Travellers, and Scottish Travellers, in addition to a growing number of European Romanichals (Roma). They each have their own language, beliefs and cultural heritage.

Travellers experience a variety of problems (see Box 5.2), which are partly attributable to the difficulty and stress of pursuing their traditional lifestyle in a hostile environment, rather than to travelling itself.[4] They are generally unwelcome in most neighbourhoods and the sites available to them are often on land that is deemed unsuitable for any other purpose, such as landfill areas or near motorways. The scarcity of play facilities and the proximity of busy roads are responsible for a high accident rate among Traveller children.

It is important for Travellers to have access to a healthcare professional that they can get to know and trust. A specialist health visitor can fulfil this role, but needs to be aware that the job will involve advocacy with other agencies as well as a wide range of healthcare issues. A dedicated general practitioner and a community paediatric service may also play a role. Lack of continuity in care is a particular challenge with Traveller families and staff need to ensure that they can be contacted easily for results, appointment dates, etc., wherever the families happen to be at the time.

BOX 5.2 Health issues for Traveller families:

- high stillbirth, perinatal and infant mortality rates compared to the settled population;
- increased frequency of consanguinity and of congenital anomalies, metabolic disorders, etc.;
- reduced life expectancy;
- high rates of depression and anxiety;
- irregular school attendance;
- high illiteracy rates; difficulty with appointments, patient information, etc.;
- lack of continuity of medical care for children with chronic disorders;
- increased rates of infections (especially gastrointestinal and respiratory) and of accidents;
- difficulty in detecting and assessing child abuse;
- difficulty in arranging access to healthcare and in receiving and keeping appointments;
- increased rates of depression and alienation when Traveller families are forced to settle in conventional housing;
- low rates of immunisation and routine health surveillance;
- the need for patient- or parent-held medical records.

MOTHERS IN PRISON

Over a quarter of women in prison were sentenced for drugs offences. These women are a largely young and vulnerable group with a high incidence of attempted suicide, and previous physical, emotional or sexual abuse. Almost half have no educational qualifications and three-quarters have a mental health problem. About one-third have a child under 5 years, and only 5% of women prisoners' children remain in their own home once their mother has been sentenced. Policies regarding female imprisonment are currently (2008) under review.[5]

HOMELESS FAMILIES

A distinction is drawn between statutorily and non-statutorily homeless people in the UK. Statutorily homeless households include people with dependent children, women who are pregnant and single people who are vulnerable, in that they cannot be expected to fend for themselves. They are entitled to permanent re-housing, but may have to wait in leased accommodation, hostels or bed and breakfast hotels until permanent social housing becomes available. Generally, single people without children do not qualify for assistance under the homelessness legislation.

The most common reason for a woman with children to be homeless is a relationship breakdown, which is often accompanied by domestic violence. Other precipitating causes include harassment by neighbours and refugee status. Financial problems and eviction only account for a small proportion.

The children and parents living in temporary accommodation suffer a variety of health problems (Box 5.3), but healthcare is difficult to provide for such families. Often the change of address is not known to the primary healthcare team and this may be deliberate because of fears of further partner violence. The family may move several times and not register with a new GP. Access is difficult for health visitors to negotiate; there is little or no privacy and often arranging appointments is impossible as the delivery of mail is unreliable. It is important to record the mobile phone number, if available, and to establish a permanent address, if possible; a grandparent or friend, for example. Close liaison with social services and housing departments, and arrangements for health visitors to give priority to homeless families, are crucial.

BOX 5.3 Healthcare issues for homeless families

There are a number of healthcare issues relevant to homeless families:

- many families become homeless on more than one occasion;
- frequent moves make it difficult to register the child(ren) with a GP or school;
- the child(ren) are unable to sustain friendships because of frequent moves;
- educational progress falls behind;
- children in homeless accommodation tend to be shorter and thinner than their peers;
- parents are often depressed and anxious;
- the children are at high risk of developmental delay and of psychological and emotional problems;
- lack of play space;
- accident and injury rates are high;
- immunisation rates are low;
- routine health checks are often missed and any problems are not followed up;
- frequently, children have been abused and/or exposed to violence involving their parent(s).

SUBSTANCE MISUSE

Substance misuse is 'use that is harmful, dependent use or use of substances as part of a wider spectrum of problematic or harmful behaviour'. The long-term effects of intra-uterine exposure are difficult to separate from the significant effects of drug misuse on family social circumstances and a parent's ability to care for a child.[6]

Some women with addiction problems book late in pregnancy or present in labour unbooked and in this situation there is likely to be a high level of concern for the infant. However, the stereotype of the 'drug addict' is not the reality for many women who continue to function socially and conceal their habit effectively. The majority of women whose substance misuse may put their own or their baby's health at risk should be identified at the antenatal clinic and a direct question should be routine. A specialist midwife for substance misuse can make a major contribution to the outcome in many ways. She can change attitudes among staff so the woman is not ostracised, but is treated like any other pregnant mother and given any additional health checks and support that are needed. Her understanding of neonatal problems associated with substance misuse and the availability of expert advice for professionals and parents are also invaluable.

Problem drinking is very common and crosses all social classes. It may occur in isolation or in combination with the use of illicit drugs. Users of illicit drugs tend to be young and many have children. Addiction to opiates (most commonly heroin) causes many problems for the child's home environment: addiction to stimulants such as amphetamines and crack cocaine may also produce adverse home circumstances. Other commonly used drugs include methadone, tranquilizers, cannabis and solvents.

Substance-abusing parents have a high risk of:

▶ poverty;
▶ criminal activity and imprisonment;
▶ chaotic lifestyles;
▶ poor nutrition;
▶ missed appointments;
▶ unsafe individuals in the home;
▶ frequent parental absences.

Many drug-abusing parents received poor parenting and suffered childhood abuse themselves. Heroin addicts face the financial pressure of obtaining typically £10–£100 daily to buy heroin; they have an increased risk of death from an overdose, infectious diseases and other causes. Addicts entering methadone maintenance programmes rapidly show substantial improvements in the time spent with their family and in time spent attending to the home. This can stabilise families, improve childcare skills and prevent removal of children into care, which proves that lack of access for addicted parents to maintenance-prescribing services affects children as well as adults.

Child outcomes

Babies born to opiate users tend to be of a lower birth weight and may also have smaller head circumference. There is a high risk of negative long-term outcomes for infants born addicted. There is an increased incidence of antepartum haemorrhage and intrauterine death.

Children of addicted parents as a group perform less well academically; they have an increased risk of emotional and behavioural problems, poor school attendance, substance misuse in adolescence and attempted suicide. They are more likely to suffer child abuse in various forms and to be taken into care. Neglect is the most common type of abuse.

Alcohol consumption in pregnancy can cause fetal alcohol syndrome (FAS). The amount of alcohol needed and the most sensitive period of the pregnancy are still uncertain. Many women report significant alcohol consumption in the early weeks of pregnancy, often before they realise they are pregnant. FAS is probably much more common than is realised. The features include a typical facial appearance and small stature, together with a wide range of neuro-developmental abnormalities; however, the latter are easily overlooked or misinterpreted if the typical facial features are absent or have not been recognised. The combination of FAS and an alcoholic parent(s) often leads to serious educational and social problems for the child.[7]

Management issues

Whenever significant substance misuse is identified, whether in pregnancy or after the child is born, a multi-disciplinary risk assessment should be undertaken. Ideally this should include child protection, psychiatry and substance misuse expertise. A plan must be drawn up to ensure the safety of the child. Box 5.4 summarises key points about substance misuse.

BOX 5.4 Alcohol and drug misuse and its effect on children

Harm minimisation:

- if neglect or abuse is suspected, act immediately according to the local Child Protection Guidelines;
- be sure that the family has sufficient funds to adequately provide for the child's physical needs;
- check that the child is not being left alone whilst the parent is out procuring drugs;
- advise the parent(s) on where to access drug treatment services and make appropriate referral where necessary;
- advise on testing and vaccination for blood-borne viral infections; make referrals for parent and child where necessary;
- give harm minimisation advice regarding injecting and safer sex in order to protect parent and child from contracting transmissible infections;
- make a risk assessment before prescribing drugs of abuse; e.g. dexamphetamine for childhood ADHD.

Parenting:

- give general advice on parenting as the parent may have only very poor role models and a poor support network;
- give advice on nutrition for parent and child, and consideration to parental drug problems as a possible contributing factor where children fail to thrive;
- give advice on the safe storage of drugs away from children, especially methadone mixture, which is attractive in appearance and has been responsible for a number of child deaths;
- make enquiries to ensure that the child has not missed the routine childhood health checks and vaccinations;
- give attention to ensuring that children are not lost to follow-up (see page 21);
- liaise with other professionals who may be involved with the family so that information may be shared in case of concern.

Pre-conception counselling:

- make enquiries to ascertain whether a further pregnancy is planned, and give contraceptive advice where appropriate;
- where a pregnancy is planned or is a possibility, give pre-conception counselling focusing on nutrition and the need to reduce or stop injecting and to keep all illicit drug use to a minimum; make a referral to drugs services at this stage, if appropriate;
- should a further pregnancy occur, early diagnosis and referral to specialist services is required;
- early counselling and testing for blood-borne virus status in pregnant woman and neonate is required.

Sources: Derived from Keen and Allison.[6] Some of this material first appeared in, and is reproduced from, Hall and Elliman[8] with permission from Oxford University Press.

REFERENCES

1 Statham J. Effective services to support children in special circumstances. *Child Care Health Dev.* 2004; **30**(6): 589–98.

2 www.scie.org.uk/publications/briefings/files/scare11.pdf (accessed 20 December 2008).

3 Singleton JL, Tittle MD. Deaf parents of hearing children. *J Deaf Stud Deaf Educ.* 2000; **5**(3): 221–36.

4 Van Cleemput P. Health care needs of travellers. *Arch Dis Child.* 2000; **82**: 32–7. *See* also www.msfcphva.org/clieffectiveness/clieffbulletins/bulletin8.pdf.

5 Black D, Payne H, Lansdown R, *et al.* Babies behind bars revisited. *Arch Dis Child.* 2004; **89**: 896–8.

6 Keen J, Alison LH. Drug misusing parents: key points for health professionals. *Arch Dis Child.* 2001; **85**: 296–9. *See* also Forrester D, Harwin J. Parental Substance Misuse and Child Welfare: Outcomes for Children Two Years after Referral. *Br J Soc Work.* 2008; **38**(8): 1518–35. *See* also Street K, Harrington J, Chiang W, *et al.* How great is the risk of abuse in infants born to drug-using mothers? *Child Care Health Dev.* 2004; **30**(4): 325–30.

7 Becker KL, Walton-Moss B. Detecting and addressing alcohol abuse in women. *Nurse Pract.* 2001; **26**: 13–23. *See* also Bradley KA, Boyd-Wickizer J, Powell SH, *et al.* Alcohol screening questionnaires in women: a critical review. *JAMA.* 1998; **280**: 166–71. *See* also Elliott EJ, Payne J, Morris A, *et al.* Fetal alcohol syndrome: a prospective national surveillance study. *Arch Dis Child.* 2008; **93**: 732–7. *See* also Giglia RC, Binns CW. Alcohol and breastfeeding: what do Australian mothers know? *Asia Pac J Clin Nutr.* 2007; **16**(Suppl 1): 473–7.

8 Hall DMB, Elliman D, editors. *Health for All Children.* 4th ed. revised. Oxford: Oxford University Press; 2006.

CHAPTER 6

Nutrition

BREASTFEEDING

Breastfeeding should be encouraged as the first choice in infant feeding, but mothers should not be made to feel guilty or inadequate if they elect not to breastfeed their babies. The greatest health gain from breastfeeding occurs in the poorest families. There are many advantages to breastfeeding:

▶ Breast milk is an ideal and complete source of nutrients for the first 6 months of life. It continues to be a valuable source of nutrients even after weaning, as part of a mixed diet, throughout the first year of life.
▶ Colostrum has a high concentration of immunoglobulins and other substances, which are thought to contribute to the infant's gut immune defences, thus safeguarding the infant against infection. These agents are also found in mature human milk, though not in such high concentrations.
▶ Breast milk is not liable to contamination by pathogenic bacteria.
▶ It is always available at the correct temperature and concentration; it is convenient and less expensive than formula.
▶ It may reduce the incidence of allergic and atopic responses in infants, particularly in families with a history of allergy and atopy, although this is controversial.

▶ It reduces the chance of hospital admission for gastroenteritis, even in a developed country like the UK.
▶ There are also benefits for the mother: breastfeeding is, for many mothers, psychologically satisfying; it stimulates uterine involution; it uses energy stores that help the mother to lose weight; and the incidence of pre-menopausal breast cancer may be reduced.
▶ Breastfed babies encounter the flavours of foods that their mothers eat during lactation and are more ready to accept them at weaning.
▶ Breastfeeding is associated with a lower risk for obesity later in childhood and in adult life.

Nevertheless, in the UK, about 76% of mothers commence breastfeeding, but only 48% continue for 6 weeks and only 34% for 4 months. This compares unfavourably with, for example, many Scandinavian countries. Failure to initiate, establish or maintain breastfeeding may be due to a variety of factors:

▶ Lack of motivation. Even mothers who are very keen to succeed with breastfeeding sometimes find it difficult and give up, albeit reluctantly, so it is not surprising that mothers who are not really committed to this from the start are unlikely to persist.
▶ Unavoidable practical difficulties, such as prescribed medication that is transmitted in significant quantities in breast milk,* or the need to return to work. In the latter case, the mother may continue to breastfeed for some feeds and could express milk.
▶ Sceptical family discouraging the mother from persevering. It is particularly important for the father to be positive and supportive about breastfeeding.
▶ Inadequate preparation and understanding. In particular, few mothers appreciate that getting breastfeeding established takes patience and may be slow and frustrating for the first week or two. Their own worries about whether the baby 'is getting enough' are often compounded by the uncertainties and ambivalence of professional staff, and confusing and contradictory advice, so they switch to the immediate reassurance offered by formula feeding.
▶ Painful nipples and breasts.
▶ Problems with the baby (ill, premature, neurologically abnormal).
▶ Breastfed babies *must* have additional vitamin K (*see* Box 6.4) and some mothers worry about this.
▶ There is an increased incidence of jaundice in breastfed babies (page 227) which can lead to mothers stopping breastfeeding if staff fail to convey the benign nature of the condition.

Public policy: a good start

Maternity units should adopt the code of practice recommended by UNICEF (*see* Box 6.1). Primary care staff should be knowledgeable about local services to help breastfeeding mothers: information leaflets, plus various organisations, such as the National Childbirth Trust, La Lèche League, etc. (*see* Box 6.2). The community needs to regard breastfeeding in public as normal. The support of the family is vital.

---

* In reality, this is rarely a problem – *see* for example www.ukmicentral.nhs.uk/drugpreg/qrg_p1.asp

In England, some PCTs collect data on breastfeeding at the time of each immunisation. In Scotland, data are collected at the end of the first week on the newborn blood spot screening card to allow calculation of breastfeeding rate by postcode and maternity unit. Information and feedback help to increase the rate.

BOX 6.1 The Baby Friendly Hospital

UNICEF will designate a hospital as 'baby friendly' if it follows the 10 steps to breastfeeding:

1 Have a written breastfeeding policy routinely communicated to all health staff.
2 Train all health staff in skills to implement this policy.
3 Inform all pregnant women about the benefits and management of breastfeeding.
4 Help mothers initiate breastfeeding within half an hour of birth.
5 Show mothers how to breastfeed, and how to maintain lactation, even if they have to be separated from their infants.
6 Give newborn infants no food or drink other than breast milk, unless *medically* indicated.
7 Practice rooming-in (allow mothers and infants to remain together) 24 hours a day.
8 Encourage breastfeeding on demand.
9 Give no artificial teats or pacifiers (also called dummies or soothers) to breastfeeding infants.
10 Foster the establishment of breastfeeding support groups and refer mothers to them on discharge from the hospital or clinic.

NB: For Baby Friendly community services, *see* www.babyfriendly.org.uk/page.asp?page=71

BOX 6.2 Support for breastfeeding mothers

Advice and support, including information and practical guidance, are most vital in the first few days. If it is delayed more than a week or two, many mothers will already have given up.

- Ask your health authority for advice about which leaflets and posters are to be used, so that consistent advice can be offered by all health professionals.
- The **National Childbirth Trust** and the **La Lèche League** are support organisations, with national headquarters and local groups in most areas. They offer information for *all* mothers and mother-to-mother support, often in liaison with midwives and health visitors. Support starts antenatally, with demonstrations, talks and classes.
- Mothers find it easier to talk to someone who has had the same experiences; coping alone at home can be difficult, but the mother often does not feel that her difficulties justify 'bothering the doctor'.
- Breastfeeding mothers may wish to continue well beyond the child's first birthday. Some mothers feel embarrassed about this and the support organisations help by acknowledging that this can be enjoyable and is perfectly 'normal'.
- Practical help includes hiring breast pumps, supplying nipple shields, fitting and selling a range of maternity bras, access to library material and sale of a range of helpful leaflets, for example, *What's in a nappy?*.

Organisations:
1 National Childbirth Trust, www.nctpregnancyandbabycare.com/home
2 La Lèche League (UK), www.laleche.org.uk
3 Association of Breastfeeding Mothers, www.abm.me.uk/
4 Breastfeeding network, www.breastfeedingnetwork.org.uk/.

What works and what doesn't work in breastfeeding[1]

There are many factors that contribute to breastfeeding:

- group, interactive, culture-specific education sessions on positioning and attachment; individually tailored to the needs of low income women;
- skilled breastfeeding support, peer and/or professional, proactively offered to women who want to breastfeed; however, a single home visit by a community nurse following early discharge is unhelpful;
- unrestricted feeding and mother-baby contact from birth onwards[*]; kangaroo care when appropriate (page 343);
- advising mothers to feed on demand; explain that increased sucking will increase the milk supply sufficiently to meet the infant's needs and that there are considerable variations in the amount of milk taken at each feed and in the time taken to complete each feed;
- preventing the provision of discharge packs containing formula-feeding information and samples;
- avoiding supplementary fluids for babies unless medically indicated;
- basing prevention and treatment of sore nipples on principles of positioning and attachment; the signs of good attachment, positioning and suckling are:
  — the baby's mouth is wide open;
  — there is less areola visible underneath the chin than above the nipple;
  — the baby's chin is touching the breast;
  — the lower lip is rolled down and the nose is free;
  — there is no pain;
  — the mother can see that the baby is suckling, and feel the breast getting softer.
- if the baby is not attaching effectively advise teasing the baby's lips with the nipple to open the mouth; try different feeding positions;
- systemic antibiotics for infected nipples (thrush infection in the breast is said by some authorities to be an important cause of nipple and breast pain[2]);
- combination of supportive care, teaching breastfeeding technique, rest and reassurance for women with 'insufficient milk';
- giving expressed breast milk by syringe or cup may help if the baby is slow to suckle;
- a self-monitoring daily log has been shown to be helpful for some mothers who are worried about their baby's intake. They should record all feeds and monitor urine output (modern disposable nappies are very absorbent so it may help to use a pad of cotton wool in the nappy as this is easier to check);
- division of the frenulum in infants with signs of congenital ankyloglossia

---

[*] For a demonstration of how a newborn infant seeks the breast, *see* www.breastcrawl.org/

(tongue tie) and breastfeeding difficulties. Ankyloglossia (a tight frenulum that limits tongue mobility) may cause problems with breastfeeding, particularly nipple pain. It is difficult to diagnose tongue tie simply by looking at the tongue and observation of the baby while feeding is more useful. Ultrasound studies suggest that frenulotomy does improve feeding;[3] however, the significance and prevalence of tongue tie are still somewhat controversial;

 ▶ prevention and treatment of mastitis, which occurs within the first 3 months and is usually unilateral. It is rarely complicated by a breast abscess. Mastitis is poorly understood, but risk factors include milk stasis due to problems with feeding technique or frequency, tight clothes, skin damage or poor hygiene, usually bacterial. Analgesics may be needed; regular breast drainage and/ or continued breastfeeding are advised. Antibiotics are required for infective mastitis.

Interventions that are *unsupported* by evidence include:

 ▶ dopamine antagonists for 'insufficient milk';
 ▶ conditioning nipples in pregnancy;
 ▶ Hoffman's exercises for inverted and non-protractile nipples in pregnancy;
 ▶ breast shells for inverted and non-protractile nipples in pregnancy;
 ▶ breast pumping before the establishment of breastfeeding in women at risk of delayed lactation.

Weighing

Some weight loss is normal in the first 2 weeks of life. The average is around 7% for breastfed babies, somewhat less than this for formula-fed babies, but most recover their birth weight by the ninth or tenth day. Some babies lose 10% or more of their birth weight; the most common reason is insufficient intake, though occasionally there may be obvious reasons, such as prematurity or illness, or anatomical abnormalities, like cleft palate. The underfed baby may be restless and irritable, but some are apparently satisfied and go to sleep after a feed and this may mislead the mother and the midwife. Excessive weight loss can be associated with serious dehydration and a high sodium level, known as hypernatraemia. This may (rarely) cause brain damage. The majority of babies found to have significant hypernatraemic dehydration have lost more than 12% of their birth weight.

Opinions differ as to whether, and how often, babies should be weighed in the first two weeks of life in order to identify this problem.[4] Many midwives fear that weighing might worry the mother and may lead her to abandon breastfeeding if the baby is not gaining weight, but there is no evidence for this. One study found that, in general, mothers whose babies were weighed were *more* confident to continue breastfeeding. Identifying excessive weight loss at the same time as the blood spot test could probably prevent most cases of serious hypernatraemia. An explicit local policy is needed on this issue, since community staff must know where to refer babies for prompt breastfeeding support, and investigation (if needed) if their weight loss is causing concern (*see* Box 6.3). Test weighing – estimating the amount of milk taken by weighing before and after a single feed – is *not* recommended because milk production varies so much between feeds.

BOX 6.3 Weighing breastfed babies – an example of a UK local policy

1   Midwives weigh babies at or around days 5, 7 and 10. Accurate weighing is vital and must be done on electronic scales that are checked and calibrated regularly.

2   If weight is less than the birth weight, the Percent Weight Loss is calculated:

$$\frac{\text{Birth weight} - \text{Current weight}}{\text{Birth weight}} \times 100$$

3   Extra breastfeeding support is available for mothers whose babies have lost 10% or more of birth weight, do not gain weight by 9 days or fail to regain birth weight by 14 days. The babies are reviewed and the sodium level checked if the weight loss is ≥12.5%; or if the babies have not regained birth weight by 21 days.

4   Medical review is offered for formula-fed babies who lose more than 10% of birth weight or have not regained their birth weight by 14 days.

See page 135, for details of weight gain patterns after the first few weeks of life and an account of how to use growth charts.

COMPLEMENTARY FEEDING

If complementary feeding is unavoidable, the formula feeds should be given after each breastfeed, but only after the baby has sucked for as long as it wishes. Extra feeds given between breastfeeds are more likely to reduce the frequency of demand feeding and ultimately lead to a fall in the supply of breast milk. It is unfair on both mother and baby to insist on continued breastfeeding if the parents are becoming anxious and distressed and the baby is not thriving. Once breastfeeding is established, additional water is very rarely needed by fully breastfed babies, even in very hot weather.

Expressed breast milk

Mothers may need to express their breast milk if the breasts are very full or uncomfortable, if the baby is small or sick, or if she needs to be away from the baby, either for a social function or going back to work. All women should be shown how to carry out manual expression of the breasts or provided with written information; for example, *Expressing Your Breast Milk*, published by UNICEF. Breast pumps can be hired from the National Childbirth Trust. Expressed breast milk (EBM) can be stored in a sterile container:

- for up to 24 hours in a domestic fridge;
- up to 1 week in the ice-making compartment of a fridge;
- up to 3 months in a deep freezer.

EBM should be defrosted in the fridge for 12 hours then reheated gently in warm water. Freshly expressed milk should not be added to thawed milk and refrozen. Human milk banks provide an alternative to formula feeds for preterm babies when the mother's milk is not available.[5]

DIET FOR LACTATING MOTHERS

Lactation increases the mother's nutritional requirements and these can be met by eating a healthy and varied diet. The mother's appetite is usually the best guide to her energy needs. Low calorie diets should be avoided because they may affect the nutritional quality of the breast milk. Vegetarians and vegans should ensure an adequate and varied diet with adequate vitamins and minerals, especially calcium, iron and vitamin B12; lactating vegans need a source of extra vitamin B12.

Vitamin supplements during pregnancy and lactation

Folic acid. There is now considerable evidence that folic acid is of crucial importance in early pregnancy to help protect against neural tube defects. The Department of Health recommends that all women planning a pregnancy should supplement their diet with 0.4 mg (400 mcg) of folic acid, continuing until the twelfth week of pregnancy.

Vitamin D. Pregnant and lactating mothers with increased skin pigmentation, women who wear concealing clothing or who live a predominantly indoor life for cultural or religious reasons may have poor vitamin D status during pregnancy and lactation, and should receive a supplement of 10 mcg vitamin D daily.

Vitamin B12. During pregnancy and lactation, vegan women will need to eat fortified food two or three times a day to obtain at least 2 mcg of vitamin B12 or take a daily vitamin B12 supplement. Some vegan foods are supplemented with B12, for example, Tastex and Barmene (however, these are high in sodium and are not suitable for infants).

VITAMIN SUPPLEMENTS FOR INFANTS

Vitamin K is vitally important for newborn infants (*see* Box 6.4).

BOX 6.4 The vitamin K story[6]

Newborn infants have very low levels of vitamin K, which is needed for normal blood clotting. The aim of prophylactic treatment is to avoid vitamin K-dependent bleeding (VKDB).

Deficiency of vitamin K can lead to haemorrhage at a variety of sites; for example, gums, umbilical cord and bowel, or during procedures like circumcision. Bleeding into the brain, though rare, is the most serious. Bleeding can occur at any time in the first few months of life. There is a higher risk of early VKDB in babies who are premature, not feeding or absorbing feeds, had a complicated delivery, are ill, or whose mothers were on medication (e.g. anticonvulsants) that may increase the risk of bleeding in the newborn. Late VKDB is more likely in babies that have liver disease or any other bleeding disorder.

For many years vitamin K was given prophylactically at birth, by intramuscular (i.m.) injection. In 1992 a link was suggested between i.m. (but not oral) administration of vitamin K at birth and an increased risk of cancer in childhood. The finding has not been confirmed in other studies; nevertheless, it was thought prudent to seek alternative means of prophylaxis, pending the results of further research.

MAKE SURE MOTHERS KNOW THAT the cancer risk has not been confirmed in any other research study; the hazards of vitamin K deficiency bleeding and the effectiveness

---

of vitamin K prophylaxis are beyond doubt; there has never been any suggestion of a cancer link with oral vitamin K. Parental refusal is a significant problem and staff must be unequivocal in their advice about the dangers of VKDB.

Vitamin K (phytomenadione – Konakion MM paediatric ® Roche) is licensed for oral and parenteral use. All babies should receive one dose of vitamin K at birth. Thereafter, babies fed on modern formula feeds will receive sufficient vitamin K, but babies who are entirely or mainly breastfed should receive effective long-term prophylaxis.

No one regimen has been shown to be ideal. Commonly used options include: a single dose of 1 mg i.m at birth; two oral doses of 2 mg at birth and at 4–7 days. For breastfed babies, a further oral dose of 2 mg is given at 1 month.

The oral regimes appear to be effective if correctly administered.

There is a risk that the second and third doses, which are usually given after the baby has left hospital, might easily be forgotten (or refused), unless the importance of this prophylaxis is stressed to the parents. If serious bleeding were to result, leading to death or permanent disability, the parent might well bring a legal action against the Trust concerned. *If oral preparations are used, a mechanism MUST be in place to ensure that babies of breastfeeding mothers receive ALL the doses specified in the policy, and there must be a means of monitoring the implementation of this policy.*

Staff should record the formulation, dose, route and date of all vitamin K administration.

Some of this material first appeared in and is reproduced from Hall D, Elliman D. *Health for All Children*, 4th ed. revised 2006, with permission from Oxford University Press.

Sub-clinical deficiency of vitamin A occurs in the UK, but symptomatic deficiency is not seen. The most important vitamin deficiencies are vitamin K (*see* Box 6.4) and vitamin D. Health professionals should be aware that cases of vitamin D deficiency have become more common, particularly in Black and Asian children. Babies may present with signs of rickets or with features of hypocalcaemia, such as neuromuscular irritability or fits.

The following recommendations[7] are based on recent (2007) guidance:

Formula-fed babies. Infant formulas are supplemented with vitamins and minerals and meet accepted standards, but infants over 6 months who drink less than 500 mL of infant or follow-on formula per day should have vitamin drops.

Breastfed babies. Breastfed infants under 6 months do not need vitamin supplements provided the mother has an adequate vitamin status. After 6 months, infants receiving breast milk as their main drink should be given supplements of vitamins A, C and D.

Vitamin A, C and D drops should be given at 1 month, if:

▶ the mother's diet is poor or was poor in pregnancy;
▶ the mother is eating a restricted dietary regimen for any reason;
▶ the mother has dark skin pigmentation, that is, she is of African or Asian origin (because of reduced synthesis of vitamin D). It is recommended that these pregnant and lactating mothers receive a supplement of 10 μg vitamin D daily.

Widely available preparations providing appropriate doses of vitamins A, C and D are Abidec and Healthy Start Children's Vitamin Drops. There is no danger of reaching toxic levels provided that only one vitamin supplement is given.

Children between 2 and 5 years

Infants' and children's appetites and diets vary considerably over a week and the routine administration of vitamin drops A, C and D will ensure regular adequate intake of these particular vitamins, especially during the winter months. Vitamin drops should be given by dropper or spoon, not added to drinks or food. The mother may need to be shown how to place the drops in the mouth, rather than at the back of the throat, which may cause inhalation.

DRUGS AND BREASTFEEDING

Alcohol and caffeine pass into breast milk and should be taken only in limited quantities. Most medication also passes into breast milk, but rarely in concentrations likely to harm the baby.[*] The combined oral contraceptive pill may depress milk production, but progestogen-only contraceptives, although measurable in very small amounts in the milk, do not suppress lactation or affect the baby. It is generally advised that HIV-positive mothers, and those at risk of HIV infection, should not breastfeed; the child's paediatrician should be consulted in such cases.

BOTTLE-FEEDING

If the mother chooses not to breastfeed or is unable to breastfeed, the infant should be given an infant formula. Infants under 6 months of age should not be fed on unmodified cow's milk ('door step milk'), because this may result in hypernatraemic dehydration and does not provide enough iron and other nutrients to meet the infant's needs. This is very dangerous and can result in convulsions and permanent brain damage.

Infant formula is manufactured from modified cow's milk and its composition is regulated by the 'Infant Formula and Follow-On Formula Regulations'.[†] There are two main types of infant formula suitable for infants: whey-based and casein-based. In general, each manufacturer produces one whey-dominant milk and one casein-dominant milk, commonly known as first and second milks. (For examples, see Box 6.5.) Whey-dominant formulas have a whey:casein ratio similar to that of human milk. Casein-dominant formulas have a whey:casein ratio approximately the same as cow's milk. Whey-dominant formulas may be preferable, in that they are more similar in composition to human milk, but there is otherwise no apparent difference between whey- and casein-dominant formulas. Due to the addition of novel substrates some of these formulas may be unsuitable for infants from families who exclude certain food groups for moral or religious reasons (e.g. halal, kosher, vegetarian or vegan). Families should be advised to check manufacturers labelling information for up-to-date information.

---

[*] For detailed guidance on which drugs are safe while breastfeeding, *see* the *British National Formulary* at www. bnf.org

[†] *See* www.food.gov.uk/multimedia/pdfs/formulaengland2007.pdf

---

BOX 6.5 Whey-based and casein-based milks used in the UK

Whey-based formulas (commonly called 'first milks'): 60% whey: 40% casein ratio
Whey-based formulas are more similar in composition to breast milk than casein-based formula and have a lower renal solute load:

Aptamil First	Milupa
First Milk from Newborn	Cow & Gate
HiPP Organic Infant Milk	HIPP Organic
Nurture Newborn	HJ Heinz
Premium	Cow & Gate
SMA Gold	SMA

Casein-based formulas (commonly called second milks): 20% whey: 80% casein ratio
Casein-based formulas have a higher renal solute load than whey-based milks. Casein forms curds, which are thought to be more slowly digested and these milks are promoted as being more satisfying for hungrier babies. There is currently no scientific or medical evidence to support this.

Aptamil Extra Hungry	Milupa
Infant Milk for Hungrier Babies	Cow & Gate
SMA White	SMA
Nurture Hungry Baby	HJ Heinz

Mothers frequently change formulas because the baby is 'not satisfied', or 'has colic' (*see* page 213) or has poor weight gain. However, there is little evidence that these manoeuvres help. There is no support for the idea that changing from a whey-based to a casein-based formula will satisfy the baby more easily or that this progression is in any way beneficial. Whey-dominant milks can be continued until the baby is 12 months old. If the baby is not satisfied, the number or quantity of feeds should be increased, and the mother reassured that it is normal for feeding patterns to change. If the baby is 17 weeks old or more, solid foods could be considered, if the infant is still not settled.

Follow-on milks

Follow-on milks should not be given to infants under 6 months of age as they have a higher renal solute load than breast milk or ordinary formulas. This increases the risk of hypertonic dehydration with the hazards of convulsions and brain damage. For infants of 6 months and over, they can be introduced if the parent wishes. They have no advantage over ordinary infant formulas, but are preferable to the early introduction of unmodified cow's milk. They are higher in iron and vitamin D than standard formula and may be beneficial for older infants in special circumstances (e.g. if the weaning diet is low in iron or the child has identified special dietary requirements). Follow-on milks include:

Aptamil Follow-On	Milupa
Follow-on Milk for Babies Six Months +	Cow & Gate
HiPP Organic Follow-on Milk	HIPP
Nurture Growing Baby Follow-on	HJ Heinz
SMA Progress	SMA

Soya infant formula

Soya infant formula has a similar nutritional content to that of a cow's milk-based formula. However, soya milk and milk products do not protect against allergic conditions and concern has been raised over the phytoestrogen content of soya infant formula and the possible long-term health implications of using these in infancy. Although further studies are required to clarify these findings and thus the safety of soya formula, parents should be informed of the potential risks of their use.

The Scientific Advisory Committee on Nutrition (SACN) has advised that there are no particular health benefits associated with the consumption of soya-based infant formula by healthy infants. They should not be recommended indiscriminately for conditions such as colic or for unconfirmed cow's milk intolerance. The advice from the Chief Medical Officer is that soya-based infant formula should not be used as the first choice for the management of infants with proven cow's milk sensitivity, or lactose intolerance, and that hydrolysed protein formula (*see* the following section) should be used instead. The diagnosis of allergy to the proteins of cow's milk is difficult and should usually be made only by a paediatrician.

Soya formula may still be used in exceptional circumstances, such as in infants with galactosaemia, infants of vegan mothers who are not breastfeeding or infants with cow's milk allergy/intolerance who refuse extensively hydrolysed formula. It should not be given to premature or low birth weight infants, or babies with impaired renal function. Available soya infant formulas are:

Enfamil Prosobee	Mead Johnson
Infasoy	Cow & Gate
Isomil	Abbott
Nurture Soya	HJ Heinz
Wysoy	SMA Nutrition

If a soya formula is indicated, only soya formula specifically designed for infant feeding should be used. Ordinary soya milk drinks are not suitable as most are lower in energy, calcium, iron and vitamins; they should never be used in infants of less than 12 months. Soya infant formulas should be continued until the child is at least 1 year of age, and preferably throughout the pre-school years for vegan children. If children on a milk-free diet are consuming ordinary soya milk drinks, they should be calcium-fortified, otherwise a calcium supplement should be recommended. Vitamin drops are also advised.

Hydrolysed protein formula

These are lactose-free milks in which the protein has been extensively hydrolysed so that it is no longer allergenic and is more easily digested. They should only be used under medical and dietetic supervision. They are nutritionally complete and are available on prescription for infants with proven cow's milk intolerance/allergy. Examples are:

Pepti Junior	Cow & Gate
Prejomin	Milupa
Peptide	Scientific Hospital Supplies
Nutramigen 1	Mead Johnson
Nutramigen 2 (suitable from 6 months)	

Preterm discharge formula

Preterm or very low birth weight babies may require additional calories, fat, protein, vitamins and minerals on discharge from the Neonatal Unit. In response to this, a nutrient-enriched post discharge formula, Nutriprem 2, (Cow & Gate) has been developed as an alternative to term formula for infants who are not breastfed. This product is available on prescription for up to 6 months-corrected age

High-energy formulas

Specialised high-energy formulas can be prescribed on medical grounds for infants with disease related to malnutrition, malabsorption, growth failure or high-energy requirements. These formulas must only be used under medical and dietetic supervision and include Infatrini (Cow & Gate) and SMA High Energy (SMA).

Many *specialised formulas* are more cariogenic than standard formula because of the type of sugars they contain. Good dental hygiene is essential and parents should be advised to encourage a feeder cup rather than a bottle from 6 months old, to limit the risk of dental caries.

Feed thickeners and pre-thickened infant formula

Feed thickeners such as Carobel (Nutricia) or Nestargel (Nestlé) can be used in infants who have gastro-oesophageal reflux. The thickeners are manufactured from starch, guar gum or carob bean gum. They may be prescribed by a paediatrician, GP or paediatric dietician. Mild to moderate regurgitation during or after feeds can be common and is often harmless. In the absence of other symptoms, mild to moderate reflux does not need therapeutic interventions. However, if the infant is failing to thrive, experiencing feeding difficulties or is in pain during feeding then referral should be made for further investigation.

Pre-thickened infant formulas are available over the counter and it is claimed that they may help with posseting and minor digestive problems. Parents should be discouraged from using them without first seeking medical advice. They include:

Enfamil AR   Mead Johnson
SMA Staydown   SMA Nutrition

Modified formula for minor digestive problems

New formulas have been introduced that claim to help with minor digestive problems, but there is no sound medical evidence to recommend them. Mothers should be advised to seek advice from a health professional before changing the formula. They include:

Aptamil Easy Digest (Milupa)
Comfort 1 (Cow & Gate)
Nurture Gentle Newborn (HJ Heinz)

FORMULA-FEEDING: PRACTICAL ASPECTS

Newborn babies may take very small volumes frequently, but once established most infants ingest approximately 150–200 mL/kg per day in the first 4 months. Formula-fed infants should be demand-fed and parents should be reassured that it is normal for feeding patterns to change and a change is not necessarily an indication to introduce complementary foods. Mothers should be encouraged to feed their babies as much and as often as the baby demands.

Reconstituting feeds

Hygiene is crucial for safe formula feeding.[8] The hands should be thoroughly washed before preparing the feed. The bottles and teats must be washed carefully with a brush and then both bottle and teats must be immersed totally in a sterilising solution.*

Dried milk formula

Packet instructions should be followed at all times. Formula milks available in the UK are reconstituted by the same method. The feed should be prepared with one scoop to 1 fl. oz/30 mL of water using freshly boiled water. Do not use water that has been repeatedly boiled as this may result in an over-concentration of minerals. Formula milks purchased in other countries may be reconstituted differently and individual packet instructions should therefore be followed carefully. Feeds that are too strong or too weak result from careless preparation. The Department of Health advises that feeds should be made up as required and not in advance. Any leftover feed should be discarded.†

Ready-to-feed milks

Some milks are available in a ready-to-feed form, either in bottles or tetrapaks. They are more expensive than powder milks, but may be useful when travelling or on holiday. Mothers should be careful to avoid contamination when opening tetra-pak cartons, by wiping the outside before opening and ensuring that clean scissors are used.

Water softeners

Softened water from proprietary water softeners should not be used for infants because the exchange resin is impregnated with sodium. This exchanges sodium ions for the calcium and magnesium ions in the water and may cause hypernatraemia.

Water filters

Filters reduce the hardness of the water, but the sodium level is not altered. Some water filters use a cartridge containing silver, and traces of silver from the cartridge may be found in the filtered water. Whilst no adverse effects have been found from ingestion of traces of silver, water filtered in this way should not be used for infants until its safety has been confirmed. As different water filters use different cartridges, people are advised to check with manufacturers on their suitability for infants.

Mineral, spa and spring water

The suitability of these waters depends on the concentration of various electrolytes and minerals. Suitable bottled waters are Evian, Spa, Highland Spring Water, Volvic and Sainsbury's Natural Scottish Spring. When travelling abroad where the standard

---

* *See* www.babyfriendly.org.uk/pdfs/sterenglish.pdf for useful instructions on sterilisation. These can be downloaded in different languages.

† Useful information is available on the reconstitution of powdered formula feeds at www.babyfriendly.org.uk/pdfs/botenglish.pdf

of water supply is suspect, parents should use bottled water. Bottled water is not sterile and it should always be boiled before use for infants of less than 6 months.

Microwave ovens

Microwave ovens are hazardous if used to heat bottle feeds as heat distribution is uneven; the baby's mouth can be severely burnt by the milk unless it is shaken vigorously and checked carefully. They are not suitable for the sterilisation of feeding equipment unless a purpose-made microwave steam sterilising unit is used.

Cow's milk

Weaning and the Weaning Diet[9] advised that pasteurised whole cow's milk should be used as the main milk drink only after 1 year of age. It should not be used in the first year as it has two disadvantages:

- iron is too low at a time when demands are high;
- vitamins A, C, D and E are all too low.

Doorstep milk is microbiologically safe[*] and does not require boiling. Unmodified cow's milk and products made from cow's milk can be included in the weaning diet, e.g. custards, yoghurt. Unpasteurised milk is not safe and has been associated with many outbreaks of gastroenteritis.

Some health-conscious parents are eager to introduce semi-skimmed or even skimmed milk early in the child's life, but there is no evidence that fat restriction in the first 5 years of life reduces the risk of heart disease and it may result in a serious deficiency of energy and failure to thrive. Whole (full-fat) milk should be given at least until 2 years of age. Semi-skimmed milk may be used after 2 years, provided that fat and calorie requirements are met from other food sources.

Goat's and ewe's milk

Goat's and ewe's milk are not suitable for children under 6 months and should not be given before the child is 1 year old. They are not less allergenic than cow's milk. A goat's milk product is marketed under the name 'Nanny' by Vitacare. There is no known advantage to using this rather than cow's milk formula; it is more expensive than ordinary formulas and there are no data on the growth of infants fed on this diet. Fresh goat's and ewe's milk is not always pasteurised. It is a potential source of infection and should not be given to young children. It should always be boiled for 2 minutes before using.

WEANING

Weaning is a gradual process that begins when breast- or bottle-feeding starts to be replaced by a mixed diet. Problems of slow weight gain associated with weaning and feeding difficulties are discussed on page 139. Two useful DVDs are available to help parents and professionals understand weaning.[10]

---

* Doorstep milk is only safe if the cap is intact. Birds pecking the bottle tops can introduce *Campylobacter* infection.

Reasons for weaning

There are a number of reasons for weaning:

- milk does not satisfy all the nutritional requirements for a baby from age 6 months onwards;
- there is a natural progression from sucking to chewing;
- it is important to introduce new tastes and textures, and new skills (the use of feeding beaker, cup, cutlery).

Developmental and behavioural aspects of weaning

In the early months of life, the infant is likely to enjoy any foods given by the parent. Food preferences can be developed with only a tiny amount of food, so interventions that provide foods for experience rather than nutrition can be effective even while tube feeding is still needed. Therefore, the first weaning food should be offered in very small quantities, on a small soft teaspoon. The infant needs to become accustomed to spoon-feeding, so food should not be added to the milk in the bottle.

If the family diet is nutritionally sound, the parents should be encouraged to give the baby family foods; the food can be puréed using a food processor, sieve, or spoon and fork. If home foods are used, there should be no added salt or sugar until the baby is at least 12 months old. If the baby refuses a food after several attempts, the food should simply be removed without any fuss. Force-feeding must never be attempted as it will inevitably lead to severe feeding difficulties. The parent should try to create a relaxed sociable atmosphere and should feed the baby at *his* pace.

By the end of the first year the child has clear food preferences and each food is liked in the form in which it is normally eaten: taste, smell, texture and appearance. At this stage the child begins to group food into categories with a label and may reject food on sight without testing it. From the age of 12–14 months new food is more likely to be tried if an adult is seen to be eating it.

The regulation of food intake depends on gastric emptying and from central control by the brain. However, adults eat according to extrinsic social cues; for instance, they finish up what is on the plate even though they may be satisfied and eat at meal times whether or not they are hungry. Young children tend to eat when they feel hungry, but parents often override this self-regulation, by encouraging infants and toddlers to finish a bottle or meal, for example.

Weaning: nutritional aspects

There is a great deal of individual variation in when an infant is ready for solids and there needs to be some flexibility in the advice given, as the evidence on which this is based is not robust. Exclusive milk feeding (breast or bottle) is recommended for around the first 6 months (26 weeks) as this provides all the nutrients an infant needs. For infants who are breastfed, exclusive breastfeeding has significant health benefits for the infant and mother and there is no evidence of any harm to the infant as long as the mother is well nourished and the baby is gaining weight appropriately. Seventeen weeks is regarded by professionals as the earliest age at which complementary foods should be introduced, but in the UK most mothers have already started offering solids by this age, most commonly because they perceive their babies to be hungry.[11] The infant's developmental readiness, feeding pattern, and growth should be considered.

However, many breastfeeding mothers will be unable to or will choose not to follow the advice on exclusive breastfeeding up to 6 months, and some breastfed and formula-fed infants may need solids earlier than 6 months. Parents should be supported in their decision and given the appropriate advice on complementary feeding. The issues associated with early weaning should be discussed with parents. There may be a slight increase in minor illnesses in infants who are weaned earlier, but in general the evidence regarding age of weaning is equivocal. Infants weaned nearer 6 months will need to be moved on to a mixed diet more quickly than those weaned earlier, to ensure adequate nutrition and continued development of normal feeding behaviour.

Stages of weaning

There are four stages of weaning.

▶ **Stage 1** (by 6 months): puréed vegetables, puréed fruit, baby rice, mashed potato.
▶ **Stage 2** (by 7 months): increase the variety and quantity of food offered; food should be mashed rather than puréed. Introduce meat, chicken, fish, beans, lentils. Wheat products (bread, wheat cereals, pasta) and egg can be introduced from 6 months.
▶ **Stage 3** (by 9 months): infants should now be having 2–3 meals a day and more variety. Introduce lumpier foods and finger foods to encourage chewing. As the quantity of solids increases, the amount of milk taken will decrease. Protein from milk will gradually be replaced with meat, fish, eggs, cheese, lentils, beans and cereals. Water, diluted unsweetened fruit juice, or diluted baby juice can replace some of the milk feeds, but breast milk or formula milk should still be continued up until 1 year. Drinking from a cup or beaker can be introduced.
▶ **Stage 4** (by 1 year): infants should be eating minced and chopped food and a wide variety of foods such as cereals, fruit, vegetables (meat, chicken, fish, pulses, dairy products and eggs). Encourage three regular meals and two to three milk drinks (about 1 pint of milk per day). Additional fluids should be water and diluted unsweetened fruit juice. Warn parents about the dangers of nuts and similar foods, which can cause choking in babies.

Cultural considerations

Advice given to any ethnic group should take into account their cultural beliefs about food, cooking and mealtimes, as well as the types of food acceptable to and eaten by the family. Many problems can be avoided if families use their family foods for weaning. Mothers can be advised how to modify family foods to suit the infant and avoid giving highly spiced foods; for example, dishes containing ginger, cloves or chilli. Plain baby rice is a suitable base to which mothers can add foods from their own diets. Vegetables and dahls/lentils can be boiled, without the addition of salt. Manufactured baby foods do not introduce the flavour of traditional family meals to the infant. Furthermore, in some ethnic groups there may be concern about the religious acceptability of these foods; this may severely restrict their choice. In order to avoid using non-halal meat dishes, Moslem mothers may purchase only sweet foods, such as fruit purées. However, there is an increasing variety of manufactured vegetarian baby foods available, so choice need not be restricted to desserts in order to avoid non-halal meat dishes.

By 6–8 months an Asian baby should have tried:

▶ fruit, vegetables, dahl, rice;
▶ cereals: bread, chapatti, wheat cereals;
▶ semolina;
▶ natural yoghurt;
▶ cheese (paneer);
▶ lean meat, chicken and fish (if permitted).

If the family is vegetarian, the child should have 1 pint of milk daily and should be offered dahl, cereals and vegetable protein foods. Discourage excess intake of milk (more than 1.5 pints daily) as this will depress the appetite at meal times and the diet will become unbalanced.

Although the risk of *Salmonella* in eggs is much less than it was a few years ago, it is still wise to ensure that eggs are well cooked. Raw eggs should not be used.

Vegetarian baby

Definitions:

▶ **Partial vegetarians** exclude some, but not all, animal products; for example, they may eat poultry or fish;
▶ **Lacto-ovo-vegetarians** exclude all meat, poultry and fish products, but include milk and eggs;
▶ **Lacto-vegetarians** exclude all meat, fish, poultry and egg products, but include milk in the diet;
▶ **Vegans** exclude all animal products, including milk. These diets can be nutritionally adequate, but careful planning is needed to ensure that serious deficiencies of minerals and vitamins do not occur.

A vegetarian or vegan diet does not preclude normal growth and development, although the more extreme the dietary restriction the greater the risk of poor nutrition. Protein from animal sources contains all essential amino acids and is of high biological value; that is, it is utilised efficiently by the body. Protein from plant sources lacks certain essential amino acids. To utilise the protein efficiently, a mixture of these foods should be eaten together to complement each other. For example, pulses and grains can be eaten as dahl and rice, baked beans on toast; and pulses and seeds as hummus. Energy density of many vegetarian foods is low, due to low fat and high fibre content. Infants may have difficulty consuming the necessary volume of food, and growth should be monitored to check that energy intake is adequate.

Parents should be advised to:

▶ offer food at least four times a day;
▶ include energy-dense food at each meal;
▶ avoid diluting nutrients in foods by adding too much fluid.

Vitamin B12 deficiency can occur in breastfed infants if the maternal diet is not adequate. Vegan mothers who do not take additional vitamin B12 have low concentrations of the vitamin in their breast milk. After breastfeeding is discontinued, vegan babies should be given an infant soya formula at least until 1 year of age. Children's vitamin drops (A, C and D) should be given to breastfed vegetarian infants from 4–6 weeks and to all infants on introduction of weaning foods at least until the age of 2 years, and preferably until 5 years. It will be difficult for infants to achieve adequate calcium intake unless they are fed sufficient calcium-fortified milk. It is essential that vegetarian infants receive vitamin D supplementation so that calcium utilisation is maximised.

OTHER ASPECTS OF NUTRITION
Iron
By 6 months the infant's iron stores are becoming depleted. Iron is included in infant formulas, but unmodified cow's milk does not contain enough for the infant's needs. Iron absorption is increased by vitamin C, but is impaired by the tannins in tea. Families should be advised on iron-containing foods to include in the infant's diet: liver, red meat, corned beef, iron-fortified cereals (e.g. Weetabix), wholemeal bread, dahl and other pulses (e.g. baked beans) and green vegetables. Non-haem iron, found in cereal foods, is not as well absorbed as haem iron. It may be advantageous to give a source of vitamin C, such as fruit juice, with meals.

Iron deficiency is common in early childhood, particularly in children living in poor circumstances and in those born prematurely. The symptoms are often non-specific, but there is good evidence that iron deficiency does not only cause anaemia, but also affects neurological functioning, behaviour and perhaps also development, at least in the short term. These adverse effects are reversed by iron long before there is any rise in haemoglobin level, suggesting that the effect is mediated directly on brain enzymes. Prevention by good diet is preferable to screening, although a case has been made for screening infants or toddlers for iron deficiency in inner city areas. There should be no hesitation in giving infants a 1-month course of ferrous fumarate or similar iron preparation. A child with iron deficiency may also be at risk of vitamin D-deficient rickets.

Iron preparations are poisonous in excessive dosage; therefore it is important to warn parents to keep them in a safe place.

Sugar
Refined sugar is not required as part of a healthy diet. The addition of sugar to food should be avoided because it contributes to dental decay and may promote overweight and obesity. Parents should be encouraged to give children a diet that is low in sugar, both in volume and frequency of sugar intake.

Parents should be advised against putting sugary drinks into feeding bottles or reservoir feeders, especially for the child to hold or take to bed. Such practices result in almost continuous bathing of the teeth enamel with sugars. The use of sweetened dummies should also be avoided. Sugary drinks, many of which are marketed specially for young children, can very quickly lead to severe tooth decay, pain and distress. A general anaesthetic will then be required to remove the damaged teeth. This scenario should be avoided at all costs. Milk and water are the only 'safe' drinks for teeth. However, prolonged bottle feeding should not be encouraged as even lactose contained in milk can eventually lead to caries. The prolonged administration of sugar-containing medicines can also have a devastating effect on the teeth and sugar-free preparations should be prescribed wherever possible (*see* page 122 for more details).

Adding sugar to a feed in order to relieve constipation is not effective and should be discouraged. Fruit juice (diluted 50:50), puréed fruit or vegetables will be equally effective in treating constipation. However, over-use of fruit juices (many of which contain non-milk extrinsic sugars) can cause tooth decay. In addition, fruit juices are acidic and contribute to 'tooth erosion' (chemical wearing away of the tooth surface). This is very different from tooth decay, but a recognised problem among young children in the UK. Natural fruit juices, if used, should be diluted.

Salt

Salt should not be added to food cooked for a baby of less than 6 months because of the risk of hypernatraemia (high blood sodium levels, often in association with dehydration, which lead to cerebral damage). When the baby is more than 6 months and is eating family foods, salt should not be added during cooking or at the table. There has been concern about the role of salt intake in the development of hypertension, although there is no definite evidence in support of this hypothesis.

Fibre

An excessive intake of wholegrain cereals and pulses may lead to diarrhoea. Parents should be warned against becoming too obsessed with high fibre diets. High fibre diets are very bulky and have low energy content per unit volume. The infant's stomach may not be able to deal with the large volumes he needs to yield an adequate energy supply. Parents who persist with such diets may eventually find that their children are failing to thrive and may become malnourished. Unprocessed bran should not be given to children because it contains phytate, which binds with some minerals and inhibits absorption.

Drinks for infants

Often milk intake is reduced when the mother begins to offer alternative drinks, but milk is nutritionally valuable in a child's diet and an intake of 1 pint of milk daily is recommended. However, an excessive intake (over 1.5 pints) can depress the appetite for other foods. Many commercial fruit juices and herbal drinks contain large quantities of carbohydrates in various forms, not necessarily described as 'sugar', and these should be avoided. Offer a parent the following advice:

- drinks – preferably water – should be offered *after* meals;
- from the age of 6 months, drinks can be given from a feeder cup or beaker;
- take the drink away once the child has drunk all he requires;
- tea is not encouraged because the tannins in tea impair iron absorption and are a significant factor in causing anaemia.

Additives

The prevalence of intolerance to food additives in the population as a whole is very low, perhaps only 0.03–0.15%. Food additives are added to food:

- to prevent food contamination, increase shelf life, allow a wider variety of food to be available all year round, prevent food poisoning;
- to aid processing; for example, raising agents in cakes;
- to enhance the colour or flavour of food;
- to replace nutrients lost in processing.

Convenience foods and processed foods are part of our modern diet and lifestyle, but some additives, such as colouring agents, are not necessary. Children do tend to eat foods with unnecessary additives; for example, fruit squash, fizzy drinks, instant puddings and sweets. The evidence that these additives do any harm is limited, though they may be involved in *some* cases of hyperactivity and migraine. Nevertheless it is understandable that parents should wish to limit the child's intake. Advise them to:

▶ use fresh foods;
▶ use home-baked dishes instead of bought pies, cakes, packet soups, etc., which have a high number of additives;
▶ avoid highly processed foods (additive cocktails);
▶ look at the label (the ingredients are given in order of quantity).

'E' numbers

Permitted food additives, other than flavourings, are given a number to aid in labelling. Additives without an 'E' prefix are either awaiting approval or have not gained approval in the EC. Additives are grouped according to their function:

▶ E100–199: permitted colours;
▶ E220–321: preservatives and antioxidants (to keep food fresh);
▶ E322+: processing aids; for example, emulsifiers, stabilisers, and aerating, gelling and thickening agents.

There is no point in trying to avoid all E numbers. Some E additives are naturally occurring substances, for example:

▶ E101 (riboflavin)
▶ E140 (chlorophyll)
▶ E170 (chalk)
▶ E260 (acetic acid)
▶ E270 (lactic acid)
▶ E300 (vitamin C)

Hair analysis

Analysis of hair for mineral content is undertaken, by certain practitioners, as a measure of the 'mineral composition and deficiencies of the body'. Unfortunately, hair mineral content does not accurately reflect the composition of the body and this procedure has no scientific validity.

COMMON PROBLEMS
Premature babies

There are no official UK guidelines on the timing of introduction of complementary foods to the preterm infant and more research is needed to provide a basis for recommendations. As with term infants, developmental readiness should be considered as there will be considerable variation in the rate at which premature infants acquire the motor feeding skills that are a pre-requisite for safe feeding. Head control has to be sufficiently mature to maintain a suitable position for the safe taking of food from a spoon. It is difficult to give an age or age range, but as 17 weeks is considered the right developmental stage for the term infant, around 17 weeks developmental age could be used as a guide for the preterm infant.

Some parents see the introduction of solids as a sign of progress and may be eager to introduce solids much earlier; this may lead to feeding problems if the infant is not developmentally ready. Poor weight gain should not be used as a sign to start solids as it may reduce the amount of milk taken and no advantage is gained; however, it may be helpful for infants with poor sucking skills who may do better with spoon feeding. Premature infants who have problems with feeding should be referred to a paediatric dietician and speech and language therapist for more detailed assessment and advice.

Premature babies should receive iron supplements of 1–2 mg/kg/day to a maximum of 15 mg/day, and multivitamin supplements.

Food 'allergy'

Food allergy and food intolerance have received considerable publicity in recent years. Only a small number of reactions to food are true allergic responses; that is, involving immune reaction in the body. Adverse reactions to food can be classified into three areas (excluding food poisoning, which is caused by microbial or chemical contamination of food):

▶ **food aversion** is a psychological avoidance of certain foods;
▶ **food intolerance** is an abnormal reaction to food, due to a digestive enzyme deficiency, for example;
▶ **food allergy** is an abnormal reaction to food involving the immune system.

Food intolerance is commonly suspected by parents and a bewildering variety of complaints have been attributed to an 'allergy' to milk, gluten, yeast and many other foods. Only rarely can these 'diagnoses' be confirmed by any scientifically valid procedure, but this fact does not reduce the faith of parents in the power of diet to solve their child's difficulties. The removal of foods from the diet of a young child has to be carried out with care. If the suspected food is a major source of nutrients, alternatives must be included to make good any deficiency. Advise the parents to obtain a specialist opinion before embarking on such experiments.

Children who have a genuine confirmed food allergy usually become less allergic as they get older and the offending food can often be re-introduced. However, they may occasionally become extremely ill when the food challenge is given, so if the original reaction was severe, this should be done under expert medical supervision.

Allergy to peanuts and other nuts

Reactions to nuts are among the most common food allergies and this seems to be an increasingly common problem. Deaths from nut allergy are rare but appear to be more common in children with asthma.[12] The diagnosis of allergy to peanuts and tree nuts such as cashews is difficult; the clinical history is often unclear and IgE tests are not reliable. Children seen in primary care settings should preferably be referred to a paediatrician. A definitive diagnosis is useful as true nut allergies are probably life-long and have significant implications for lifestyle. Direct challenge under expert supervision in hospital may be the best way to establish or exclude the diagnosis.

Dietary avoidance of peanuts can be difficult as peanuts can often be hidden in food and foods are not always clearly labelled. Prevention is important and current advice is:

▶ Pregnant or lactating mothers from allergic families should avoid nuts in their own diets. The introduction of peanuts and other nuts to the diet of their infants should be delayed until the age of 3 years unless otherwise advised by an expert in the field (for updated guidance, *see* www.food.gov.uk).
▶ These precautions are not necessary for non-allergic or non-atopic families. Peanuts of a suitable texture (e.g. smooth peanut butter) can be introduced from 6–8 months of age.
▶ Whole nuts should not be given to children under 5 due to the risk of choking.
▶ These restrictions are only of any nutritional consequence if the family is vegetarian or vegan, in which case dietetic advice should be obtained.

There is also some evidence that children with inflamed skin (e.g. eczema, nappy rash) may be sensitised to peanuts from the use of creams containing peanut oil. There may also be a link between exposure to soya protein and peanut allergy. Although further research is needed in this area it would be sensible to avoid the use of creams containing peanut oil in the management of eczema or other inflammatory skin conditions and also to follow the CMO advice on the use of soya formula (*see* page 107). Some medicines and vitamin drops (including Abidec) contain arachis (peanut) oil. It is uncertain whether there is any significant risk involved with any of these preparations. Specialist advise should be obtained from a paediatrician and/or dietician if parents are concerned about a family history of allergy or if the child has suffered a serious reaction. Injectable adrenaline may be prescribed for emergency use but it is only part of the strategy needed to deal with serious allergic reactions.

Cow's milk protein intolerance

This is a well-recognised but uncommon condition and is certainly over-diagnosed. The most common symptoms are vomiting, diarrhoea and failure to thrive. Mild cases may present later and the symptoms are varied. Colic without other symptoms is unlikely to be due to cow's milk protein intolerance. Children suspected of having this condition should be referred to a paediatrician to confirm the diagnosis. Dietetic advice should be sought on weaning diets suitable for an infant with cow's milk intolerance, as many commercial baby foods contain milk powder.

Family history of allergic conditions

Infants with a family history of atopy or allergic disease (at least one affected parent or sibling) are at an increased risk of developing food allergy and exclusive breast-feeding for 6 months may be protective. If breastfeeding is not possible or the mother cannot continue until 6 months, an extensively hydrolysed formula may be recommended for high risk infants. Soya formula is not suitable.

If weaning is started before 6 months the following foods should be avoided:

▶ wheat-based foods and foods containing gluten (rusks, bread, chapatti, pasta, wheat containing breakfast cereals);
▶ eggs, including scrambled eggs, egg custards;
▶ fish and shellfish;

- nuts and seeds;
- citrus fruits, including juices;
- soya and soya products;
- mustard;
- celery;
- cow's milk, including infant formula or in weaning foods.

Currently, there is no evidence that delaying the introduction of high allergenic foods much beyond the age of 6 months is beneficial to the high-risk infant. However it is recommended that potentially allergic foods are introduced one at a time, starting with a small amount and leaving a week between each new food. This allows identification of any food that may have caused a reaction. If cow's milk is tolerated in weaning foods, then the gradual introduction of formula can be considered, if appropriate.

Infants with a suspected or proven food allergy should be referred for specialist medical and dietetic advice.

GASTROENTERITIS

Milk feeds should be stopped in babies who develop diarrhoea, with or without vomiting, but breastfeeding should be continued. Small amounts of bland solids may be offered if the child is hungry and can tolerate them. Antibiotics should not be given unless there are special indications. Anti-diarrhoea drugs and anti-emetics are potentially hazardous in young children and should not be used. One of the standard glucose and electrolyte mixtures (oral rehydration solutions (ORS)) should be prescribed. The parent gives this by bottle, beaker, or, if necessary, by cup and spoon. Although the correct amount can be calculated, in practice the child usually regulates his own intake. Many babies vomit if given several ounces of the solution at once, but will tolerate it if it is spooned slowly, but continuously, into the mouth.[13]

ORS should be used to prevent and treat dehydration. It is not a treatment for the underlying condition. In normally nourished children with mild or moderate dehydration in the Western world, the traditional 24-hour period of starvation does not speed the process of recovery. Current advice is that breastfeeding can be continued throughout an episode of diarrhoea. ORS should be given for 3 or 4 hours and other feeds should then be cautiously resumed. If diarrhoea returns when feeding commences, hydration can be maintained with ORS, but there is little or no benefit in further starvation. Flat cola and similar drinks are not recommended as a substitute for ORS.

ORS is highly effective but there are several dangers for the unwary:

- The solution is simply a means of making good the losses of water and electrolytes. The parent should be told the rationale for its use and should appreciate that it is not a treatment for the underlying condition. The diarrhoea and vomiting will not necessarily cease at once.
- Diarrhoea and vomiting can be features of illnesses other than gastroenteritis. Every case should be kept under frequent review until the baby has recovered. Each year babies die from conditions such as intussusception and appendicitis because the initial symptoms were identical to those of gastroenteritis.

▶ Most mild cases of gastroenteritis are viral; nevertheless, a stool sample should be sent if diarrhoea persists, or is severe, or is accompanied by blood, in order to identify other organisms including *Campylobacter, Salmonella, Shigella* and *Cryptosporidium*.

▶ Gastroenteritis in a healthy child rarely leads to severe dehydration, but this can occur. If the baby is becoming too lethargic to take the replacement solution, or is clinically dehydrated, or is acidotic (rapid deep breathing often mistaken for pneumonia), hospitalisation should be arranged.

▶ Do not continue with replacement solution if the symptoms are not improving. The nutritional content is negligible and babies can become undernourished very quickly, perhaps pre-disposing to more serious infections. Do not hesitate to get specialist advice in such cases.

▶ Monitor growth after a severe episode of gastroenteritis, until it is clear that weight gain is satisfactory.

Assessing dehydration

There are a number of things to consider when assessing dehydration:

▶ **mild**: minimal physical signs (thirst, dry mouth, slightly sunken eyes, normal pulse and circulation);

▶ **moderate**: reduced urine output, raised pulse rate, skin turgor reduced, definitely sunken eyes, depressed fontanelle;

▶ **severe**: restless or drowsy, rapid weak pulse, deeply sunken eyes, skin turgor obviously reduced;

▶ **acidosis**: indicated by deep 'air-hunger' breathing, sometimes mistaken for pneumonia; can occur with any degree of dehydration; needs hospital care.

NB: Combinations of signs vary; do not expect to find all the signs in every case. The severity of dehydration is easily underestimated in hypernatraemic dehydration.

DANGER SIGNS: any of the following are indications to consider referral to hospital: tender or distended abdomen; bile-stained vomiting; bloody diarrhoea; disturbed consciousness.

There may be transient lactose intolerance after severe gastroenteritis. A lactose-free milk product can be used in such cases; for example, Nutramigen or Pepti Junior would be suitable. However, if the symptoms are sufficiently troublesome to merit consideration of such measures, it is probably wise to obtain specialist advice.

TODDLER DIARRHOEA

Toddler diarrhoea is the most common cause of chronic loose stools in early childhood. It is also known as peas and carrots diarrhoea because the presence of these undigested foods in the stool is often noted by parents. The onset is often difficult to time precisely, though it may follow an episode of gastroenteritis. The motions vary in consistency from day to day and may be accompanied by mucus, but not by blood. Sometimes they are so loose that toilet training is difficult. The crucial diagnostic feature is that the child is absolutely well in every other respect and putting on weight normally. No treatment is necessary. If the symptoms are troublesome, it may help to increase the fat and fibre content of the diet; reduce the amount of fruit juice (especially clear apple juice); and control the amount of fluid drunk between meals. Paediatricians often prescribe loperamide, though most parents prefer to use this for outings or special occasions rather than regularly. It is not licensed for children or recommended by the manufacturers for children under 4 years, but nevertheless it is safe even when used over longer periods. Remind parents to keep it in a safe place as overdose is hazardous.

VOMITING, POSSETTING AND REGURGITATION
Vomiting
Vomiting may be associated with diarrhoea in acute gastroenteritis as discussed in the previous paragraphs. The sudden onset of vomiting *without* diarrhoea may be due to a simple viral infection, but more serious infections, intestinal disorders and metabolic conditions may also present in this way. Repeated forceful or 'projectile' vomiting in the first few months of life may be due to pyloric stenosis. Such cases should be referred promptly.

By far the commonest cause of repeated small vomits in an otherwise well baby is possetting or regurgitation, associated with reflux of stomach contents up the oesophagus. This varies from an occasional mouthful of milk with wind to severe reflux leading to growth impairment and/or respiratory disorders. To make a diagnosis of uncomplicated regurgitation you need to establish that:

▶ the baby is well in all other respects;
▶ the problem is chronic rather than acute;
▶ the baby is thriving;
▶ the baby's development is within normal limits;
▶ there are no respiratory complaints (which might suggest aspiration of stomach contents into the lungs);
▶ the stools are normal;
▶ there is no blood in the vomit.

If there is doubt about any of these points, referral is advisable.

Management
There are various ways to manage possetting and regurgitation:

▶ Review the feeding regimen. The baby may be very hungry and feeding too quickly, or the mother may be giving the baby more milk than he can tolerate.
▶ If the baby is difficult to feed, a home visit to observe feeding and handling may be undertaken by the health visitor, community paediatric nurse or community dietician.
▶ The feeds can be thickened using an agent such as carobel.
▶ The introduction of solids often leads to improvement.
▶ Infant Gaviscon® may help.
▶ Changing the brand of milk formula rarely helps.
▶ Gradual improvement usually occurs as the baby is weaned.
▶ Monitor weight gain until you are happy that the baby is thriving.

FOOD AND POVERTY

For some families, purchasing food even for the next meal is a constant headache (*see* page 16 for 'food insecurity'). Poor families reduce expenditure on food whenever times are hard. This can have a serious effect on the nutritional status of low income families. Advice given to individual families must be appropriate to their social circumstances (finance, housing, education, partner support, cooking facilities, cooking skills, ease of access to shops and interest in food preparation). Fuel costs are also an important consideration. The gas and electricity boards provide leaflets and information on economic use of fuel during cooking.

Emphasis should be placed on eating an adequate diet within the budget and ability of the family. Encourage family meals, as cooking for a family is easier and cheaper than cooking individual meals. Poverty and poor living conditions are factors linked with the incidence of iron deficiency. Low income families should be told about cheap food sources of iron:

- cheap cuts of meat have as good an iron content as more expensive cuts;
- sardines and pilchards have an appreciable iron content;
- other useful low-cost foods are pulse vegetables and baked beans, dahl and lentils;
- iron-fortified cereals (e.g. Weetabix).

Vitamin C in the diet and in vitamin supplements helps the body to utilise iron from cereal sources more efficiently.

The Welfare Food Scheme has been replaced in the UK by the Healthy Start programme; this provides vouchers for qualifying families that can be exchanged for fresh fruit and vegetables as well as milk.[14]

PREVENTION OF DENTAL DISEASE

The first tooth is a milestone for parents and they may want to know when and in what order the teeth appear (*see* Figure 6.1). The appearance of the first teeth is a good opportunity to discuss prevention of decay and disease. The government set an objective that by 2003 the average DMF (total number of decayed, missing and filled teeth) index in 5-year-olds should not exceed 1 and that 70% of 5-year-olds should have no experience of tooth decay. This target was not achieved – the 2005/6 survey showed a DMF index in England of 1.47; across Wales it was 2.38; and in Scotland 2.16. This represents significant progress in Scotland but only a small improvement in England and Wales.[15]

Poor dental health has a strong relationship both with poverty and with non-fluoridated water supplies, though the link is stronger with poverty. Prevention of tooth decay and promotion of oral health are important and potentially achievable targets for child health programmes. The dental health of young children from an Asian background is poorer than that of White or African Caribbean children. It seems that Asian families are less likely to register their child with a dentist and need additional guidance.

Tooth development

Upper teeth	Primary erupt	Permanent erupt	
Central incisor	8–12 mos	7–8 yrs	
Lateral incisor	9–13 mos	8–9 yrs	
Canine	16–22 mos	11–12 yrs	
First premolar		10–11 yrs	
Second premolar		10–12 yrs	
First molar	13–19 mos	6–7 yrs	
Second molar	25–33 mos	12–13 yrs	
Third molar		17–21 yrs	
Lower teeth			
Third molar		17–21 yrs	
Second molar	23–31 mos	11–13 yrs	
First molar	14–18 mos	6–7 yrs	
Second premolar		11–12 yrs	
First premolar		10–12 yrs	
Canine	17–23 mos	9–10 yrs	
Lateral incisor	10–16 mos	7–8 yrs	
Central incisor	6–10 mos	6–7 yrs	

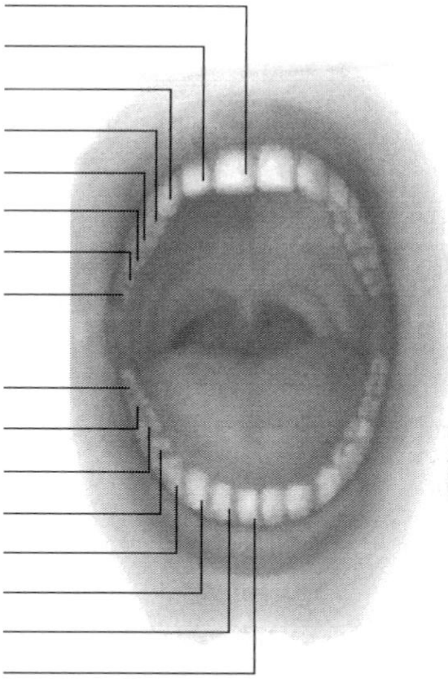

FIGURE 6.1 Picture of teeth eruption.

BOX 6.6 Age of eruption of teeth. Reproduced
with the kind permission of Dr Bunn[16]

Primary teeth are also called baby teeth, milk teeth, or first teeth. Baby teeth are very important as place holders for permanent teeth. There are some simple rules that usually apply to the eruption of baby teeth:

- lower teeth usually erupt before upper teeth;
- girls' teeth usually erupt before boys' teeth of the same age;
- teeth usually erupt in pairs.

Permanent teeth usually start to erupt at about 6 years of age. A special note here is that often the first molar, or 6-year molar, erupts before the front tooth. Additionally, the first molar erupts *behind* the last baby tooth and does not replace a baby tooth in contrast with what occurs for front teeth. Often lower front teeth come in behind, on the tongue side, and give the appearance for a while (can be many months) as if there are two rows of teeth.

Common dental diseases

The two main dental diseases are tooth decay (dental caries) and gum disease (periodontal disease). Caries causes most concern in young children and can be prevented. Unfortunately, many children do not attend a dentist until dental disease is well established. Disease levels vary throughout the country but between one-third and one-half of the nation's children have experienced caries on entry to school at 5 years of age. An increasing problem is damage to teeth caused by acidic drinks and juices, which de-mineralise teeth causing erosion (thinning of enamel).

Baby teeth are important and should not be neglected. If they are badly decayed, and develop an abscess and/or become painful, the permanent teeth may be damaged. It is important to promote healthy diet and good teeth cleaning from an early age as it is difficult to unlearn bad habits (*see* Box 6.6 for examples of local initiatives). Dental caries in children can be prevented by:

▶ **diet**: reducing the consumption and especially the frequency of intake of sugar-containing food and drink;
▶ **tooth brushing**: cleaning the teeth thoroughly twice every day with a fluoride toothpaste;
▶ **strengthening teeth**: the use of a fluoride toothpaste is recommended;
▶ **dental attendance**: attending a dentist every year for an oral examination;
▶ **avoiding** other sources of sugar, such as sugar in medicines.

BOX 6.6 Prevention of dental disease in children

The 'Brushing for Life' scheme was a project funded by the Department of Health in those health authorities in the UK with the poorest levels of dental health. Fluoride toothpaste (with a middle range of fluoride content at 1000 ppm) and toothbrushes were distributed by health visitors to the parents of infants and advice was given, not only about oral hygiene and twice-daily brushing with a fluoride toothpaste, but also on sugar-free weaning and early dental registration. An evaluation in Barnsley showed positive benefits, but many parents dropped out of the scheme.

The MANCIT* project was targeted at 5000 children in central Manchester. Health visitors who had extra training in oral health promotion first saw the children at 8 months old with their parents. The parents were given a feeder cup to substitute for a bottle and a leaflet (available in seven languages) on oral hygiene. At the 18-month visit, the health visitor gave each child a tube of fluoride toothpaste and a toothbrush and demonstrated how to use them properly. A new toothbrush and another tube of toothpaste were given to the children at 3 years of age and again at school entry.

Other examples of good practice include:

• integration of oral health considerations into all local weaning and infant feeding policies;
• review of samples, vouchers and advertising promotions of sugary foods and drinks – especially samples of foods in, for example, Bounty packs†;

---

* Manchester Action against Nursing Caries in Teeth (MANCIT).

† The Bounty packs are bags of free samples and information for expectant and new mothers, and provide a range of samples for the mother, baby and family.

- promoting the availability of healthier choices, by the provision of sugar-free snacks and drinks in crèches, pre-school playgroups, mums and tots groups, private, education and social services nurseries, child and family centres, for example (the 'Smiling for Life' programme and materials are designed to assist in this);
- promoting the use of sugar-free medicine through the primary healthcare team and pharmacy team.

A healthy diet

This is the most important factor in preventing tooth decay. The volume, and especially the frequency of sugar ingested, should be kept to a minimum. The number of times that sugars enter the mouth is the most important factor in determining the rate of decay. Each time sugar is eaten or drunk, acid is rapidly generated in dental plaque on teeth within seconds, and within 1–2 minutes plaque pH has fallen to levels at which enamel dissolution can occur. The return to neutrality can take between 20 minutes and 2 hours. If a high frequency of sugar intake occurs, this will not allow time for the pH to recover and for a large proportion of the day, teeth are under attack. Dental caries can quickly develop. Poor dietary habits include:

- adding sugar to feeds or drinks;
- frequent sugary snacks and/or drinks;
- the use of sweetened comforters or dinky feeders.

Ideally, sugary foods and drinks should be consumed only in conjunction with mealtimes as most meals contain some 'hidden' sugar. Sugary snacks are best avoided between meals. It is important to note that many foods and drinks marketed as 'healthy' or 'for babies and young children' can cause serious damage to teeth because of their high sugar content. Parents should be encouraged to read product labels carefully. Moslem mothers in particular need advice about suitable foods (*see* page 114).

Effective tooth-brushing

Tooth-brushing *per se* does not prevent dental caries. Its purpose is to remove plaque and keep gums healthy and, to be effective, it must be carried out regularly and thoroughly. Every surface of every tooth needs to be cleaned carefully, paying special attention to the junction between the tooth and gum.

Parents should be encouraged to commence cleaning their child's teeth with a pea-sized amount of a fluoride toothpaste once teeth appear (from approximately 6 months). This can easily be carried out with the parent positioned behind their child, steadying his/her chin with their left hand while brushing with their right hand (vice versa for left-handed people). Children will require assistance to ensure effective tooth-brushing up to the age of about 8 years, although they should be encouraged to practise brushing their teeth themselves. Effective tooth cleaning is more important than frequent cleaning. Twice a day is sufficient and it is important that teeth are thoroughly cleaned last thing at night.

Tooth-brushing is an important method of applying fluoride to strengthen teeth (*see* below). If excess fluoride is ingested when teeth are forming, it can cause mottling or staining of teeth, so care must be taken to ensure that this is avoided by making sure that children are not swallowing large amounts of high fluoride toothpaste, particularly if they are receiving fluoridated water or supplements. Particular caution in the type and amount of toothpaste used (and swallowed) should be exercised if a child is taking fluoride supplements or the local water supply is fluoridated. In such cases, a pea-sized blob of a low fluoride children's toothpaste should be used.

Fluoride

'Fluoridation gives poor kids rich kids' teeth!'[*] Fluoride strengthens teeth against caries. If it is present systemically when teeth are forming (from fluoridated water or fluoride supplements) it will be incorporated into the growing teeth. Its presence makes teeth more resistant to acid attack and tooth decay. Fluoridation of the water supply is the most effective way of getting fluoride to the general public. At a concentration of 1 part per million it can reduce decay by about 50%. This occurs naturally in the water in some areas of the UK; in other areas, fluoride has been added to bring levels up to the optimum for dental health. Water authorities can provide information on the fluoride levels in local water supplies.[17]

The majority of people in the UK do not receive fluoridated water. After teeth have erupted (appeared in the mouth) they can benefit from fluoride acting topically on the surface of the teeth from fluoridated water or toothpaste. The use of a fluoride toothpaste is an effective method of strengthening teeth. Virtually all toothpaste now contains fluoride. The optimum concentration is 1000 ppm; lower amounts reduce the benefit, whereas higher concentrations may be more likely to cause mottling of the enamel.

Benefit is obtained by taking fluoride supplements from 6 months through to adolescence in areas of low/no water fluoridation. Fluoride supplements can be prescribed by both doctors and dentists. However, compliance with a regimen that requires daily fluoride tablets/drops to be taken for about 15 years has been shown to be a problem, particularly among sections of the population where disease levels are highest. In addition, parents may be rather lax with diet if they feel that their child's teeth are protected by fluoride. Healthy eating should be the main emphasis in preventing tooth decay.

Rather than using a blanket approach to the prescription of fluoride supplements, there is benefit in targeting their use towards individual children with special needs. These include children at high risk of developing dental caries or who have a medical condition where dental disease would prove deleterious to their health. Therefore, dentists are best able to determine individual and family risk and take the decision about prescribing fluoride supplements and advising on their concentration based on risk and the local level of water fluoridation; hence the importance of early dental attendance.

Dental attendance: registering with a dentist

All children are now encouraged to register with a family dentist from birth, as dental care moves from a predominantly treatment-based approach to a preventive one. If a child attends regularly,[†] there is the opportunity for the prevention of dental disease.

---

[*] A public relations slogan from the early days of fluoridation in the USA.

[†] NICE recommend an interval of not less than 3 months and not more than 12 months between routine visits. (*Dental recall – recall interval between routine dental examinations*. NICE, 2004.)

In addition, children become accustomed to attending a dentist (which can be fun!) and build up trust so that if treatment should be required, it will be easier for the child, parent and dentist. Early detection and simple treatment of dental disease will be possible if dental attendance is regular. Parents experiencing problems in finding an NHS dentist may contact their primary care organisation or the Community Dental Service for advice and support in finding appropriate care.

Teething

Many symptoms have been attributed to teething.[18] Tooth eruption is likely linked to pain, inflammation of the mucosa overlying the tooth, irritability, disturbed sleep, facial flushing, drooling, gum rubbing, loss of appetite, ear rubbing (on the same side as the erupting tooth); but other symptoms such as fever or diarrhoea may have more serious causes and parents should not automatically attribute them to teething. Popular treatments include teething rings (chilled), hard sugar-free teething rusks, bread-sticks, oven-hardened bread, peeled cucumber, frozen items, pacifier, and massaging the gums. Oral paracetamol may be effective. Lignocaine gels or gels containing choline salicylate are available. Parents must follow the instructions precisely otherwise there is a risk of over-dosage. In particular, several cases of severe toxicity from choline salicylate gels have been reported and we would no longer recommend their use.

Children with other medical problems

Children with frequent illness or chronic disease may require regular medication. Sugary medicines can cause serious tooth decay and sugar-free medicines should be used where possible. Children with congenital heart disease and a 'heart card' should be reviewed regularly by a dentist because of their increased risk of endocarditis.

The SIGN* guideline summarised best evidence on dental care for children at increased risk of dental disease.[19]

Dental trauma

Trauma to the mouth and teeth is common in young children and is most often due to falls, although the possibility of non-accidental injury must always be considered. Complete avulsion of a tooth may occur. Generally, no attempt is made to replace primary teeth. In the case of permanent teeth, the avulsed tooth should be held by the crown (not the root); washed in clean water and replaced in the socket or, if necessary, transported in milk; and the child should be seen by a dentist as soon as possible.[20]

---

* The Scottish Intercollegiate Guidelines Network.

REFERENCES

1 National Institute for Health and Clinical Excellence. *The Effectiveness of Public Health Interventions to Promote the Duration of Breastfeeding*, 2005. Available at: www.nice.org.uk (accessed 22 November 2008). *See* also National Institute for Health and Clinical Excellence. *Promotion of Breastfeeding Initiation and Duration*; 2006. Available at: www.nice.org.uk (accessed 22 November 2008). *See* also Renfrew M, Fisher C, Arms S. *Bestfeeding: why breast feeding is best for you and your baby*. Berkeley, Cal: Celestial Arts; 2004.

2 www.breastfeedingnetwork.org

3 Geddes DT, Langton DB, Gollow I, *et al*. Frenulotomy for breastfeeding infants with ankyloglossia: effect on milk removal and sucking mechanism as imaged by ultrasound. *Pediatrics*. 2008; **122**(1): e188–94. Epub 23 June 2008.

4 McDonald PD, Ross SRM, Grant L, *et al*. Neonatal weight loss in breast and formula fed infants. *Arch Dis Child Fetal Neonatal Ed*. 2003; **88**: F472–6. *See* also van Dommelen P, van Wouwe P, Breuning-Boers JM, *et al*. Reference chart for relative weight change to detect hypernatraemic dehydration. *Arch Dis Child*. 2007; **92**: 490–4; *See* also Crossland DS, Richmond S, Hudson M, *et al*. Weight change in the term baby in the first 2 weeks of life. *Acta Pædiatrica*. 2008; **97**(4): 425–9.

5 www.ukamb.org *See* also Baumer JH. Guidelines for the establishment and operation of human milk banks in the UK. *Arch Dis Child Educ Pract Ed*. 2004; **89**(1): 27–9.

6 For a useful guideline and links on use of vitamin K *see* www.ich.ucl.ac.uk/clinical_information/clinical_guidelines/cpg_guideline_00003 (accessed 22 December 2008)

7 Leaf A. Vitamins for babies and young children *Arch Dis Child*. 2007; **92**: 160–4. *See* also www.dh.gov.uk/en/Healthcare/Maternity/Maternalandinfantnutrition/index.htm *See* also (for infants hospitalised and/or with health problems) www.ich.ucl.ac.uk/clinical_information/clinical_guidelines/cpg_guideline_00048/ (accessed 22 December 2008).

8 Renfrew MJ, McLoughlin M, McFadden A. Cleaning and sterilisation of infant feeding equipment: a systematic review. *Public Health Nutr*. 2008; **1**(11): 1188–99.

9 Department of Health. Weaning and the weaning diet. *Report on Health and Social Subjects no. 46*. London: HMSO; 1994.

10 Rapley G. *Baby-led weaning* [DVD]. Available at: www.babyfriendly.org.uk/items/resource_detail.asp?item=422 *See* also *Tuning In to Mealtimes* [DVD]. Available at: http://henry.org.uk/resources.html#Mealtimes-DVD

11 Wright CM, Parkinson KN, Drewett RF. Why are babies weaned early?: a prospective population-based cohort study. *Arch Dis Child*. 2004; **89**: 813–16.

12 Macdougall CF, Cant AJ, Colver AF. How dangerous is food allergy in childhood?: the incidence of severe and fatal allergic reactions across the UK and Ireland. *Arch Dis Child*. 2002; **86**: 236–9. *See* also Dixon V, Habeeb S, Lakshman R. Did you know this medicine has peanut butter in it, doctor? *Arch Dis Child*. 2007; **92**: 654. *See* also Armstrong D, Rylance G. Definitive diagnosis of nut allergy. *Arch Dis Child*. 1999; **80**: 175–7. *See* also Colver A, Hourihane J O'B. Are the dangers of childhood food allergy exaggerated? *BMJ*. 2006; **333**: 494–8.

13 *Royal College of Paediatrics and Child Health*. Evidence-based guidelines for the management of children presenting to hospital with diarrhoea, with or without vomiting. Available at: www.rcpch.ac.uk/doc.aspx?id_Resource=1544 (accessed 30 December 2008).

14 www.healthystart.nhs.uk

15 Pitts NB, Boyles J, Nugent ZJ, *et al*. The dental caries experience of 5-year-old children in Great Britain (2005/6). *Community Dent Health*. 2007; **24**(1): 59–63.

16 www.drbunn.com/erupt.htm

17 McDonagh M, Whiting P, Bradley M. *A Systematic Review of Public Water Fluoridation*. NHS Centre for Reviews and Dissemination, University of York; 2000. Available at: www.york.ac.uk/inst/crd/pdf/fluorid.pdf (accessed 22 December 2008).

18 McIntyre GT, McIntyre GM. Teething troubles? *Brit Dent J*. 2002; **192**: 251–5.

19 www.rcpch.ac.uk/doc.aspx?id_Resource=1689
20 Zamon EL, Kenny DJ. Replantation of Avulsed Primary Incisors: A Risk–Benefit Assessment *J Can Dent Assoc.* 2001; **67**: 386. Available at: www.cda-adc.ca/jcda/vol-67/issue-7/386.html (accessed 30 December 2008). *See* also Mori GG, Castilho LR, Nunes DC, *et al.* Avulsion of permanent teeth: analysis of the efficacy of an informative campaign for professionals from elementary schools. *J Appl Oral Sci.* 2007; **15**(6): 534–8. Available at: www.scielo.br/pdf/jaos/v15n6/a15 V15n6.pdf (accessed 22 November 2008).

WHAT DETERMINES HOW A CHILD GROWS?

The growth of the foetus and its size at birth depend on:

▶ the health and nutritional status of the mother;
▶ her height and weight;
▶ whether or not she smokes;
▶ whether she has any illness;
▶ the uterine circulation and placenta;
▶ problems and disorders in the baby (e.g. premature birth, chromosomal disorders, intrauterine infections).

After birth, the growth of the baby depends on different factors. Assuming that he does not have any medical disorder or serious illness, the most important factor is nutrition. Babies also need loving care and attention, and if they are neglected or abused this affects their physical growth as well as their personal and social development. As the baby gets older, the rate of growth is increasingly affected by genes that

---

* This chapter first appeared as Chapter 5 in *The Child Protection Reader: Recognition and Response to Child Protection.* London: Royal College of Paediatrics and Child Health; 2007. The publisher and authors are grateful to the RCPCH for their kind permission to reproduce the text.

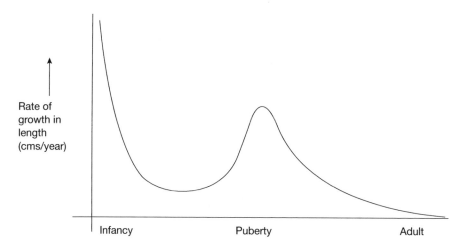

FIGURE 7.1 This chart shows the growth velocity of a male infant from birth to the end of puberty. Note that the fastest period of growth in length is in infancy and the rate is decreasing thereafter until puberty, but even in the puberty growth spurt the rate is never as fast as it is in infancy.

affect height and body build (whether he is lean, a normal build, or has a tendency to get overweight).

In the first year or two of life, growth hormone (GH) is thought to play only a small part in the pattern of growth, but gradually this increases. During the rest of childhood GH is the most important single factor – other than nutrition – in determining growth. As puberty approaches, there is an acceleration in growth and further alterations in body-build associated with hormonal changes, although GH is still important.

The fastest growth is in the first year of life. After a transient weight loss (*see* page 102), birth weight is usually regained by the end of the second week and thereafter the average baby gains 150–200 g per week. A baby who weighs 3 kg at birth will probably double that by 5 months (6 kg) and treble it by a year (9 kg) but will only add 2 or 3 kg in the whole of the third year, though he will certainly get taller. After that the rate of growth slows down and then speeds up again at puberty, but is never again as fast as in the first year (*see* Figure 7.1).

MEASUREMENT

The two most important measurements are height and weight. Babies should be weighed naked whenever possible, in a warm room. Scales need to be checked and calibrated at regular intervals. Accurate scales are vital, particularly for infants and young children* and should meet EC standards (Directive 90/384/EEC). If nude weighing cannot be done, because the child is wearing a bandage or splint, for instance, the state of undress should be recorded. Weights may vary by several hundreds of grams depending on the contents of the stomach, bladder and bowel.

---

* Equipment and charts referred to in this chapter can be obtained from http://shop.healthforallchildren.co.uk/pro.epl?SHOP=HOME

Weight changes more quickly than height. Weight loss through dehydration can occur in a matter of hours and any acute illness can cause weight loss in a few days or weeks. This means that the weight gives information about the child's health in recent days or weeks. In contrast, height is an index of health over a long period of time: months or, more usually, years. Growth in height may be slowed or stopped by chronic illness or neglect, but this will not become obvious until eventually someone realises either that the child is shorter than his younger siblings or his peer group, or that he is not growing out of his clothes. By the time parents are worried about the child's height and think he is not growing, the chances are that they are right.

It is important always to measure the child's height and weight, or length and weight, whenever there is concern about his general health or well-being. By comparing height and weight, one can sometimes get an idea of the time over which a child has become unwell. The child who has been undernourished for many years and is short in stature is said to be *stunted*. The child who has obviously lost a lot of weight is said to be *wasted*. Stunting and wasting often co-exist in the same child. These terms are widely used in resource-poor developing countries.

Growth charts

Conventional growth charts compare parameters such as height, weight, and rate of growth, with what is observed in the whole population. This makes it easier to decide whether or not the pattern is normal. New charts developed by the WHO describe how children *should* grow. These are being adopted in many countries including the UK. (*See* Box 7.1 for more details.)

It might be expected that the perfectly proportioned baby would be on the same centile for both the height and the weight, but it can be perfectly normal for a child to be lean or 'skinny' or to be chubby or 'fat' and in such cases he would be on a different centile for his weight as compared to his height. Tall, lean parents are likely to have tall, lean children. Charts may help professionals, but they can worry parents, particularly if their child grows more slowly, or is thinner or fatter than the growth chart suggests is 'normal'. Though it may seem obvious to professionals, it may be necessary to explain to a parent that just because their child falls above or below the 50th centile, it does not mean that they have a growth problem.

BOX 7.1 Growth charts

There are two ways of making a growth chart:

1 Measure a large number of children at different ages, all at roughly the same time. This gives the distribution of weight for children of various ages at the particular point in time when the data were gathered. This kind of chart is called a *cross sectional* chart. The best known example in the UK is the 1990 nine-centile chart.

2 The other way of making a growth chart is to measure the same children on many different occasions. This takes much longer, but gives more information about the growth of individual children and how it varies. This kind of chart is called a *longitudinal* chart.

Both types of chart have conventionally been descriptive; they show how children grew in the community at the time the data were collected, irrespective of how they were fed or cared for. The new WHO charts show how children *should* grow when given healthy

---

environments that promote good diets, adequate healthcare, prevention and control of infections, and no exposure to smoking in pregnancy or after birth. They illustrate the weight gain pattern of breastfed babies as the norm.

What the charts show

Suppose that at the age of 5 months the average weight of children is six kilos. Put another way, half of all children weigh more than six kilos and half weigh less than six kilos. This point on the chart is called the 50th centile. To determine the other centiles, one may find, for example, that out of every 100 babies of a certain age, 10 weigh more than nine kilos, but the other 90 weigh less than nine kilos; and out of every 100 babies, 10 weigh less than four kilos and 90 weigh more than four kilos. These two points on the chart are called the 90th centile and the 10th centile, respectively.

Repeating this process for each age group, or for every month of age, produces a growth chart with a range of centile lines. Knowing the age and weight of a baby allows one to determine what centile he is on.

The 98th and 2nd centiles mark the point where only 2 out of every 100 children are respectively bigger or smaller than this, but this does not necessarily mean that they have anything wrong with them. There are also 99.6 and 0.4 centiles, where only 1 in 250 children is bigger or smaller than this. So it is quite unusual for a child to be this big or small and there is more likely to be some underlying cause that may need to be identified.

Ethnic charts

Attempts to develop charts for individual ethnic groups have not been successful. There is too much variation even within apparently homogeneous groups (for instance, children from different parts of the Indian sub-continent might need different charts). After emigrating to a Western country, a family may experience an increase in height and weight in several successive generations. Gathering data on enough children would be difficult or impossible and the number of different charts needed would be impossible to sustain. The new WHO charts are based on data from six countries and show how children from any ethnic background should grow.[1]

Secular trend and obesity

Over the past century children have become taller and heavier; this is called the 'secular trend'. The increase in height has now more or less levelled off for European children. But weight is still increasing and there is now much worry about the 'obesity epidemic'. This cannot be monitored if the charts are adjusted every few years to keep up with the epidemic, so the 1990 figures for weight for those over 4 years are used as a permanent reference, so that children's weights can be compared with the same fixed standard.[2]

Plotting measurements on a growth chart

When plotting measurements on a chart, make a small mark with the point of a pen or pencil; *do not* make a large blob as this reduces accuracy. Plot exactly what the measurement is (it is easy to let the mark drift up or down to come into line with previous measurements). The measurement should be signed and dated on the chart or at the relevant place in the notes. Then consider if the chart and what one observes are compatible. If the chart shows something unexpected; for instance, if the child has apparently shrunk in height or a child who looks small for his age seems to be on the 98th centile, the measuring or plotting may be wrong. It should not automatically be accepted; the measurement must be repeated.

Growth charts are sometimes presented as evidence in child protection cases. If a growth chart is to be displayed at a child protection conference or in Court, every length, height, weight and age must be double checked to make sure that they have been correctly plotted. (It may even be necessary to create a new chart and enter the data correctly. If so, it must be clearly indicated that this is what has been done. Keep, but do not alter, existing charts in the records.) Check also whether the baby was weighed in the same state of undress and on suitable scales that are regularly checked or re-calibrated.

Correction for any prematurity should be applied before plotting the results. This should be done up to the first birthday. After that, the measurement error in relation to the rate of change in height and weight means that the prematurity correction becomes less important.

How to measure length and height

Length and height should be measured using a device designed for the purpose (*see* Figure 7.2); tape measures and biro marks on a sheet or a wall are unacceptable. The current best buy for general use is probably the Leicester Height Measure. Box 7.2

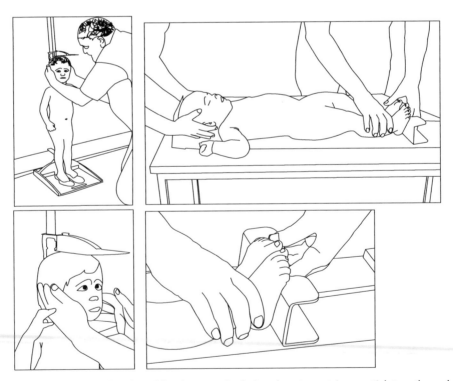

FIGURE 7.2 Measuring length and height: properly designed equipment is essential. Length can be measured using the Rollameter; for height, the Leicester Height Measure is recommended. Illustrations courtesy of Harlow Printing (www.harlowprinting.co.uk).

summarises the optimal measuring technique.[3] Different observers or different equipment will produce different results. It is important always to be as accurate as possible but there is no such thing as absolute precision. Measurement error and imprecision are two different things. Errors arise through bad technique, poor equipment and wrong plotting. Imprecision is unavoidable because children are not rigid objects and do not have an exact height.

Supine length is measured up to the age of 2 years; *standing height* thereafter. Standing height is about 0.7 cm less than supine length on the new WHO charts. It is often possible to obtain an acceptable measurement of *height* as early as 18 months, but reliable measurement of young children depends on securing their cooperation, which is usually easier in 3- and 4-year-olds. Standing height varies during the day: it falls on average by 0.3 cm by mid-morning, another 0.2 by lunch time, and very little thereafter.

BOX 7.2 Correct measurement of height

Measuring procedure:

- remove the child's shoes;
- ask him to stand with heels against wall or plate;
- ask an assistant to hold the feet on the ground, so that the child's heels do not rise when you ask him to stand as tall as he can;
- make sure the child is standing straight; press the thighs and pelvis gently backwards against the surface of the wall or measuring device;
- ensure that the upper margin of the auditory meatus is in a horizontal line with the angle of the orbit (the 'Frankfurt plane');
- steady the child with support under the angle of the jaw, but do not apply pressure in order to stretch him upwards (different observers apply varying amounts of pressure, so stretching does not increase the reliability or repeatability of the measurement);
- measure with your eye in line with the scale to avoid parallax errors;
- plot carefully on the chart; your chart may one day be required by a specialist colleague, or may even be examined by a Court!

Regular weighing

Breastfed babies: growth patterns

Breastfed babies show a slightly different growth pattern from formula-fed babies. In the first few months, fully breastfed infants are slightly heavier than shown on the 1990 UK growth charts and they cross centiles upwards to reach +0.3 SDs (standard deviations) at 2 months old, but subsequently cross centiles downwards to –0.2 SDs by 12 months. The new WHO charts (*see* Box 7.1) are based on the growth pattern of breastfed babies.

Weighing after the first few weeks

The regular weighing of babies may help in the detection of various disorders, although it is also capable of causing needless worry and unnecessary referrals. More importantly, mothers like their babies to be weighed as a reassurance that the baby is well, particularly in the first few months of life and with their first baby. Weighing often acts as an entrance ticket to the clinic and an initial focus for the consultation; this might be about feeding or growth, but could be about an entirely separate issue. For these reasons, facilities for weighing should be readily available in primary care clinics.

Weight worries

If the weight is plotted regularly during the first 2 years of life, the result is the growth curve for that particular child. If that curve is exactly parallel to the centile lines on the chart, everyone is happy, but in the first year or 18 months of life, babies do not necessarily follow the centile lines. If the baby is growing faster than the centile lines suggest, parents are usually pleased, but if the baby's growth curve indicates that he is growing more slowly than the growth centiles would suggest, the parents and their health visitor are likely to get worried.

This phenomenon of crossing over centile lines, rather than growing along them, mainly occurs in the first 2 years of life. The reason is simple: the size of an older child or an adult is determined mainly by the size of his or her parents and big tall

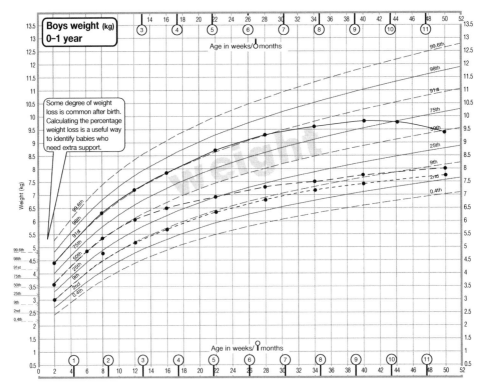

FIGURE 7.3 Interpreting infant growth charts. The *dashed* line shows the growth curve of a healthy baby who was on the 50th centile at birth; however, his parents are small and the curve gradually moves down towards the 2nd centile line. The *dotted* line is the growth curve of a baby who was small at birth and grows steadily along or just above the 2nd centile. The *continuous* line is suggestive of a significant problem – the baby stopped gaining weight at around 6 months and is now losing weight (UK-WHO 2008 and Royal College of Paediatrics and Child Health).

parents are likely to have big tall children, but the size of the baby when he is born is more related to various maternal factors. These two influences might have a very different effect on the weight gain pattern. So for example consider a baby who has grown well in utero and is on the 75th centile at birth. If the parents are small, the child might be on the 10th centile for height and weight by the time he is 3 years old. This means that it is common for a normal infant's measurements and growth curve to cross the growth chart lines (*see* Figure 7.3).

There is a tendency for very large babies to show a downward trend in their growth curve, whereas small babies tend to show an upward curve. It is as if babies born at the extreme end of the weight distribution, that is, unusually big or small, 'try' to make their way back towards the average line. This mathematical phenomenon is known as 'regression to the mean', but some normal big babies show an upward trend and some small babies show a downward trend.

Weight loss

A short period of weight loss, followed by rapid catch-up, happens quite often if the baby has a viral illness, gastroenteritis or respiratory infection. If the baby is *continuing to lose weight*, as opposed to simply gaining weight more slowly than the centile lines suggest is normal, further investigation is needed as there are many possible causes.

INFANT GROWTH PATTERNS: CONCEPTS AND TERMINOLOGY

A common problem for primary care staff is the baby or child whose chart suggests that he is not gaining weight at the 'expected' rate but there is no other evidence of anything wrong. It can be very difficult to decide whether the growth pattern is abnormal for that particular child. It is possible to determine how *unusual* a child's pattern of weight gain is by using 'thrive line' charts,[4] but *unusual* does not necessarily mean *abnormal*. Some people use the term 'failure to thrive' to describe babies whose pattern of weight gain is less rapid than one expected; others refer to 'growth faltering'. Both terms suggest that there is a problem with the baby and can be used where one suspects that the baby's food intake is insufficient (the most common explanation) or that there may be an underlying illness, disorder or syndrome that merits investigation. The term 'slow weight gain' may be preferable when one is simply referring to a finding on the growth chart, but has not come to any conclusion about the reason.

The term 'non-organic failure to thrive' has been used to describe the situation where there is thought to be poor parenting and inadequate feeding, although these cases are often more complicated than they appear at first sight and the division between organic and non-organic causes is probably unhelpful.

Outcomes

It has been suggested that slow weight gain or growth faltering in the first year of life may lead to poor outcomes later in childhood; for example, smaller adult height or lower intelligence.[5,6] However, in general, the outlook for these babies seems to be satisfactory. There may be an increased risk of developmental difficulties in some babies with slow early weight gain, but this does not necessarily mean that the slow weight gain is *the cause* of these difficulties.

Growth in premature and small for gestational age babies

Infants who were of very low or extremely low birth weight (ELBW) have an increased risk of poor growth in height and head circumference, particularly if they also have other problems such as lung disease. Babies who were small for gestational age (SGA) at birth often show catch-up growth, but some will not attain their predicted adult height.

There has been much interest, initiated by Barker's research, into how weight gain and growth before and after birth might affect the health of the child when he grows up to be an adult. Slow weight gain may adversely affect brain growth, but rapid weight gain in infancy may increase the risk of high blood pressure and obesity. These are controversial topics and primary care staff should be very cautious in raising them with parents. Paediatric and nutritional guidance may be advisable for ELBW and SGA babies.

PROBLEMS WITH WEIGHT GAIN

Slow weight gain

Slow weight gain is a frequent cause for concern. The first step is to decide if there really is a problem.[6] If the parent is anxious, it may be useful to demonstrate on the chart how little weight is actually gained by the normal child in the second year, in contrast to the gain in height. The baby's overall health and well-being are as important as the growth chart. A baby who has lots of energy, is sleeping and eating well, is developing satisfactorily and is happy and smiling, is unlikely to have anything seriously wrong. Similarly, the mother who is relaxed, competent and caring, is managing her baby well and there is good communication between them, is unlikely to be behaving completely differently when she is at home alone with the child. Conversely, when the parent is unhappy or depressed, or is making negative comments about the baby, or has strange ideas about how he should be fed, or does not show any anxiety even when the health visitor is obviously concerned, there may be problems that need investigation.

Thin babies

Parents sometimes worry if their baby is thin, but provided linear growth is satisfactory and the baby is otherwise well, thinness is very rarely a sign of serious disease.

Fat babies

Professionals worry about fat babies in the light of increasing evidence that infant obesity can be a predictor of adult obesity. If a baby is gaining weight rapidly, advice should be offered about healthy eating habits and encouraging physical activity. Be sympathetic and supportive to mothers when raising this issue as it is not easy to reduce the food intake of hungry babies! Conversely, some parents can become obsessed about 'healthy eating' and obesity.

FEEDING PROBLEMS ASSOCIATED WITH WEANING

Developmental and nutritional aspects of weaning are discussed on page 111. Eating problems in 3- and 4-year-olds are reviewed on page 327.

Difficulties with weaning can arise for many reasons:

▶ The late introduction of solids may result in preference for a more limited range of food; this may occur because of illness, early tube feeding, oro-motor dysfunction or general developmental delay.
▶ Delays in learning to chew food, from lack of early experience, may lead to a gag response when solid or lumpy food is given. However, such difficulties may also be the result of oro-motor dysfunction, which may have been the *reason* for late weaning.
▶ Early unpleasant experiences affecting the mouth and pharynx may also lead to food refusal; for example, tube feeding, gastro-oesophageal reflux, repeated vomiting, unpleasant medicines.
▶ Aversion to food could be due to abdominal pain and nausea, reflux or constipation.

Iron deficiency may result from weaning problems. There is some evidence that it can also be the cause of behavioural changes and difficulties.

There is a tendency to blame parents for these problems, but that is often a simplistic explanation. Several sets of interacting factors may be involved:

▶ parental knowledge, personal resources and mental health; disappointment with the child's behaviour or appearance; pre-occupation with other children or other worries;
▶ insecure infant, disturbed emotional affect in the parent, lack of mutual attachment and enjoyment;
▶ child characteristics such as undemanding or unresponsive behaviour, poor appetite and immature feeding skills;
▶ family relationships and tensions, social isolation, lack of support and misconceptions about diets due to lifestyle or culture;
▶ management problems, such as difficulty in establishing predictable mealtimes, allowing unrestricted access to food at all times, no effective cues, prompts or rewards for age-appropriate eating.

BOX 7.3 Feeding problems: how to offer practical advice to carers

- *Never* force-feed.
- Don't aim to solve problems all at once; plan small steps to build up parents' confidence and competence.
- Teach parents to tolerate mess. Discuss the child's need to learn to feed himself. Help the child to become more involved in the feeding process by encouraging touching and playing with food, even if it is very messy. Show parents how to be a positive model for the child; for example, putting their own fingers in the food and licking them, then eating a tiny amount, then increasing the quantity.
- Start with food that is familiar to the child; don't worry if interest is initially only shown in a limited variety of foods.

- Food that is withheld seems more desirable; food that the child is rewarded for eating is less desirable than food that is given as a reward!
- Some children have a small appetite. Offer a small portion of food to start with and if readily eaten, offer more.
- If weight is a concern, try to increase caloric intake by 'sneaking in' extra calories. High calorie foods are important for growth in young children; for example, use full fat milk, cheese, yoghurt and butter. These can be added to mashed potato, pasta, etc.
- Some children fill up on drinks throughout the day. This can take the edge off their appetite, so offer food first. Reduce excess fluids, particularly juice and milk.
- Try to provide a relaxed, calm atmosphere at mealtimes.
- Advise parents to avoid battles and aversive experiences. Don't use anything that has become a focus of fear (e.g. spoon or high chair).
- Encourage social eating. Ensure seating is comfortable and appropriate to the child's age and size. Eat with the child as children learn by example. Make meal times social, enjoyable occasions. The child may show interest in what other older children or adults are eating, so allow them to share it.
- Don't prolong the mealtime unduly. In general, 20–30 minutes is the longest a child should take to eat a meal (45 minutes was the longest observed mealtime in a study of 'normal' infant care). Remove food without comment. Allowing mealtimes to go on for longer than is necessary rarely results in food being eaten.
- Ignore unacceptable behaviour at mealtime by turning away from the child; praise the child for eating, but don't over-do it. Give praise for finishing the plate even when there is very little on it.
- Some children find a dummy comforting, but frequent daytime use may affect food intake and language development.
- Remind parents that it's better for a child finish a very small amount than to have an imaginary target that is unrealistic.

A THREE-PRONGED APPROACH TO ASSESS AND MANAGE EATING PROBLEMS

In assessing and managing eating problems and poor weight gain, it is helpful to consider three aspects: (i) evaluation of medical, dietary and nutritional issues; (ii) mealtime management; and (iii) dealing with family problems.

Medical, dietary and nutritional issues

In the first instance, a psychosocial and medical evaluation is required. If 'medical' causes (e.g. chronic illness or oro-motor delay that can affect chewing and swallowing) need to be excluded, this is best done early on, so that the anxiety of the parent or health professional can be set aside; but it is also vital to explain right at the start that usually in such cases, no disease or disorder will be found and that the focus will be on approaches to feeding and family issues.

Look for behavioural and emotional difficulties in the child. Be aware of unusual behaviour that may give a clue to major feeding and management problems: extreme hunger drive, searching for food, eating or drinking from unlikely places, such as animal feeding bowls, begging for food or stealing food and scavenging.

Mealtime management

A home visit to observe a mealtime is the best basis for providing support and provides an opportunity to give advice about feeding (*see* Box 7.3). An account of the baby's diet and feeding practices given to health professionals in a clinic may not relate very closely to what is happening at home. For example, few parents will admit to feeding their baby by leaving a bottle propped on the pillow. Video recordings made in parents' homes showed how many parents have enormous difficulty in feeding their young child.[7] There were battles over feeding, lack of any routine, too many distractions and no understanding of the social aspects of mealtimes. In most cases, there had been no suspicion in the clinic regarding the extent of the difficulties these mothers were experiencing. These feeding and management difficulties are, of course, not confined to babies with slow weight gain.

A few children are extremely fussy eaters – a trait that sometimes seems to run in families. The difficulties usually begin around 18 months and growth is generally satisfactory. These children tend to be more difficult in temperament, more cautious and often very shy. Some show a dread of new food, express contamination fears between foods they like and dislike, smell the food before eating it, and are visibly disgusted at foods they do not like. They can distinguish even between different brands of the same food. Some also show disgust in other ways, like hatred of getting dirty or standing barefoot on grass. A few of these children are in the autism spectrum or have semantic pragmatic disorder, but others are normally socially competent.

Family problems

When there are issues with eating and poor weight gain in a child, often there are family issues to consider:

- The mental health of the parents. Depression, social isolation, substance abuse and domestic violence may all affect their ability to cope.
- Understand their response to the feeding problems. Parents often feel as if they are being blamed and expect to be criticised so appointments with health professionals and social workers are not always kept. They become preoccupied with getting the child to eat. They may feel defeated and rejected by the child, become impatient, angry, or anxious; or give up and retreat into neglect and emotional indifference.
- Start by aiming to reduce parents' anxiety. Worries about eating can take over their lives. Identify depression, parental conflict, family violence and lack of interest in the child. A community psychiatric nurse or a play therapist may be able to help.
- Nursery placement can be very beneficial. The parent is relieved of the continuous stress and children often eat better in this social setting.
- Liaise with other professionals who may have important information that can help in addressing the difficulties.

Approaches to intervention are summarised in Box 7.3. Monitoring weight gain is usually essential, but frequent weighing inevitably reveals random fluctuations in weight and must be managed carefully, otherwise parents will dread the next clinic visit and will feel pressured to get more food into the child. They may resort to forced feeding, which invariably makes matters worse.

141

It may be necessary to get specialist professional help.[8] If necessary, consult a psychologist for guidance on behavioural management and a dietician for advice on increasing calorie density. As an extreme measure, it may be necessary to consider tube feeding during the night to reduce the pressure on daytime mealtimes.

GROWTH AND CHILD PROTECTION

In general, the child who is healthy and happy will also be growing normally, but the reverse does not necessarily apply. It is possible for a child to be of normal length and weight, yet still have a chronic illness or be suffering abuse or neglect. However, assessment of growth is an important part of any child protection assessment.

Sometimes there is such obvious neglect and unacceptable parenting that action is imperative; more often, there is tension between the wish to help and support the family (which community staff fear might be made more difficult by involving social services) and anxiety as to how much the child's safety is threatened. Iwaniec's monograph[9] contains many accounts of children who failed to thrive in association with management problems. The complexity of the family circumstances in most of these cases emphasises the vital importance of consultation with colleagues (e.g. the health visitor, the named or designated doctor or nurse and an experienced social worker). Occasionally, parents' accounts of feeding problems seem incompatible with what is observed in the clinic or during an admission to the children's ward and one then needs to consider the possibility of fabricated illness.

The most extreme examples of child neglect and under-nutrition are found in situations of war, famine or extreme poverty. Mercifully, these are rare in the Western world, though cases of extreme neglect are occasionally seen where the family has managed to conceal their child from all statutory services. Serious under-nutrition occurs in some chaotic or dysfunctional households. In such cases, there will usually be other evidence that the child is not receiving adequate care and attention, and that the parent is not providing good enough care.

WORRIES ABOUT HEIGHT

Parents are more likely to worry about short stature than about excessive growth in height. Children with hormonal deficiencies and other disorders affecting growth need treatment as early as possible. Each year that passes without appropriate therapy may represent some loss in final adult height. Tallness or excessively fast growth is a rare complaint before puberty and one for which parents usually seek advice, particularly where daughters are concerned. It merits immediate specialist referral. The same applies to unusually early signs of puberty; do not attribute these to the child having got hold of the mother's contraceptive pills!

Height and weight should be measured, and plotted on a chart whenever a question is raised by parents or professionals about the child's general health or growth and this should be a routine procedure in the follow-up of children with chronic disorders or disabilities. A more difficult question is whether and when to measure children who are thought by their parents to be well and growing normally; that is, a screening test (see page 177). A single measurement will identify children who are extremely short or tall – outside the limits of the 0.4 and 99.6 centiles, for example – and in the UK every child should have their height measured and plotted at school entry.

A single measurement cannot identify those who are within the normal range for height, but are growing more slowly than normal. This could be due to a wide variety of disorders (*see* page 144) and can only be detected by a series of measurements over time. However, serial measurements as a way of detecting children with occult growth problems is difficult because:

▶ children do not grow at the same rate all the time;
▶ the rate may slow in the few years immediately before the onset of puberty; it is very difficult to interpret such measurements as one does not know exactly when puberty will begin;
▶ the precision of each measurement is crucial: two or more measurements of high quality, taken on proper equipment by the same competent observer, showing that the child's height line is crossing centile channels, may well justify referral and investigation; however, when serial measurements are taken on poor equipment by different untrained observers, such a finding is very common and the chance of it being significant is very much less.

For these reasons, monitoring the growth of all children by repeated measurements over time is currently not recommended as a routine community-wide procedure.[10]

BOX 7.4 Could a child's unusually short or tall stature be due to having short or tall parents?[11]

Common sense suggests that one might reasonably be more worried about the short child who has tall siblings and tall parents. If parents themselves raise this issue they should be taken seriously.

There are several ways of adjusting a child's height measurement to take account of the parents' and/or siblings' heights; however, there are several points that must be taken into consideration:

1   You need to be sure that both 'parents' are the biological parents!
2   A parent's estimate of their own height is unreliable, and estimates of their partner's height even more so. Their heights must be checked.
3   The relationship between a child's expected height and the heights of his or her parents are not constant for all members of every population at all times. Parents may be short because of deprivation and poverty in childhood, or one or both of them may have a condition that is also affecting the child.
4   The child's growth may need to be carefully monitored for at least a year if there is significant concern, even if the parental height correction is reassuring. Correcting the heights of short children for their parents' heights may result in not referring several children who, in fact, have a growth disorder.

Correcting for parental height is useful but it is not straightforward and rarely provides sufficient evidence to *dismiss* concerns about short or tall stature in the child. If the primary care team or the parents are concerned about a child's growth, consider referral to a paediatrician for further assessment.

IMPORTANT CAUSES OF IMPAIRED GROWTH
Genetic and familial

By definition, 2% of children are below the 2nd centile in height (i.e. more than 2 SDs from the mean). The vast majority are healthy and are normal, short children and in many cases the parents are also short (*see* Box 7.4). When the height is below the 0.4 centile line there is more likely to be a specific cause.

Intrauterine growth retardation

Intrauterine growth retardation (small for gestational age, SGA) is an important cause of short stature. Many SGA babies have lost weight acutely in the last few weeks of gestation and these are likely to catch up by two years of age, and attain a height above the 2nd centile. Those who have suffered more prolonged malnutrition may remain small. Some of these babies are difficult to feed and care for. In such cases, it is easy to assume that poor growth is the parents' fault. A child who was SGA, and is still below the 2nd centile at age 3, should be referred for paediatric assessment.[12]

Neglect, abuse and malnutrition

In developed countries, neglect, abuse and malnutrition are usually associated with psychosocial deprivation, which may lead to impairment of linear growth as well as failure to gain weight. Often this is associated with other evidence of neglect and in this situation parents do not usually seek medical advice. Identification of children who are growing poorly because of under-nutrition combined with adverse social circumstances is more likely to be achieved by alert observation (by community staff or teachers) than by routine height monitoring, as explained on page 142.

Poverty is associated with under-nutrition – both obesity and under-weight (*see* page 122 for further discussion). Under-nutrition also occurs when parents develop fixed ideas about food allergies or health food enthusiasts offer their children highly unsuitable diets with too much fibre and insufficient energy content (e.g. using skimmed milk for young children). Such misguided feeding practices can cause serious malnutrition.

Some parents develop distorted ideas about feeding and present their child with repeated complaints about poor growth. This can be one manifestation of fabricated and induced illness (previously called Munchausen syndrome by proxy or Meadow's syndrome) and such complaints can even mislead paediatricians into embarking on naso-gastric feeding.

Occasionally, children respond to chronic stress and distress in the home with a characteristic behavioural syndrome, involving hyperphagia and polydipsia, together with growth failure, normal BMI and impaired growth hormone deficiency.[13]

Other causes

Important treatable causes of short stature include hypothyroidism, growth hormone deficiency (isolated GH deficiency, multiple pituitary hormone deficiency) and Turner's syndrome. Occasionally some serious diseases, such as renal failure and inflammatory bowel disease (mainly Crohn's) can present with poor growth, but no other symptoms or signs. Coeliac disease should always be considered in any child with unexplained poor growth as there are often no other obvious clues to this diagnosis. Milder forms of dysmorphic and short-limbed, short-stature syndromes are easily missed if one does not look carefully at the child's appearance and proportions.

OBESITY

Obesity is rapidly becoming a major health problem in both developed and developing nations. Both obesity and under-nutrition affect the lower social groups and poorer section of the community more than the prosperous middle classes, although the difference between them is reducing. The number of children who are overweight or obese (*see* Box 7.5 for definitions) has increased steadily over the past decade. The probability that an obese child will become an obese adult increases with the age of the child, the degree of obesity and having obese parents. Obesity in childhood is linked with lower self-esteem and a variety of emotional and psychological sequelae, and markers that predict future type 2 diabetes and heart disease are commonly present. Indeed, type 2 diabetes is now being recognised in the paediatric age group.

The underlying cause of the obesity 'epidemic' is a changing balance between energy intake and energy expenditure, though it is not easy to decide how much each contributes. Intake has probably gone up, with easy access to attractive energy-dense fast foods, snacks and drinks. Expenditure has gone down with fewer opportunities for outdoor play, walking to shops, doing domestic duties, etc. Watching TV or playing computer games is associated with low energy expenditure, exposes children to advertising of attractive foods and is often an occasion for continual snacking.

Body Mass Index (BMI) is the most readily available measure of obesity for community and public health use and is currently the most practical measure for individual children, though it must be interpreted with care (*see* Box 7.5). An example of a BMI chart is shown in Figure 7.4. The chart illustrated in this figure shows extreme centiles which are useful in the management of individual obese children. Waist circumference is sometimes used as a measure of obesity, though its value as a routine measurement is uncertain.

BOX 7.5 The Body Mass Index – BMI

BMI is derived by the formula: weight in kg/height in metres squared.

For example, weight = 25 kg, height = 120 cm = 1.2 metres.

BMI is $25/(1.2 \times 1.2) = 17.4 \, \text{kg/m}^2$

BMI is best regarded as weight corrected for height. It correlates reasonably well with direct measures of the proportion of body fat although this can vary by ethnicity and body build. It is the best measure of obesity for community and public health use; for example, it is used in surveys to monitor the spread of the obesity 'epidemic'. However, it is not a direct measure of body fat and two children with an identical BMI may have a very different body composition, different amounts of fat and different risks of future obesity and disease. This means that any BMI cut-off point for overweight or obesity is arbitrary. (The same applies to children whose BMI is at the low end of the range – they are not

---

necessarily 'underweight'). Staff should exercise caution when interpreting BMI results to parents, particularly when the Index is in the borderline overweight zone.

In infancy, BMI increases rapidly from a median of 13 at birth to 17 by the first birthday; it dips to a low point of 15 between 4 and 7 (the inflection point is called the point of adiposity rebound) and then starts to rise again to a median of 21.

Overweight is defined for the National Child Measurement Programme as BMI over the 85th centile and obesity as BMI over the 95th centile.[14] (However, many clinicans regard a BMI over the 91st centile as overweight and over the 98th centile as obese.)

Different cut-offs, based on the adult definitions of overweight and obese as 25 and 30 kg/m² respectively were proposed by the IOTF (International Obesity Task Force).[15]

Specialist referral and management for obesity should be considered for parental and child distress, sleep apnoea, severe obesity in children under 2 (there are several rare genetic causes) and obesity with short stature (as this may indicate a syndrome or endocrine cause).

Neither parents nor professionals reliably recognise obesity, perhaps because perceptions have changed of what is 'normal'. It is difficult to prevent or treat obesity, particularly where young children are concerned. There is some evidence that a growth trajectory towards obesity is established very early in life.[16] In the pre-school years, much depends on the motivation of the parents as one cannot expect young children to understand the issues or cooperate readily with demanding dietary changes. Advice to parents on reducing the risk of obesity may include:

- babies should be breastfed for at least six months;
- the intake of fruit and vegetables should be increased early in life (the 'Eatwell Plate' offers a pictorial approach to understanding healthy eating);[17]
- encourage a wider variety of flavours and textures in the diet;
- encourage family mealtimes and discourage grazing and snacking;
- water instead of high energy drinks should be provided;
- examine the family's lifestyle for opportunities to reduce TV viewing and computer time, and increase the child's (and parents') activity level; sport and physical exercise are just one aspect of this and developing lifestyle habits such as walking instead of using the car, or climbing stairs instead of using the lift, may all play a part.

An important goal is to prevent obesity starting early in life; however, health visitors often find it difficult to raise the issue of obesity and it may be useful to utilise the communication approaches discussed on page 31 onwards. HENRY (Health Exercise Nutrition for the Really Young) is a programme that offers training to community and health practitioners to enhance their skills and help them work more effectively with parents and carers. It focuses on the five key lifestyle areas: parenting, healthy eating patterns, nutrition, physical activity and emotional well-being, and utilises a toolkit depicting the Glugs, a group of animals who live on an island and are used to convey fun lessons about healthy living.[18] The HENRY handbook is available from the CPHVA.*

---

* Community Practitioners' and Health Visitors' Association; www.amicus-cphva.org/

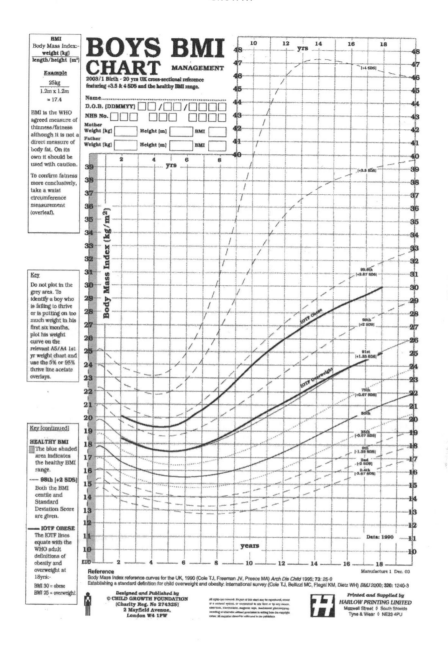

FIGURE 7.4 This chart was created using the 1990 nine-centile charts. The population is getting fatter and in order to provide a fixed standard against which to monitor this trend the BMI charts are 'frozen' using the data from which the 1990 charts were derived. The chart shows the cut-offs proposed by the International Obesity Task Force for obesity and overweight. These correspond to the adult cut-offs at age 18, which are BMI ≥ 30 for obesity and BMI ≥ 25 for overweight. The chart also shows +3.5 and +4 SDs for use in obesity clinics. Courtesy of Harlow Printing Ltd. © Child Growth Foundation.

NB: BMI charts based on the new WHO growth standards are in development but were not available at the time of going to press.

Schools are being encouraged to provide healthier meals and control the availability of high energy snacks. In order to monitor the progress of the obesity epidemic, all children are to be weighed and measured at age 4–5 years (reception year) and at 10–11 years (year 6), unless their parents opt out. Their parents will be informed of the BMI result, with an explanation of what it means and advice as to what action, if any, they should take.[14]

In a few cases, obesity can be so severe as to be a serious health hazard to the child. Often, the parents, who are frequently seriously overweight themselves, seem not to cooperate with efforts to control or reduce the child's weight, and in such cases the question may arise as to whether this is a child protection issue. This is an extreme step to take, and should only be contemplated where there is other evidence of neglect and there is concern that the obesity is life-threatening.

GROWTH AND THE BRAIN
Early brain growth: why it matters

The infant's head circumference (HC) increases from a median of 25 cm at 28 weeks gestation, to 35 cm at term and 45 cm by 8 months. The brain weighs on average 400 g at birth and increases to 1000 g (70% of its adult weight) by the baby's first birthday. There is a corresponding rapid increase in brain protein and nucleic acid. During this time there is dramatic growth and remodelling of synaptic connections. These processes need input from the environment and can be adversely affected by deprivation and negative or stressful experiences.

Modern magnetic resonance (MR) scanners can measure the volume of the whole brain and of specific parts of the brain. Brain volume shows a stronger relationship with IQ than does HC; this may be partly because HC measurement cannot take account of variations in the shape (especially the height of the head, which is not normally measured) and the thickness of the skull.

The HC is a crude, but useful, proxy for brain size and growth. It should be measured as part of the newborn examination, but preferably not in the first 2 days as it may be increased by scalp oedema or decreased by moulding. A second measurement should be taken at 6–8 weeks. The HC should be measured using a paper tape such as the Lasso.* It is important to take the maximum circumference, since this is the only repeatable reading. Some babies are upset by this procedure and it is wise to leave it until near the end of the examination. The measurement is meaningless unless it is plotted on a chart.

After 8 weeks of age, the value of routine HC monitoring in the community is limited. Routine measuring seems to have very modest benefits that are probably outweighed by the unnecessary referrals and anxiety that result. The HC should of course be measured, recorded and monitored over time in any child with a previous or current neurological or developmental problem, or if the head looks large or small.

Measurement of the HC is helpful in clinical practice for several reasons:

▶ In the newborn, head size may help in the assessment of infants who are small for gestational age. An infant who is small in length, weight and HC is likely to

---

* Charts and the Lasso are available from: http://shop.healthforallchildren.co.uk/pro.epl?DO=USERPAGE& PAGE=Site

have suffered prolonged under-nutrition *in utero*, whereas one who has grown well in length and has a normal HC, but has a disproportionately low weight, is likely to have suffered a shorter period of under-nutrition towards the end of pregnancy. This distinction is not always as simple as it sounds, because genetic disorders, intrauterine infections and hypoxic ischaemic injury to the developing brain may complicate the picture.

▶ Many disorders are associated with abnormal size (and sometimes shape) of the head. This may be apparent at birth, but sometimes only becomes obvious later in infancy or childhood.

▶ Measurements at birth and in the first two months of life provide a baseline for future measurements in the event of suspected deviant developmental progress or abnormal growth of the head as may occur, for example, in hydrocephalus. Monitoring head growth can also be useful when an infant appears to have suffered severe brain injury at birth or in the early days of life. In these circumstances, a declining rate of growth (i.e. the HC crosses centiles downwards) is ominous as it suggests that the brain has sustained significant damage. Conversely, if the HC was already small at the time of birth, this may suggest that any damage occurred long before the baby was born.

▶ In individual cases, HC measurements are mainly useful if they are abnormally big or small or changing at an abnormal rate. Within the normal range, a single measurement is usually unhelpful for clinical purposes. Generally, the HC has a weak relationship to the child's IQ. There are familial variations in head size and in some individuals a very small head may be associated with high IQ and vice versa.

▶ In population research, HC can be very useful; for example, in follow-up studies on the effects of early malnutrition.

Impact of poverty and neglect on brain growth

Infants who suffer chronic malnutrition, neglect or abuse are at risk of permanent effects on the developing brain. The impact may depend partly on the nature of the adverse experiences; for example, they may include physical deprivation such as under-nutrition, emotional neglect, failure to teach the infant basic skills and concepts, living in a hazardous and impoverished environment, or actual physical abuse. It seems unlikely that all adverse experiences would have the same impact on the developing brain or lead to the same behavioural and cognitive outcomes in later life. Differences in the volume of key cortical brain structures can be demonstrated by MR scans in children who have suffered various forms of abuse.

Observations in poor countries

In resource-poor countries, where severe under-nutrition is common in the early years of life, children who have been undernourished and neglected often have persisting deficits in growth. In extreme situations, such as severe poverty and under-nutrition in the first year or two of life, the growth of the brain and therefore of the head is affected and this is reflected in a lower IQ and lower educational attainment. Infants who have spent the critical early months of life in such conditions can, to some extent, recover if they are placed in a more normal environment, but the later this happens, the less complete the recovery.

Observations in Western countries

In most cases of child neglect in Western countries, deficits in height and weight are more common than measurable impairments of HC and brain volume. Improvement in these parameters after placement in a foster family is more readily demonstrated. Children who have been removed from their home because of child protection concerns and placed with foster carers often show some catch-up growth in height and weight, although it is unusual for these children to be so short or underweight that they could have been identified solely by their growth patterns. Deficits and subsequent catch up in HC are less commonly seen except in the most extreme cases. In premature and low birth weight infants there is an association between reduced growth in HC, neglect and cognitive outcome.

Summary

Deprivation, neglect and abuse are linked with, and may cause, reduced and probably sub-optimal brain growth and development. However, it may also work the other way round: babies who are born with neurological deficits, or are less responsive, or have difficult temperaments, are more likely to be neglected or abused, and perhaps elicit less care-giving from their parent(s).

LARGE HEADS

If the growth line is crossing the centile lines in an upwards direction, or if the measurement is above the 98th centile, but the baby is entirely well and normal, measure the parents' heads, particularly the father's. A large head is commonly a familial feature and in some families not only the size of the head, but also its rate of growth are increased, relative to standard growth charts.

Abnormal growth of the head may present at any age, but is most commonly a cause for concern in the first year of life. There are many causes, of which the two most familiar are hydrocephalus and subdural haemorrhage (haematoma, effusion). In the great majority of cases there will be other clues that there is something wrong, such as poor weight gain, delayed or abnormal development, irritability, vomiting, seizures or signs of raised intracranial pressure: separated sutures, a bulging anterior fontanel, downward deviation of the eyes (sunset sign), squint and prominent veins on the forehead. If you are in doubt about the tension of the fontanel, particularly if the baby is crying, sit the baby up and feel it again. If you are still uncertain, it is probably abnormal.

Note that hydrocephalus, subdural haematoma and raised intracranial pressure can occur in a head of any size – not just in big ones! In infancy the sutures are not yet fused and the head can expand easily, so the intracranial pressure, the size of the head and the effect on the baby depend on how quickly the underlying disorder is developing.

Never remark to the parents that their baby's head is big or small without explaining exactly what you mean and how you intend to find out whether the fact is significant. If in doubt, it is best to refer the child to a paediatrician. There is no justification for repeated measurements, either in hospital or in primary care settings, as this leaves parents in a state of chronic anxiety. Modern ultrasound allows rapid, safe investigation of unexplained head enlargement in a baby whose anterior fontanel is still open.

SMALL HEADS

Microcephaly simply means a small head. *Pathological microcephaly* cannot be defined purely on the basis of size. HC measurements below the 2nd centile do not necessarily imply abnormality. A HC which is *far* below the 2nd centile line is often associated with pathology and developmental or neurological disorder, but this is not the case invariably. The measurement may be less significant if the baby is small or if one or other parent has a small head.

Microcephaly may be obvious at birth as an isolated finding or as part of a syndrome or systemic disorder, or it may occur as a result of severe perinatal or postnatal brain damage (e.g. after meningitis or non-accidental injury). These babies should be under specialist care so they should not present problems for primary care staff.

Routine measurements of HC by community staff occasionally result in a referral to the paediatric clinic regarding the possibility of microcephaly. In the absence of any evidence of developmental problems or dysmorphic features, it is difficult for the paediatrician to deal with this situation. Imaging techniques do not always help. As with big heads, it is important to check the parents' HC to see if this might be a familial feature. It may be necessary to observe the head growth for several months to decide whether the rate of growth is abnormally slow. The developmental problems associated with mild degrees of microcephaly may not be apparent for 12 or 18 months.

REFERENCES

1 WHO charts – www.who.int/childgrowth/standards/en/

2 Hall DMB, Cole TJ. What use is the BMI? *Arch Dis Child*. 2006; **91**: 283–6. *See* also Prentice AM. Body mass index standards for children. *BMJ*. 1998; **317**: 1401–2.

3 Hall DMB, Voss LD. Growth monitoring. *Arch Dis Child*. 2000; **82**: 10–15. *See* also Voss LD, Bailey BJ. Diurnal variation in stature: is stretching the answer? *Arch Dis Child*. 1997; **77**(4): 319–22.

4 Cole TJ. Conditional reference charts to assess weight gain in British infants. *Arch Dis Child*. 1995; **73**(1): 8–16. NB: New thrive line charts utilising the WHO standards are currently (December 2008) in preparation and will be available from Harlow Printing Ltd (www.harlowprinting.co.uk).

5 Rudolf MC, Logan S. What is the long-term outcome for children who fail to thrive?: a systematic review. *Arch Dis Child*. 2005; **90**(9): 925–31.

6 Raynor P, Rudolf MC. Anthropometric indices of failure to thrive. *Arch Dis Child*. 2000; **82**(5): 364–5. *See* also Wright C. Identification and management of failure to thrive: a community perspective *Arch Dis Child*. 2000; **82**: 5–9.

7 University of Leeds. *Clues from Children's Mealtimes: a video and teaching manual on eating difficulties in young children*. Leeds: Media Services, University of Leeds; 1998 – *order from:* http://mediant.leeds.ac.uk/vtcatalogue/ *See* also Raynor P, Rudolf MC, Cooper K, *et al*. A randomised controlled trial of specialist health visitor intervention for failure to thrive. *Arch Dis Child*. 1999; **80**(6): 500–6. *See* also Raynor P, Rudolf M, Cottrell D, *et al*. An RCT of focused intervention and its effect on mealtime and eating behaviour in families with children diagnosed as failing to thrive (NOFTT). *Arch Dis Child*. 1999; **80**(Suppl. 1): A62.

8 Douglas J. Psychological Treatment of Food Refusal in Young Children. *Child and Adolesc Ment Health*. 2002; **7**(4): 173–80.

9 Iwaniec D. *Children Who Fail to Thrive: a practical guide*. Chichester: John Wiley; 2004.

10 Cole TJ. Growth monitoring with the British 1990 growth reference. *Arch Dis Child*.

1997; **76**(1): 47–9. *See* also Grote FK, van Dommelen, P, Oostdijk W, *et al.* Developing evidence-based guidelines for referral for short stature. *Arch Dis Child.* 2008; **93**: 212–17. *See* also Fayter D, Nixon I, Hartley S, *et al.* Effectiveness and cost-effectiveness of height screening programmes during the primary school years: a systematic review. *Arch Dis Child.* 2008; **93**: 278–84. *See* also Mei Z, Grummer-Strawn LM, Thompson D, *et al.* Longitudinal Data From the California Child Health and Development Study. *Pediatrics.* 2004; **113**: e617–27.

11 Cole TJ. A simple chart to identify non-familial short stature. *Arch Dis Child.* 2000; **82**: 173–6.

12 Clayton PE, Cianfarani S, Czernichow P, *et al.* Management of the Child Born Small for Gestational Age through to Adulthood: *J Clin Endocrinol Metab.* 2007; **92**(3): 804–10.

13 Skuse D, Albanese A, Stanhope R, *et al.* A new stress-related syndrome of growth failure and hyperphagia in children, associated with reversibility of growth-hormone insufficiency. *Lancet.* 1996 Aug 10; **348**(9024): 353–8.

14 The National Child Measurement Programme. Available at: www.dh.gov.uk/en/Public health/Healthimprovement/Healthyliving/DH_073787 (accessed 24 November 2008).

15 Cole TJ, Bellizzi MC, Flegal KM, *et al.* Establishing a standard definition for child overweight and obesity worldwide: international survey *BMJ.* 2000; **320**: 1–6.

16 Gardner D S-L, Hosking J, Metcalf BS, *et al.* The contribution of early weight gain to childhood overweight and metabolic health: a longitudinal study (EarlyBird 36). *Pediatrics.* 2009; **123**: e67–73.

17 www.eatwell.gov.uk/healthydiet/eatwellplate/

18 Hunt C, Rudolf M. *Tackling Obesity with HENRY.* London: Community Practitioners' and Health Visitors' Association; December 2008. *See* also the e-learning course available at: www.ukvirtual-college.co.uk/Childhood_Obesity_and_HENRY (accessed 24 November 2008). *See* also www.HENRY.org.uk

CHAPTER 8

Prevention of infectious diseases

IMMUNISATION

A general practice perspective on immunisation

It is good practice to aim for a high uptake of immunisation so that protection is provided for the whole population, including those who cannot be immunised. This is 'herd immunity'. Everyone who is likely to be concerned with immunisation and children should be familiar with the vaccines, their indications and contraindications (*see* page 157). There are very few contraindications and it is important that any misconceptions amongst practice personnel about them should be dispelled as parents rank advice from GPs, health visitors and practice nurses as their most trusted source of information. Incorrect or conflicting advice is very difficult to remedy and once doubt has been introduced into a parent's mind, it is very difficult to reassure them.

In a general practice, accurate records should be kept and regularly reviewed so that children who have missed immunisation can be recalled. Paradoxically, those children who are frequently in the surgery or attend hospital are those who are most likely to miss immunisation. If their records and their parents' and siblings' records are marked, the immunisation can be offered when they attend with another member of the family. Another group who have a low immunisation uptake are those who are highly mobile. They are frequently seen by their GP before their records arrive. It should be practice policy that as children are registered, they are seen by the practice nurse and information is collected about immunisation status. As a last resort a practice may consider immunising children in the home.

In the 1990 UK Contract for General Practice, two target take-up levels were set for payment purposes. To achieve the lower level of remuneration, an average of 70% of children aged 2 years should have been immunised with three groups of vaccines: diphtheria, tetanus and polio; pertussis; and MMR (mumps, measles and rubella). To achieve the higher level, 90% would need to be immunised. Since then there have been many changes to the immunisation schedule and to the GP Contract. These targets, including meningococcal C vaccine, have now been incorporated into the 2004 GP Contract.

Importance of childhood vaccination

The vaccination of children has been shown to be a highly effective form of preventive care and also saves money. Many vaccines have been in use for decades, but the take-up rates are still, on average, below target figures set by the WHO. The latest figures (2006–07) show that the average take-up, by 2 years old, of the triple (diphtheria, tetanus and pertussis), polio, *Haemophilus influenzae* type b (Hib) and *meningococcal C* (Men C) immunisation was 94%, whereas that for MMR was only 86%, though this had risen from 81% in 2004/5.

The primary source of information about vaccination in the UK is *Immunisation Against Infectious Disease* from the Department of Health ('the Green Book'). The last hard copy was issued in 2006–07 and it is updated at intervals on the Department of Health web sites.[1] The current recommendations are summarised in Box 8.1.

BOX 8.1 The recommended schedule of vaccines in the UK (as at 2008)

Age	Vaccines	Comments
Birth	BCG	Only to those in high risk groups (*see* page 173)
	Hepatitis B	Only to those babies whose mothers were hepatitis B surface antigen-positive or had an acute episode of hepatitis B during pregnancy
4 weeks#	Hepatitis B	(As above) – second dose
8 weeks#	Hepatitis B	(As above) – third dose
	DTP/IPV/Hib	One injection
	PCV	One injection
12 weeks#	DTP/IPV/Hib	One injection
	Men C	One injection
16 weeks	DTP/IPV/Hib	One injection
	Men C	One injection
	PCV	One injection

(*cont.*)

Age	Vaccines	Comments
12 months	Hepatitis B	(As above) – fourth dose
	Hib/Men C booster	One injection
13 months	MMR	One injection
	PCV booster	One injection
3 years 4 months	DTP/IPV or d*TP/ IPV	One injection – 'pre-school booster'
	MMR†	One injection – second dose
School year 8 (12-13 years old) girls only	HPV‡	Three injections over 6 months
13-18 years	dT/IPV	One injection – 'school leavers' booster

BCG = *Bacillus Calmette-Guérin*; **dT** = low-dose diphtheria with normal dose tetatnus; **dTP** = low-dose diphtheria with normal dose tetatnus and pertussis; **DTP** = diphtheria, tetanus, pertussis; **Hib** = *Haemophilus influenzae*; **HPV** = human papilloma virus; **IPV** = inactivated polio vaccine; **Men C** = meningococcal C; **MMR** = measles, mumps and rubella; **PCV** = pneumococcal conjugate vaccine.

* 'd' indicates low dose diphtheria vaccine.

† The second dose of MMR can be given earlier. In a child under 18 months old, a gap of 3 months is necessary to achieve an optimum immune response. This can be shortened to 1 month when protection is needed urgently, but, in these circumstances, a further dose is necessary at the time of the pre-school booster. A child over 18 months old can receive a second dose at any time after the first, as long as at least 1 month has elapsed.

The intervals between the three doses of primary course of DTP, Hib and polio should not be reduced below the recommendation of 4 weeks. Any further reduction might impair efficacy and should only be undertaken on the advice of an expert.

‡ HPV vaccine was introduced in 2008–09. The vaccine supplied by NHS (Cervarix) is active against the HPV types (16 and 18) associated with 70% of cervical cancer. It is to be given to all girls in school year 8 (age 12-13 years). In 2008–09 it will also be given to girls of an age to be in Year 13 (whether or not in school) and in 2009–10, there will be a catch-up programme for the remaining school age girls. The vaccine will be given predominantly in school. At this stage, it is not planned to offer the vaccine to older women or boys.

Source: *Immunisation Against Infectious Disease* from the Department of Health ('The Green Book').

CONJUGATE VACCINES

The Hib vaccine was introduced into the routine vaccination schedule in the UK in 1992; Men C in 1999; and pneumococcal conjugate vaccine (PCV) in 2006. These three are conjugate vaccines, that is, a protein has been tagged onto the polysaccharide capsule of the organism, thus improving immunogenicity in young children. Experience has shown that while a primary course of vaccinations in infancy produces immunity, it is short-lived and therefore it is important that children receive a booster against each disease in the second year of life. As yet there is no vaccine available against meningococcal B disease, although the results of trials are promising. In addition, the PCV does not cover all *Streptococcus pneumoniae* serotypes. Therefore, parents should be warned that vaccines do not protect against all possible causes of meningitis, so they must not ignore suggestive symptoms and signs in their child.

The MMR vaccine has been in use in the USA since 1972, in some parts of Scandinavia since 1982 and in the UK since 1988. Over this period the incidence of measles has fallen dramatically. However, the vaccine has an efficacy of only 90–95% for the measles component and less for the mumps. For this reason, most countries using the vaccine recommend a two-dose schedule. There is considerable evidence that MMR is highly effective and rarely gives rise to serious adverse reactions (*see* Box 8.2).

In 1998, concerns were raised in a *Lancet* paper about a possible link between the vaccine, autism and inflammatory bowel disease. It was suggested by one of the researchers that any such risk could be reduced by giving the MMR antigens separately and many worried parents requested these for their children. There is now a large body of research that has shown no evidence of a link between MMR and autism and no country has withdrawn the vaccine on this basis. In 2004, 10 of the 13 authors of the *Lancet* paper made it clear that they did not believe there was a link between the MMR vaccine and autism or bowel disease:

> We wish to make it clear that in this paper no causal link was established between MMR vaccine and autism as the data were insufficient. However, the possibility of such a link was raised and consequent events have had major implications for public health. In view of this, we consider now is the appropriate time that we should together formally retract the interpretation placed upon these findings in the paper, according to precedent.

Use of the single antigen vaccines is not recommended and is not in the best interests of the child because:

- mumps, measles and rubella infections can cause serious problems, even in industrialised countries;
- a regimen of single measles, mumps, rubella vaccines has NEVER been used so there is NO evidence about its safety and efficacy;[2] however, it inevitably means that there is a longer period during which the child is not protected;
- such a regimen would allow continued circulation of diseases in the community, thus putting more children at risk.

Does it matter if vaccine uptake rates fall?

The fall in uptake of MMR has resulted in an increase in measles cases, particularly in London. In 2006, there were 740 confirmed cases of measles in England and Wales (the most since salivary viral confirmation testing was introduced in 1996) and the first death from measles in over 14 years occurred. In 2008, the figure had risen to 1348 confirmed cases of measles. There was a further death in May 2008. Both deaths were in immuno-suppressed teenagers, emphasising the importance of high uptake levels to achieve herd immunity. A child died from diphtheria in April 2008; the child had not been immunised and had not been abroad recently, so must have been infected from another recent traveller.

OTHER VACCINES

Other vaccines may need to be given in special circumstances. Hepatitis B vaccine should be given to those at risk by nature of disease-state or contacts. Those with some chronic disorders (severe asthma, cystic fibrosis, bronchopulmonary dysplasia, cyanotic congenital heart disease, etc.) should be given influenza vaccine. It should also be considered in all children with Down's syndrome and those with major neuro-developmental problems. Rabies, yellow fever, hepatitis A, typhoid, Japanese encephalitis and tick-borne encephalitis vaccines may be appropriate in some individuals as may the plain polysaccharide meningococcal (A, C, W135 and Y) and pneumococcal vaccines.

CONTRAINDICATIONS TO VACCINATION

There are very few contraindications to vaccination, but many myths abound. Asthma, eczema, hay-fever, snuffles, treatment with antibiotics or locally-acting steroids, being breastfed, mother being pregnant, a history of neonatal jaundice, previous clinically diagnosis of infection with pertussis, measles, mumps, rubella or polio, failure to thrive, stable neurological conditions such as cerebral palsy and spina bifida and Down's syndrome have all been cited as reasons for withholding vaccinations. None of these are contraindications to any vaccination.

The true contraindications are set out below:

▶ Any vaccination should be postponed for any child who is **acutely unwell** with a fever or systemic upset. A mild illness without these features can be ignored. As soon as the child is well the vaccination should be given. Treatment with antibiotics is not, in itself, a contraindication.
▶ In individuals with an evolving neurological condition, immunisation should be postponed until the condition has stabilised. This does not include static conditions such as Down's syndrome and cerebral palsy. Any such postponement should be reviewed at regular intervals in order that the child can be immunised as soon as appropriate.
▶ Children who are known to have had an **anaphylactic response to a constituent of a vaccine** should not receive that vaccine. Minor allergic reactions to eggs or antibiotics are not relevant. Although MMR vaccine contains trace quantities of egg protein, it can be given safely to children who have had an anaphylactic reaction to egg. Influenza and yellow fever vaccinations are contraindicated in those who have had an anaphylactic reaction to egg.
▶ Children who are **immuno-compromised**, whether due to disease or treatment, or are **HIV-positive**, should be referred to their consultant for advice. Depending on the circumstances, live vaccines may be contraindicated, due to the risk of adverse effects, whereas killed/inactive vaccines should be given, but may be less effective.

▶ **No allowance should be made for prematurity.** The timing of the vaccination programme dates *from birth*, not the expected time of delivery.

Whenever a vaccination is postponed, the decision should be reviewed after a suitable interval, depending on the reason for postponement, to ensure that it is not overlooked.

A severe local or systemic reaction to a previous dose of vaccine is no longer a contraindication to any routine childhood vaccination, except if accompanied by an anaphylactic reaction.

SITE OF INJECTION AND TECHNIQUE

Apart from BCG, all routine childhood immunisations should be given by intra-muscular injection. There is evidence that more superficial injections are likely to give rise to a greater number of significant local reactions. Except for premature or very small babies, a 25 mm needle should be used for the intramuscular route and the injection should be given at a right angle to the skin to ensure that the vaccine is given deeply enough.

All intramuscular and subcutaneous injections should be given into either the deltoid region of the upper arm or the anterolateral aspect of the thigh. Vaccines should never be given into the buttocks as the efficacy may be reduced and there is a small risk of sciatic nerve damage. Intradermal injections should only be given by those who have had the requisite training and who use this route regularly. Two injections can be given in the same limb as long as they are at least 25 mm apart and the needle is inserted at 90 degrees/vertically.

The skin may be cleansed with soap and water if visibly dirty, but vigorous attempts at sterilisation are not needed. If alcohol is used, it should be allowed to dry before the injection is given; otherwise it hurts and may inactivate live vaccines.

STORAGE OF VACCINES

A breakdown in the 'cold chain', the system of keeping vaccines at the correct temperature during transfer from manufacturer to patient, is potentially as great a problem in the UK as it is in the tropics. Vaccines that are incorrectly stored may lose potency. If frozen, glass vials may develop hairline cracks and become contaminated.

The following points are important wherever vaccines are given:

▶ one named individual should be responsible for monitoring the refrigerator temperature at least once on every working day, and ensuring that the correct action is taken in the event of a breakdown or error;
▶ vaccines should be stored at 2–8°C;
▶ an overfull refrigerator will have a wide temperature range within it because air cannot circulate; there should be spaces between vaccine packages to allow free air circulation;
▶ the temperature should be monitored with a maximum/minimum thermometer placed in the middle of the refrigerator;
▶ the refrigerator should be defrosted regularly if it has no automatic defrosting

facility; during defrosting the vaccines should be kept in another refrigerator or in a cool box;

▶ food and specimens should not be stored in the same refrigerator as vaccines;
▶ reconstituted vaccines must be used within the specified period; partially used multi-dose vials must be discarded at the end of a session;
▶ vaccines should be kept in a cool box for transport from district pharmacies or between practice premises.

ANAPHYLAXIS
Prevention is better than cure
Check for a history of anaphylaxis or sensitivity to antibiotics. If in doubt, do not simply advise against immunisation; consult the Green Book or call the local immunisation coordinator. You may find it useful to copy the protocol below, and place it where vaccination is carried out. The drugs and equipment mentioned should be easily accessible.

Treatment of acute anaphylaxis
Anaphylaxis is very rare. Most staff will never see a true case, so occasional rehearsal of its management is good practice. This can form part of the regular cardio-pulmonary resuscitation training and updates that all staff should undergo. Whenever vaccines are in use, there should be a tray with resuscitation equipment available. It should include adrenaline 1/1000, together with 1 mL syringes, needles and airways.

Diagnosis
Anaphylaxis may present with a variety of symptoms:

▶ pallor, limpness and transient apnoea are the most common signs in children;
▶ upper airway obstruction: hoarseness and stridor as a result of angio-oedema involving the hypopharynx, epiglottis and larynx;
▶ lower airways obstruction: subjective feelings of retrosternal tightness and dyspnoea with audible expiratory wheeze from bronchospasm;
▶ cardiovascular: sinus tachycardia, profound hypotension in association with tachycardia; severe bradycardia;
▶ skin: characteristic rapid development of urticarial lesions – circumscribed, intensely itchy weals with erythematous raised edges and pale, blanched centres;
▶ also, consider the possibility of reflex anoxic seizures (*see* page 271).

Management
The UK Resuscitation Council has provided guidance on the management of anaphylaxis:[3]

▶ **Distinguish acute anaphylaxis from a simple faint.** Feel for a carotid or femoral pulse: if present, and of a normal rate and strength, this is probably a faint; if absent or very weak assume this is anaphylactic shock. If in doubt, assume anaphylaxis: fainting is rare in infants.
▶ **Place patient in the recovery position**, with the head down. Insert an **oral airway** (size 00 or 0 if 0–1 year, 0 or 1 if 1–5 years, 1 or 2 if 5–12 years and 2, 3 or 4 if an adult).

▶ **Summon help if readily available**, but not if this will delay treatment for more than a minute or so.
▶ **Administer adrenaline** (1/1000; i.e. 1 mg/mL) by intramuscular injection in a dose depending on age:
  — 0–6 years: 150 micrograms IM (0.15 mL).
  — >6–12 years: 300 micrograms IM (0.3 mL).
  — >12 years and adults: 500 micrograms IM (0.5 mL) – 300 micrograms IM (0.3 mL) if child is small or prepubertal.
  — Further doses can be given at 5-minute intervals according to the patient's response.
▶ *Chlorpheniramine* (Piriton®) may be given intramuscularly after the acute episode has been treated. The evidence in favour of its use is poor, but there are logical reasons to suspect it may help. The usual preparation is a 1% solution; i.e. 10 mg in 1 mL. The following are appropriate:
  — <6 months: 250 micrograms/kg IM or IV slowly.
  — >6 months to 6 years: 2.5 mg (0.25 mL) IM or IV slowly.
  — >6–12 years: 5 mg (0.5 mL) IM or IV slowly.
  — >12 years and adults: 10 mg (1 mL) IM or IV slowly.
▶ **Always admit the patient to hospital** after treatment, as there is sometimes a recurrence of symptoms within the first 24 hours.
▶ **Consult the local immunisation coordinator** about further immunisations.

Children with a documented history of cerebral damage, a personal history of convulsions or a family history of febrile convulsions or idiopathic epilepsy are at increased risk of a febrile fit following vaccination, in particular pertussis and MMR. Such children are also at greater risk of complications associated with natural infection. The benefits of vaccination outweigh the risks; they are not at any greater risk of permanent adverse effects from the vaccines and should receive them. Parents of such children may give them paracetamol or ibuprofen for 36–48 hours following vaccination with the infant vaccines; however, while it may reduce the fever, there is no evidence that it will prevent a convulsion. As the pyrexia following MMR vaccine occurs at an interval of 5–10 days after vaccination, prophylactic paracetamol is not appropriate. The parents should be told what to do in the event of a fever occurring. If such a child is under the care of a paediatrician and there is any doubt as to whether either vaccine should be given, the paediatrician ought to be consulted first.

TABLE 8.1 Notifications (and deaths) from vaccine-preventable diseases reported to ONS 1990–2004. Deaths (where data are available) are shown in brackets: (–) indicates that data are not available.

Disease	Year			
	1990	1995	2000	2004
Diphtheria	2(0)	12(1)	19(1)	10(0)
Hib meningitis	431(26)	51(0)	43(–)	45(–)
Measles	13 302(1)	7768(1)	1213(0)	2356(0)

(cont.)

Disease	Year			
	1990	1995	2000	2004
Meningococcal meningitis and septicaemia	1415(–)	1853 (–)	2778 (195)	1245 (84)
Mumps	4277(0)	1936(0)	2162(0)	16 367(0)
Pertussis	15 286(7)	1869(2)	712(2)	504(3)
Rubella	11 491(0)	6196	1653	1287
Tetanus	9(1)	6(2)	2(1)	12(0)
Tuberculosis	5204(390)	5608(447)	6572(373)	6723(344)

WHY ARE HIGH RATES OF VACCINATION NOT ACHIEVED MORE OFTEN?

Bearing in mind the very few contraindications to the primary course of vaccinations, uptake rates of over 99% are theoretically possible. Why is this level so rarely attained? There are a number of reasons:

- **Low priority.** Acute illnesses and child abuse attract publicity and hence resources at the expense of vaccination programmes.
- **Perceived low risk of diseases.** Many of the diseases against which vaccination is carried out are perceived as being rare. For diphtheria, polio and tetanus and (until recently) measles, this is true, but for others, such as whooping cough, the illnesses are still very common, frequently distressing and sometimes fatal. Table 8.1 shows how commonly these diseases occur in England and Wales. Encephalitis follows measles at between 0.1% and 0.2% of cases and can result in permanent disability. Mumps is the most common cause of aseptic meningitis and is a significant cause of sensorineural hearing loss in children.
- **Vaccination not seen as a positive activity.** Undue attention has been given to the very rare adverse effects of vaccination without pointing out the hazards of the diseases. Professionals seem to worry about being blamed for the adverse effects of a vaccination they have given, but are unconcerned by the far more common situation of a vaccine being withheld for spurious reasons and the child suffering the ill effects of a preventable disease.
- **Lack of responsibility.** Vaccination is undertaken by GPs and the Community Child Health Services. Until the appointment of district immunisation coordinators (DICs) in the late 1980s, no-one had overall responsibility; thus low uptake rates could be, and often were, blamed on someone else. With the appointment of DICs, this was no longer the case. Amongst their responsibilities, the DICs offered any practice advice on setting up or improving an immunisation programme and help in individual 'problem' cases where there was doubt as to whether or not a child should be vaccinated. With the demise of health authorities, DICs no longer exist and it is up to each Primary Care Organisation (PCO) to ensure there is someone with overall responsibility for its immunisation programme. Unfortunately many PCOs do not have someone with this role, and responsibilities are unclear.
- **Poor education.** The abundance of mythical contraindications and their propagation by professionals and public alike has caused understandable confusion for some parents. Better training of the professionals and

161

adherence to official guidelines should help to dispel many of these myths. With this in mind, the Health Protection Agency has developed national minimum standards and a core curriculum for all those involved in providing immunisation.* Many PCOs provide courses for doctors and nurses. The Department of Health provides useful information and there are a number of good web sites. Ready access to a local expert who can offer speedy advice is often found to be helpful. Some districts have immunisation advice clinics where children can be referred if there is doubt as to what vaccinations they should be given, and where parents can have their concerns explored in more depth.

▶ **Poor information transfer.** Many parents will bring their children for vaccination with little prompting. However, a significant number forget or are reluctant and therefore need reminding. This cannot be done unless accurate records are kept and there is adequate transfer of data between all the professionals involved (i.e. PCOs, GPs, health visitors, etc.). Only in this way can individual parents – and their doctors – be reminded of overdue vaccinations. Without efficient and speedy feedback, it is impossible to monitor the service being provided and attend to any inadequacies. Feedback to professionals at the grass roots allows them to monitor their own performance in comparison with others and to be alerted to any decline in uptake. All immunisations should be recorded in the Personal Child Health Record (PCHR) as this should follow the child wherever they go for healthcare.

▶ **Inflexibility.** Vaccinations should be performed not only by the doctor at set times during the day or week, but also by any suitably trained person, doctor or nurse, whenever and for whatever reason a child is brought to see that professional, assuming the child is due for vaccination and no real contraindication exists. Practice nurses, clinic nurses and health visitors should all be trained to advise about and give vaccinations, without a doctor being present. If a child is a few days early for a vaccination it should not be put off. On any occasion that a child is seen, the vaccination history should be ascertained and any gaps in the programme completed. All vaccines can be given together. Opportunistic vaccination is one of the best ways of increasing uptake rates. Hospital paediatric units should ensure they have policies in place for opportunistic immunisation, as children attending hospital are less likely to be fully immunised.

CHILDHOOD VACCINATION: A CHECKLIST FOR STAFF
All vaccines
This checklist should be followed for all vaccines.

▶ Is the child acutely unwell with a fever or systemic upset? If so, postpone the immunisation until the child is better.
▶ Has the child had an anaphylactic reaction to a previous dose of one of the

---

* Health Protection Agency. *Immunisation Training Resources for Healthcare Professionals.* www.hpa.org.uk/ (accessed 31 December 2008).

vaccines about to be given, or to one their constituents? If so, discuss with local paediatrician or immunisation coordinator.
▶ Has the child an evolving neurological condition? If so, defer immunisation until the condition is stable.

For MMR vaccine
This checklist should be followed for MMR vaccines.

▶ Is the child immunosuppressed (excluding due to HIV)? If so, the vaccine should not be given. It is important that all other family members are immune.
▶ Has the child been given another live vaccine (including BCG) within the last 4 weeks? If so, postpone until a full 4 weeks have elapsed.
▶ Has the child received immunoglobulin within the last 3 months? If so, postpone until a full 3 months have elapsed.
▶ Is the child allergic to gelatin or neomycin? If so, discuss with local paediatrician or immunisation coordinator.

NB: Any female receiving MMR should be advised that pregnancy should be avoided for 1 month, although the risk of any adverse effect is negligible.

For BCG vaccine (not usually performed in general practice)
This checklist should be followed for BCG vaccines.

▶ Does the child need a Mantoux test prior to BCG? (Consult current edition of the Green Book.) If so, ensure this takes place and is read 48–72 hours later.
▶ Is the child HIV positive? If so, the vaccine should not be given.
▶ Is the child immunosuppressed? If so, the vaccine should not be given.
▶ Has the child been given another live vaccine within the last 4 weeks? If so, postpone until a full 4 weeks have elapsed.

PATIENT GROUP DIRECTIONS (PGDs)
Where nurses are to give immunisations without a prescription it is essential that they are covered by a 'Patient Group Direction' (PGD).[4] These are written instructions for the supply or administration of medicines to groups of patients who may not be individually identified before presentation for treatment. They replace the need for individual prescriptions and are ideal for allowing opportunistic immunisation by professionals who cannot themselves prescribe. Patient safety must not be compromised and PGDs should not *normally* include: new drugs under intensive monitoring and subject to special adverse reaction reporting requirements (the Black Triangle scheme[*]); unlicensed medicines (e.g. the current Mantoux preparation in use in UK); medicines used outside their licensed indications; medicines being used in clinical trials.

Development of the PGD
The PGD should be drawn up by a group, including a doctor, pharmacist and at

---

[*] Black Triangle products are new drugs and vaccines which are being intensively monitored in order to confirm the risk/benefit profile of the product. *See* www.mhra.gov.uk/index.htm

least one representative of each of the professional groups likely to be involved in giving the immunisations covered. This will usually include health visitors, school nurses and practice nurses. It should be approved by the relevant local professional advisory committees and clinical managers.

The content

The content of the PGD should comprise:

- the qualifications and training required of staff (e.g. a nurse giving immunisations should hold a basic qualification and have attended a course on immunisation);
- necessary updating;
- the criteria for eligibility for vaccination and any exclusions;
- all the vaccines included in the PGD should be listed, along with their presentations, dosage and route of administration;
- details of the means by which the administration of the vaccine is to be recorded;
- action to be taken where a vaccine is refused;
- identification, management and follow-up of adverse events;
- arrangements for regular review, monitoring and audit;
- the names of the professionals drawing up the PGD and the professional advisory groups and managers giving approval to it;
- the PGD should be dated and signed.

Implementation

The implementation of the PGD should follow the following process:

- all professionals operating under the PGD should be named and have evidence of competence in the relevant skills and knowledge;
- participants should be approved by their professional managers;
- participants must not act beyond their professional competence;
- participants should sign a copy of the PGD and be provided with written evidence that they are authorised to operate under the PGD;
- a copy of the PGD should be available in the clinical setting in which it operates;
- arrangements must be in place to modify the PGD in the light of any new data or recommendations.

NB: With the expansion of nurse prescribing in the future, PGDs will become unnecessary in many settings.

FREQUENTLY ASKED QUESTIONS

Q. A child is adopted and the family history is not known – what immunisations should he receive?

A. He should receive all the vaccinations appropriate to his age. The only factor that may be of relevance is the HIV status of the mother. If there is any evidence to suggest that the mother may be HIV-positive, before giving BCG, the adoption agency should be consulted.[*]

Q. A child comes from abroad and the immunisation status is unknown – what vaccinations should he receive?

A. Assume the child has only received those vaccinations for which there is documentary evidence and give full courses of the remainder.[†]

Q. A course of vaccinations is interrupted by a longer interval than is recommended – should the course be restarted?

A. A course never needs restarting. The remaining dose(s) should be given at the same intervals as would have been appropriate had the course not been interrupted.

Q. Should a child receive all his primary immunisations before he is allowed to go swimming?

A. It is not necessary for any immunisations to be given before a child can go swimming. This myth arose when oral polio vaccine was used and even then it was not appropriate. Polio has not been transmitted via swimming pools in the UK.

Q. A child has had a disease – should he receive the vaccination against that disease?

A. BCG should not be given to someone who is known to have had TB or has a positive Mantoux test. Apart from this single exception, no harm will come to a child who is vaccinated when already immune. In many cases, vaccination will boost immunity and in some cases provide it when absent. If a child has definite evidence of having had hepatitis A or B, vaccination would be wasted and is therefore not indicated. For all other diseases, however strong the evidence of past infection, vaccination should still be given.

Q. Can more than one vaccine be given at the same time?

A. The only combination of vaccines that *cannot* be given at the same time are the Hib/Men C and PCV boosters. There are currently no data on the safety and immunogenicity of these vaccines when given at the same time. No vaccines should be mixed in the same syringe, unless specifically indicated in the manufacturer's literature.

Q. The Department of Health guidelines are different from the manufacturer's literature. Which is correct?

A. The manufacturer's literature is based on the original product licence and is often very conservative. The Department of Health guidelines are more likely to take account of experience since the vaccine was introduced and should be followed in preference to anything else.

---

[*] For further guidance *see* www.hpa.org.uk/web/HPAwebFile/HPAweb_C/1194947406156

[†] Ibid.

Q. A child develops a nodule at the site of a DTP injection. Is this a contraindication to further doses?

A. Such nodules are quite common and may take months or, less frequently, years to resolve. They are not a contraindication to further doses. They may be more common with injections given too superficially and extra care should be taken with subsequent injections.

Q. A parent had a 'bad reaction' to a particular vaccine. Should her child receive the vaccine?

A. There is no convincing evidence that reactions to vaccines run in families and, in any case, it may be difficult to be sure that an event happening at the time of a vaccination is in any way related to the vaccination. Therefore, a family history is not relevant unless the suspected reaction was a fit, in which case it would be appropriate to recommend that the child should receive an antipyretic after immunisation (although there is no direct evidence that this prevents post immunisation convulsions).

Q. Is recent immunisation a contraindication to surgery such as tonsillectomy?

A. No.

Q. Is there a risk of MMR vaccine causing meningitis?

A. There were some cases of mild transient meningitis with the Urabe strain of mumps vaccine virus, which was withdrawn in 1992. The MMR vaccines now in use in the UK contain the Jeryl Lynn or a closely related strain. The rate of meningitis due to this strain of mumps virus is very low. Note that meningitis occurs in 80% of natural mumps and can be severe; vaccine cases have been mild and have left no sequelae.

Q. A relative has inflammatory bowel disease or autism. Should the MMR vaccine be withheld?

A. The hypothesis that measles or MMR vaccines are linked to inflammatory bowel disease and autism has been disproved. This family history is not relevant and the vaccine should be given.

Q. Should childhood immunisations be made compulsory, as in the USA?

A. In many parts of the USA it is compulsory for a child to be immunised before school entry. Overall uptake rates are no better than those in Scandinavian countries where immunisation is voluntary. More importantly, for a long time, the uptake rates in 2-year-old children in the USA were significantly lower than in the UK. Professional knowledge and enthusiasm are much more effective than compulsion.

Q. Is there any tissue or protein from cattle in BCG?

A. No.

Q. Don't all these vaccines overload the immune system?

A. There is good evidence that children who have been fully immunised are no more susceptible to other infections or to develop atopic or autoimmune diseases than unimmunised children.

HOW TO ACHIEVE HIGH RATES OF VACCINATION

This list provides pointers on achieving high rates of vaccination:

▶ Give it a **high priority**. Devote time to organising it within the practice. Give someone overall responsibility for vaccination within the primary care team.

▶ Be **enthusiastic** and convince parents that it is important. **Emphasise the benefits.**

▶ Be **well-informed** (*see* Box 8.2) and know the true contraindications, which are very few.

▶ **Never say that a child should not receive a vaccination without being absolutely certain that this advice is correct.** There should be very strong grounds for denying a child the benefits of vaccination. If in doubt, seek further advice from a paediatrician (community or hospital), a consultant in communicable disease control or the PCO's immunisation lead.

▶ Know where to seek further advice locally.

▶ Be **flexible** and vaccinate whenever the opportunity arises.

▶ **Liaise** closely with all others involved in vaccination in the district. This includes health visitors, clinic doctors and the PCO's immunisation lead.

You are probably more likely to be sued in future for withholding a vaccine than for giving it.

BOX 8.2 Useful sources of information about immunisation

- The Department of Health web site, from which can be accessed the 'Green Book', other publications and useful links: www.dh.gov.uk/en/Publichealth/Healthprotection/Immunisation/index.htm
- Jefferson N, Sleight G, MacFarlane A. Immunisation of children by a nurse without a doctor present. *BMJ.* 1987; **294**: 423–4. A very useful article showing that a suitably trained nurse can carry out immunisation without a doctor being on the premises.
- Royal College of Paediatrics and Child Health. *Manual of Childhood Infections*. London: WB Saunders; 2001. A concise guide to childhood infections. It includes details of diagnosis, management and prevention of infectious diseases in children.
- Booy R, Sengupta N, Bedford H, *et al.* Measles, mumps, and rubella: prevention. *Clin Evid.* 2006; **15**: 448–68. A review.
- Bedford H, Elliman D. Concerns about immunisation. *BMJ.* 2000; **320**: 240–3. Available at: www.bmj.com/cgi/reprint/320/7229/240 A review of how to talk to worried parents.
- Elliman DA, Bedford HE. MMR: Where are we now? *Arch Dis Child.* 2007; **92**: 1055–7. A review of the current evidence in relation to the MMR vaccine.
- Muscat M, Bang H, Wohlfahrt J, *et al.* Measles in Europe: an epidemiological assessment. *Lancet*, Early On-line Publication, 7 January 2009. Reviews rise in measles infections across Europe.
- Great Ormond Street Hospital/Institute of Child Health (www.ich.ucl.ac.uk/immunisation/) An independent web site for parents and professionals.

- Health Protection Agency. Immunisation web site: www.hpa.org.uk/infections/ topics_az/vaccination/vacc_menu.htm
- Health Protection Agency. Vaccination of individuals with uncertain or incomplete immunisation status: www.hpa.org.uk/infections/topics_az/vaccination/ algorithm_2006_Septl.pdf
- Offit PA, Quarles J, Gerber MA, *et al.* Addressing parents' concerns: do multiple vaccines overwhelm or weaken the infant's immune system? *Pediatrics.* 2002; **109**(1): 124-9. Available at: http://pediatrics.aappublications.org/cgi/reprint/109/1/124 A review.
- Offit PA, Hackett CJ. Addressing parents' concerns: do vaccines cause allergic or autoimmune diseases? *Pediatrics.* 2003; **111**(3): 653-9. Available at: http:// pediatrics.aappublications.org/cgi/reprint/111/3/653 A review.
- Offit PA, Jew RK. Addressing parents' concerns: do vaccines contain harmful preservatives, adjuvants, additives, or residuals? *Pediatrics.* 2003; **112**(6 Pt 1): 1394-7. Available at: http://pediatrics.aappublications.org/cgi/reprint/112/6/1394 A review.

OTHER ASPECTS OF PREVENTION OF INFECTIOUS DISEASES
Prophylaxis for contacts of meningococcal and *Haemophilus* infections
Prophylaxis will usually be arranged by the hospital where the patient is admitted, or by the consultant in communicable disease control (CCDC), but the GP may be asked to write the prescription and anxious parents will expect him to know what should be done.

The spectre of meningitis always strikes fear into the hearts of parents. In fact it is unusual for secondary cases to occur, even within families. Remember that it is the septicaemic form of meningococcal disease that has the high mortality, rather than meningitis. What follows is advice that is current at the time of writing. **Before treating contacts with antibiotics or vaccine, always consult the local CCDC.**

Meningococcus
The highest attack rates are in the age group of 0–4 years. Antibiotic treatment should be offered to all household contacts and boy/girl friends as soon as possible. This includes boarders in the same dormitory, but not other school or nursery contacts.

The antibiotic of choice is rifampicin: 10 mg/kg every 12 hours for 2 days (5 mg/ kg if <1 month old) to a maximum 600 mg/dose.* Ciprofloxacin is an unlicensed alternative. Rifampicin or intramuscular ceftriaxone (a single dose of 250 mg) should be used in pregnant women.

Antibiotic prophylaxis is usually only given to a wider group when two or more cases of the same strain have occurred within the same setting over a short period of time. This should never be done except on the advice of the CCDC, who will often wish to seek national guidance.

If the organism is found to be serogroup A, C, W137 or Y, the appropriate vaccine should also be given.†

---

* Don't forget to warn women that rifampicin inactivates the oral contraceptive pill for the rest of the cycle.

† For more details *see* HPA guidance at www.hpa.org.uk/web/HPAwebFile/HPAweb_C/1194947389261

Haemophilus

All unimmunised children under 10 years should be vaccinated as soon as possible.

In households where one or more individuals are at risk (e.g. under 4 years old, immunosuppressed or asplenic), all household contacts and the index case should be given antibiotic prophylaxis.

The antibiotic of choice is rifampicin: 20 mg/kg once daily for 4 days (10 mg/kg if <1 month old) to a maximum of 600 mg/dose.[5]

Antibiotic prophylaxis is usually only given to contacts at playgroup, nursery or crèche when two or more cases have occurred within the same setting within 120 days. This should never be done except on the advice of the CCDC, who will often wish to seek national guidance.

Needlestick injuries

Children may find needles on rubbish tips or even in their own gardens. The parents will be concerned that they may have been discarded by drug users and might therefore cause AIDS. The risk of hepatitis B and C is much greater than that of AIDS, but all are unlikely.[5] The current advice is to offer an accelerated course of hepatitis B vaccine if there is thought to be a high risk. It is probably sensible to refer such children to the nearest A&E department, where advice can be offered on testing for HIV and post-exposure prophylaxis (PEP) with multiple agents. This probably needs to be given within 1 hour of exposure to be most effective, but can be given up to 2 weeks after the injury. If PEP is to be given, the advice of a paediatrician experienced in HIV should be sought.

Visits to farms and zoos

These are a potential source of infectious diseases, especially gastrointestinal infections, and accidents are also a hazard, but simple precautions can increase safety. It is undesirable and unnecessary to prevent children from handling the animals, but they should be under close supervision. Food and drink should not be consumed in close proximity to animals and the children *must* wash their hands first. The Health and Safety Executive has produced advice on farm visits for farmers and teachers.[6]

Preventing infections in nurseries and primary schools

Skin diseases, infestations, diarrhoeal illnesses, hepatitis A, congenital cytomegalovirus infections and meningitis may worry parents. Many areas have guidelines to minimise the risk of infection. These may be obtained from the community paediatrician or department of public health medicine. The Department for Education and Employment offers guidance on infection control in schools and nurseries.[7] This includes whether, and how long, children should remain away from school if they have an infectious disease. Once a child is well and non-infectious they should be allowed to return; however, they should not return early as they may infect others and cause unnecessary disruption.*

---

* At the time of writing, this advice is being revised. The updated guidance will be available on the HPA (www.hpa.org.uk/) and RCPCH (www.rcpch.ac.uk/) web sites.

Food hygiene and prevention of gastroenteritits

The incidence of gastroenteritis could be reduced by better food hygiene in the home. The health visitor may be able to provide the appropriate health education:

- All carers should wash their hands with soap:
  — before breastfeeding;
  — after using the toilet;
  — after changing the nappies of other infants or wiping toddlers' bottoms;
  — after handling raw meat, poultry or eggs.
- Raw meat, *particularly poultry*, often carries bacteria, so advise that:
  — such foods should be prepared on a separate surface if possible OR the surface should be cleaned, preferably with bleach, before preparing other foods which are not going to be cooked;
  — raw foods, *particularly poultry*, should be stored at the bottom of the fridge, and covered; cooked foods should be at the top;
  — eggs should be well cooked;
  — poultry must be well cooked; (i.e. not bloody in the middle).
- Unpasteurised milk should NOT be given to babies or young children.
- Toilet handles and taps are a potential source of infection, particularly in day nurseries or large households; they should be wiped with a cloth soaked in diluted bleach.
- Barbecues are a particular hazard: burgers must be well cooked; when preparing and handling food beware of using the same implements for raw and cooked meat.

Foreign travel*

Ideally, preparations for travel abroad should be made well in advance so that any immunisations can be performed. Apart from travel immunisations, all routine immunisations should be up to date. Where appropriate, malaria prophylaxis should be arranged. This is as important for babies as it is for older individuals. Depending on the destination, extra care will need to be taken with the care of food and fluids. A common misunderstanding is that bottled water is sterile. This cannot be assumed to be so and all water used for making up formula feeds should be boiled and allowed to cool.

INFECTIOUS DISEASES: IMPORTANT TOPICS FOR PRIMARY CARE STAFF

Children die or suffer avoidable damage each year because healthcare staff forget that infections can still kill. This section highlights some potentially lethal conditions that are uncommon in the experience of the individual GP, yet need prompt recognition and referral.

---

* The National Travel Health Network and Centre (NaTHNaC) has useful and up-to-date information on immunisation requirements and anti-malarial precautions for individual countries as well as other aspects of travel health (www.nathnac.org/index.htm). Prescribing details for vaccines for travel should be obtained from *Immunisation Against Infectious Disease* (Department of Health) (www.dh.gov.uk/en/Publichealth/Healthprotection/Immunisation/Greenbook/index.htm) and for anti-malarial prophylaxis from the British National Formulary for Children (available at http://bnfc.org/bnfc/ or via www.library.nhs.uk). *See* also www.hpa.org.uk/publications/2006/Malaria/guidelines.htm?submit=Accept

Recognising the sick baby

Parents often notice that there is something wrong with their baby, based on a change in behaviour, but they may not be able to put this into words. NICE has produced a guideline on the management of fever in the child under 5 years.[8] To assess fever, health professionals should only use an electronic or chemical dot thermometer in the axilla or an infra-red tympanic thermometer. Any child under 3 months old with a fever ≥38°C should be referred to hospital for further assessment. On the basis of their symptoms and signs, older children can be designated a risk category on a 'traffic light system' and managed accordingly. An important part of this assessment is the measurement of capillary refill time.

Antipyretic medication should be used to make a child feel comfortable, not in the expectation that it will prevent a febrile convulsion. Either ibuprofen or paracetamol can be used to reduce a fever but, as a routine, only one should be used at a time. Tepid sponging is not recommended. Regular fluids should be offered.

Respiratory infections

These are extremely common. Simple preventative measures that can be applied by all parents include:

- washing hands thoroughly with soap and warm water and drying them thoroughly;
- washing hands thoroughly before and after touching the baby, and asking family and visitors to do the same;
- trying to keep individuals who have a cold or fever, colds and runny noses away from the baby;
- making sure the baby is not exposed to smoking.

Febrile convulsions

This topic is discussed on page 272.

A febrile convulsion is a convulsion occurring in infancy or childhood, usually between eight months and five years of age, associated with fever but without evidence of an intracranial infection or cause. They can occur as a result of any infection causing a pyrexia, or less commonly after a pyrexia due to a vaccination.

Early diagnosis of meningococcal disease[9]

Since the 1999 introduction of a conjugate vaccine against serogroup C, the number of cases of invasive meningococcal disease has fallen by 50%, and in 2007, for the first time, there were no deaths in children from meningococcal C disease. However, in the absence of a vaccination against meningococcus B, meningococcal disease, in general, is still a significant cause of mortality, which can be reduced by improved early treatment. Any child with a short history of a fever and a purpuric rash should be given intramuscular penicillin at once and transferred to hospital as an emergency. The presence or absence of classical signs of meningitis is irrelevant. The risk of anaphylaxis is tiny compared with the dangers of the disease. Crystapen® (benzylpenicillin) is stable over several years and should be kept in the emergency bag. The dose is 300 mg (1/2 m unit) for infants under 1 year; 600 mg for children aged 1–10 years.

In some children, meningococcal disease is heralded by a transient rash early in the illness, which is maculopapular and not purpuric. Unexplained limb pain may also occur. Children with an isolated petechial rash, but who are otherwise well, present a problem for parents and professionals, as this can – but usually does not – indicate early meningococcal disease. As a generalisation, when the rash is on the upper part of the body (above the nipple line), it is less likely to be associated with serious infection. It is important to avoid giving unnecessary treatment, but if there is any doubt, the child should be reviewed after a few hours.

Urinary tract infection

A urinary tract infection (UTI) in older children usually presents either with frequency and pain or as an ill child with a high fever, abdominal and/or loin pain. Diagnosis is much more difficult in the first year of life, but is also more important because of the potential to develop invasive or systemic illness and renal scars. Consider the diagnosis in any unwell infant, particularly with a temperature over 40°C, whether or not you can identify symptoms related to the urinary tract. Unless you can find some other unequivocal source of the infection (beware of a slightly red throat or ears) it is important to get a urine specimen, preferably before starting antibiotics; a blood count and blood culture may also be advised. It can be very difficult to get an adequate urine specimen in the home or in most health centres, so optimum management of the unwell infant with unexplained high fever may require a visit to the hospital emergency department. Features can be non-specific but include:

▶ any baby under 4 weeks old with a fever;
▶ any child over 4 weeks old with a fever and at least one of the following:
  — vomiting;
  — poor feeding;
  — lethargy;
  — irritability;
  — abdominal pain or tenderness;
  — urinary frequency or dysuria;
  — haematuria.

A recent review of how best to make a diagnosis of UTI in a child under 5 found that a clean voided midstream urine sample had similar accuracy to suprapubic aspiration samples when cultured, with the advantage of being a non-invasive collection method that can be used in the GP's surgery. There was less evidence for the reliability of other methods such as urine pads. A dipstick test for leucocyte esterase (LE) and nitrite is useful in guiding immediate management, but does not replace culture in making a definitive diagnosis. NICE recently produced guidance for the management of infants and children under 16 years old with a clinically possible UTI:[10]

▶ in children under 3 years old, a specimen should be collected and antibiotic treatment started;
▶ in children of 3 and over, a specimen should be collected and immediate treatment is dependent on the result of dipstick testing for nitrite and LE;
▶ nitrite and LE positive: UTI highly likely, start antibiotic treatment;
▶ nitrite positive and LE negative: UTI probable, start antibiotic treatment;
▶ nitrite negative and LE positive: may be a UTI, treatment should depend on clinical state;
▶ nitrite and LE negative: UTI excluded, antibiotics unnecessary.

Tuberculosis

Over the years, tuberculosis (TB) has become much less common in the White population, such that a policy of immunising all school age children at 12–14 years old was no longer appropriate. In 2005, this immunisation policy in the UK changed and the universal schools programme ceased. Instead, the vaccination programme is now targeted at people who are at relatively high risk. This includes:

▶ all infants born in areas where the incidence of TB is ≥40 per 1000 total population;*
▶ anyone who is going to spend, or has spent, more than 3 months in a country where the incidence of TB is ≥40 per 1000 total population;
▶ anyone under 16 years old whose parents or grandparents were born in a country where the incidence of TB is ≥40 per 1000 total population;
▶ close contacts of a case of pulmonary TB.

In young children, TB may present with TB meningitis, which often causes severe brain damage if the child survives. There have been many cases of TB meningitis that can be traced to an adult who was not noticed to be unwell. TB occurs in persons of all races and ages; it is not confined to people from the Indian sub-continent or Africa or the stereotype of the homeless alcoholic. It is common in some European countries. Energetic, urgent contact tracing is the most important means of controlling TB (more important than BCG) and is mandatory whenever a person is found to have TB. A child with TB is rarely a significant risk to other people, but contact tracing is equally vital to discover the source of the infection before more people are infected. Although this is not primarily the responsibility of the general practitioner, standards of follow-up vary. Therefore, it is important to ensure that patients get optimum management: check that the index case has been notified; that the contact tracer has visited all families exposed to the infected person; and that agreed guidelines have been followed.

Infective diarrhoea

Diarrhoea and vomiting have many causes, not all of them infectious. The management of diarrhoea and gastroenteritis is discussed on page 119.

Kawasaki disease

This infection is not rare and is easily mistaken for measles. Saliva antibody testing shows that, in the absence of an outbreak, only a small minority of suspected cases of measles actually have measles. So whenever measles is considered, it is important to also think of other conditions, such as 'slapped cheek syndrome' (parvovirus) and drug reactions. With Kawasaki disease, the child is *extremely* miserable. The diagnosis should be considered in any child with fever for more than 5 days and four of the following:

▶ bilateral conjunctival injection;
▶ changes in mucous membranes of the upper respiratory tract (e.g. injected pharynx, dry cracked lips or strawberry tongue);

---

* For a list of such countries, *see* www.hpa.org.uk/web/HPAweb&HPAwebStandard/HPAweb_C/1195733758290.

- changes in the peripheral extremities (e.g. oedema, erythema or desquamation);
- polymorphous rash;
- cervical lymphadenopathy.

Early identification and referral are vital because of the risk of coronary artery aneurysms, the chances of which can be reduced by appropriate management.

Encephalitis and encephalopathy

The important features are changes in behaviour and consciousness. Sometimes these can be quite subtle and are mistaken for the child being uncooperative or aggressive. Any child with such complaints should be seen promptly. Deterioration can be rapid and the child should be admitted without hesitation.

Head lice

Head lice cause little serious morbidity, but take up a lot of time. There are many myths surrounding their spread. They do not favour dirty hair and they are not spread exclusively at school; in fact, intra-familial spread is common as close contact is necessary. Treatment is controversial and falls into two categories: chemical treatments (organophosphates, pyrethroids, carbamate and dimeticone), and mechanical treatments. Although there is no evidence to suggest it is a problem, many parents worry about the potential for chemical treatments to cause toxic effects and, in the case of organophosphates, environmental damage. A more real concern is the development of resistance to such treatments. Dimeticone has a physical mode of action and resistance is less likely. Mechanical treatments such as 'bug busting' do not have these problems and are probably at least as effective.[11]

Croup

Traditionally, it has been advised that croup should be treated with humidification; however, there is no evidence that it is beneficial in mild croup, and indeed, it may be harmful as some commercial humidifiers harbour pathogens. In the home setting, a steaming kettle has traditionally been used, but there is the risk of scalds. A single dose of dexamethasone (0.15 mg/kg) in mild to moderate croup is effective. Prednisolone is not as effective. Nebulised epinephrine is also useful, but is usually reserved for more severe cases, and children may relapse quite quickly after it is stopped.

REFERENCES

1 www.dh.gov.uk/en/Publichealth/Healthprotection/Immunisation/Greenbook/dh_4097254
   See also http://80.168.38.66/article.php?id=401
2 www.immunisation.nhs.uk
3 www.resus.org.uk/siteindx.htm
4 www.portal.nelm.nhs.uk/PGD/default.aspx
5 Papenburg J, Blais D, Moore D, *et al.* Pediatric injuries from needles discarded in the community: epidemiology and risk of seroconversion. *Pediatrics.* 2008; **122**(2): e487–92.
6 Advice on visits to farms and zoos: www.hse.gov.uk/pubns/ais23.pdf
7 www.wiredforhealth.gov.uk/PDF/Guidance_on_infection_control_web_poster_April_2006.pdf
8 National Institute for Health and Clinical Excellence. *Feverish Illness in Young Children:*

NICE Guideline 47. London: NIHCE; 2007. Available at: www.nice.org.uk/guidance/CG47.

9 Thompson MJ, Ninis N, Perera R, *et al.* Clinical recognition of meningococcal disease in children and adolescents. *Lancet.* 2006; **367**(9508): 397–403. *See* also Wells LC, Smith JC, Weston VC, *et al.* The child with a non-blanching rash: how likely is meningococcal disease? *Arch Dis Child.* 2001; **85**(3): 218–22. *See* also Downes AJ, Crossland DS, Mellon AF. Prevalence and distribution of petechiae in well babies. *Arch Dis Child.* 2002; **86**(4): 291–2.

10 National Institute for Health and Clinical Excellence. *Urinary Tract Infection in Children: NICE Guideline 54.* London: NIHCE; 2007. Available at: www.nice.org.uk/guidance/CG54.

11 www.phmeg.org.uk/Documents/Headlice/HeadLiceStaffordRpt_2008.pdf *See* also www.chc.org.

CHAPTER 9

Screening, surveillance, monitoring and assessment

EARLY DETECTION: DOES IT MATTER?

Early identification and treatment dramatically improve outcome in some situations; for example, in children with congenital cataract or with severe or profound congenital hearing impairment. Early detection of abnormal development and disabling conditions is important even when no specific medical intervention is available, for a number of reasons:

- Some problems are mainly or entirely due to the child's social circumstances; intervention may change his pattern of development and perhaps protect him from neglect or abuse.
- Parents value early diagnosis. This is partly because it is easier to come to terms with a serious problem in a young baby than in an older child who has already acquired a personality and a shared life with the parents. It is not a kindness to keep parents in ignorance or leave them to find out for themselves that their child has a serious disorder or disease.
- Parents are generally disappointed and feel let down if the healthcare system fails to identify a problem, whether or not early diagnosis was a reasonable expectation from a professional point of view.
- Early diagnosis allows parents plenty of time to access other services and to discuss educational and social implications of the child's condition.

▶ An early diagnosis may allow genetic investigation and counselling, thus giving the parents choices as to whether they wish to have another child and if so, whether they would want antenatal diagnosis if available.

Critical and sensitive periods

Early intervention is worthwhile for all disabling conditions in childhood (for the reasons outlined above), but in some situations it is crucial because of critical or sensitive periods in brain development.

The term 'critical period' refers to a limited period of time during which the brain is primed to develop in response to appropriate stimuli. The best-known example in human infants is vision: if the brain does not receive a clear image from the eye in the early months of life (e.g. due to congenital cataract) the visual cortex does not develop normally and vision is permanently impaired even if the cataract is subsequently successfully treated.

A 'sensitive period' is a period of time when the brain is most ready to learn, but learning can take place outside this period even though it may be less efficient and more difficult. For example, a child who has suffered gross deprivation and neglect from birth, as may occur in an orphanage, can make a good recovery if adopted, but the older the child, the outcome is less good. Cochlear implants for children with profound deafness give the best results in terms of speech and language development if they are fitted in early childhood.

EARLY DETECTION, ASSESSMENT AND DIAGNOSIS

There are several ways in which early detection can be achieved:

▶ careful examination of all neonates and a repeat examination at 6–8 weeks of age; these should identify a large proportion of children with congenital disorders and syndromes;
▶ specific screening procedures: antenatal screens, newborn blood spot tests for metabolic disorders and haemoglobinopathies, hearing impairment, developmental dysplasia of the hip;
▶ specialist follow-up is important for high risk babies and children (e.g. those at risk of brain injury due to extremely low birth weight, severe intra-partum asphyxia, periventricular haemorrhage or meningitis); many of the more severe disabling conditions, such as cerebral palsy, are identified in this way;
▶ parents and others who are in regular contact with young children are often the first to suspect a problem; early detection often relies on a prompt and appropriate professional response to such concerns.

TERMINOLOGY

Screening

The term 'screening' refers to 'the examination of a whole population of apparently healthy children, using simple tests to distinguish those who probably have a condition from those who probably do not, so that the outcome can be improved by treating the condition before it produces obvious symptoms or signs'.[1] The aim of a screening programme is to examine all the children at risk. This usually means the entire population of children of a particular age group, but in some cases a programme may focus on a sub-population at particular risk; for example, ophthalmic examination of very low birth weight infants to detect retinopathy of prematurity. The role of screening tests in child health is to detect conditions that might otherwise be overlooked by both parent and professional unless a specific search is undertaken.

Although screening is an attractive concept, it is difficult to set up and run a screening programme, and maintaining high standards is expensive in professional time. With most screening tests, some cases are missed (false negatives) and some children are incorrectly identified as possibly abnormal (false positives). Both can cause anger and distress in the parents. For these reasons, there are now stringent UK standards for screening programmes.[2]

As a general rule, screening is most effective for conditions that can be identified by an objective laboratory test (such as phenylketonuria (PKU), hypothyroidism and haemoglobin disorders) and/or can be targeted at a 'captive audience' such as newborn infants (*see* Chapter 10, page 217 onwards). It works less well for conditions identified by a clinical examination procedure in which observer variability and the ease or difficulty in examining the child play a part (such as congenital dislocation of the hip or cardiac disorders). Screening works poorly for developmental difficulties such as speech and language problems or behaviour problems, such as aggression or hyperactivity.

Child health surveillance

Child health surveillance refers to a programme of regular age-related reviews that incorporate screening tests and other means of identifying problems. It is usually combined with a variety of preventive measures, such as immunisation (*see* page 153 onwards) and health education.

Opportunistic detection and screening

The term 'opportunistic detection' is sometimes used to describe the use of parent-initiated contacts between child and professional (e.g. for minor illness) to evaluate aspects of the child's health and development; these are in addition to those that the parent attended. The term 'opportunistic screening' should be reserved for situations where a formal screening test has not been performed at the usual time and is carried out when the child is seen for some other reason.

Monitoring

By monitoring we mean an activity undertaken to varying degrees by most parents and, increasingly, by competent crèche, early years and pre-school staff. It involves observing a child's development and progress over time, relating this to knowledge of and data on the range of normality and deciding whether any expert assessment or intervention is needed.

Assessment

Assessment is undertaken when concern is expressed by parents or professionals about a child in order to determine if there is a problem and define its nature and severity.

Diagnosis

Diagnosis usually means identifying the cause(s) of the problem or, if that is not possible, describing it in terms of a recognised classification system. In most cases, primary care staff refer children to specialists when there are concerns, but in some circumstances it is helpful to undertake some initial assessment before referral.

SCREENING TESTS FOR CHILDREN UNDER 5: THE NATIONAL PROGRAMME

Only a small number of procedures meet the UK criteria for screening;[2] these are summarised in Box 9.1. The conditions detected by the newborn blood spot programme are uncommon and a positive screening test normally results in direct referral to a paediatrician. The issues raised by these programmes can be complicated and confusing for parents; for example, in some cases the screening tests identify a child who is carrying just one copy of a gene for a disorder. Such a child will be unaffected by the condition, but in adult life will be at risk of having an affected child if they partner another carrier.

BOX 9.1 Screening tests recommended by the UK National Screening Committee[2]

Target disorder	Birth prevalence	Comments
Screening tests using newborn blood spot at 5–8 days		
PKU	1:10 000	PKU causes brain damage with learning difficulties and fits if not diagnosed; without screening, damage is already irreversible by the time the diagnosis is apparent clinically. Treatment is by specialised diet
Hypothyroidism	1:3000	Severe cases of congenital hypothyroidism can be recognised clinically ('cretinism') but often the diagnosis is not obvious; delayed diagnosis causes learning difficulties. The treatment is thyroxine replacement therapy
CF*	1:2500	The benefits of early diagnosis by screening are a reduction in lung damage and better growth. Without screening, children may have suffered months of ill health, unexplained chest infections and poor weight gain. The screening procedure is not straightforward as there are many genetic variants, some of which are less severe and have a better prognosis than the common form. Management of CF includes control of infection by physiotherapy and antibiotics and dietary measures

(cont.)

Target disorder	Birth prevalence	Comments
Haemoglobin disorders (sickle cell disease and variants)	1:2400	Early diagnosis of sickle cell disease reduces early morbidity and mortality. Management includes prophylaxis for pneumococcal infections and parent education about how to identify and respond to complications
MCADD*	1:10 000	MCADD can cause sudden catastrophic metabolic disturbance that may be fatal. It is often triggered by apparently minor infections, particularly if they result in the child not eating. Early diagnosis enables parents to respond appropriately to any such illnesses and is expected to reduce morbidity and mortality

Screening tests for impaired hearing and vision

Congenital hearing impairment in infancy	1:1000	Universal newborn hearing screening is now the preferred approach
Late onset and acquired hearing impairment in early childhood	1:1000 (prevalence at school entry)	School entry hearing test
Cataract in newborn and at 6–8 weeks	2–3:10 000	Red reflex when viewed through ophthalmoscope
Refractive error and amblyopia at age 4–5	Between 3% and 7% of all children	Orthoptist examination – described in Appendix 2

Screening tests that rely on clinical examination

Congenital heart disease in newborn and at 6–8 weeks	6–7:1000	Examination of cardiovascular system
Developmental dysplasia of the hip in newborn and at 6–8 weeks	Dislocation of the hip: 1.3:1000	Check for risk factors; inspection and Ortolani-Barlow manoeuvre: ultrasound for high risk groups.
Undescended testes in newborn and at 6–8 weeks	10:1000 at 6–8 weeks	Examination to check position of testes
Growth disorders	Many causes (see text)	Height and weight at school entry

CF = cystic fibrosis; **MCADD** = medium chain acyl CoA dehydrogenase deficiency; **PKU** = phenylketonuria.

* At the time of going to press, this screening test is not yet universally available, but roll-out is expected to be complete by 2009.

The role of primary care staff is to explain what the programme aims to do and why, when the blood spot test is carried out; and, in the event of a positive result, to support the parents; to ensure, if necessary, that their path through specialist services is as smooth as possible and to assist them to obtain accurate and up-to-date answers to their questions from their specialist services or the internet (*see* page 33 in Chapter 2 for advice on how to make the best use of internet resources).

Early detection of hearing and visual impairment is an important issue for primary care staff and is therefore discussed in detail. The screening procedures are imperfect; furthermore, new problems can arise at any time and are not always obvious to parents or professionals, unless a high index of suspicion is maintained at all times.

EARLY DETECTION OF HEARING IMPAIRMENT

There are two kinds of deafness:

1 **Sensorineural** or **nerve** deafness is caused by a defect in the cochlea, auditory nerve or its central connections. It affects 1–2:1000 children. It varies in severity from mild to profound.
2 **Conductive** hearing loss is very common in pre-school children. It is usually caused by external or middle ear problems; in children this is most commonly otitis media with effusion (OME), commonly known as glue ear. The term secretory otitis media (SOM) is also used, but can be confused with suppurative otitis media. The hearing loss is usually mild and transient, but occasionally it can be sufficiently persistent and severe to affect speech and language development and behaviour.

NB: Impaired or abnormal hearing responses can also occur in infants and children with impaired vision, learning disability or autism.

Significance of congenital deafness

Deafness is a hidden disability. Even a profound hearing loss may not be suspected by parents until it becomes apparent that the child is not learning to talk. Babies use visual information and communicate by body movements and facial expressions, thus disguising the impact of a hearing problem.

Children with severe congenital deafness are likely to have seriously impaired speech and verbal comprehension which, in turn, affects their educational progress, employment prospects and mental health. Early identification and intervention can substantially improve the outlook, particularly if implemented within the first 6 months of life; therefore screening programmes are necessary. The essence of early intervention is to ensure good language development. It does not seem to matter very much, from a neuro-developmental point of view, whether the first language relies on signing or on speech – the crucial issue is the acquisition of a structured language. For those severely or profoundly deaf infants who do not make good progress even with the best hearing aids and teaching, cochlear implants can dramatically transform the outlook.

Early identification

Nearly half of all newborns found to have a hearing loss have one or more risk factors (*see* Box 9.2) but a 'targeted' programme that focused only on high risk babies was found to be inefficient. A universal screening programme (i.e. one that tests all newborns for hearing loss) has now been adopted, because it is possible to find most cases, achieve high coverage and initiate intervention well before 6 months of age. The programme depends not only on good screening procedures, but also on a seamless referral pathway to an audiology service that can identify, investigate and manage very young babies with hearing loss in partnership with clinical geneticists, audiological physicians, paediatricians, ENT surgeons and educational and social services.

It is essential to maintain vigilance and to arrange for hearing assessment at any age whenever there is doubt about the child's hearing or ability to understand speech, because the newborn screening service will miss some cases. Some types of congenital hearing loss are not present at birth and evolve during the first months or years of life and some cases are acquired (e.g. following meningitis or viral illnesses). Children who have had acute bacterial meningitis or meningococcal septicaemia should have a hearing test very soon after recovery. Parents should be reminded, directly or via the Personal Child Health Record, that the child's hearing should be re-checked if they ever have any worries about it.

Infants and children at high risk of persistent conductive hearing loss or 'glue ear' should be checked regularly, that is, those with Down, Turner or Williams syndromes, cleft palate (even after repair), Pierre Robin sequence and other craniofacial malformations. Children found to have serious developmental problems, such as cerebral palsy, learning disability or visual loss should routinely be referred for full hearing assessment as these conditions are often associated with hearing loss.

All school entrants should have an audiometric test (often the 'sweep' test), and/or a speech discrimination test, according to local policy. Impedance testing is a useful tool for assessing middle ear function (*see* Appendix 1) but should not be used as a screening procedure.

Children with hearing loss

The identification and follow-up of a child with hearing loss is the responsibility of the audiology service, which is usually organised in three or four tiers:

1 primary screening;
2 community referral or second tier clinics: the precise role varies from place to place; some are fully staffed and equipped, and provide a wide range of expert services, whereas others act only as a filter and refer on any child needing further investigation or treatment;
3 consultant (third tier) clinics: these are usually based in a hospital; at district level they provide diagnostic services and support early intervention programmes;
4 regional or supra-regional centres providing specialist audio-vestibular assessment, genetic services, cochlear implantation and other specialised services; services needed for children with impaired hearing are listed on page 344.

BOX 9.2 What primary care staff should know about newborn hearing screening

Targeted screening programmes rely on risk factors for hearing loss in infancy

- Infants requiring intensive care (not merely special care) for more than 48 hours; this includes those with prematurity (gestation less than 33 weeks at birth or weight less than 1500 g), severe asphyxia or respiratory depression at birth, prolonged ventilation, meningitis, jaundice needing exchange transfusion, high levels of aminoglycosides.
- Family history of a hearing loss compatible with genetic transmission (include infants where the family history of a hearing loss is attributed to some other factor unless this is unequivocal; parents often falsely attribute the defect to measles, head injury, etc.).
- Chromosome defects and malformation syndromes; any infant with another major defect, particularly those that involve the head, face and neck.
- Children with stigmata/conditions known to be associated with hearing loss; white forelock, fetal alcohol syndrome, etc.
- Documented or suspected rubella, cytomegalovirus or other congenital infections in pregnancy.
- Consanguinity is associated with a small increase in risk.

The universal newborn hearing screening programme (NHSP)[3]

- The UK universal newborn hearing screening programme utilises two tests: automated otoacoustic emissions AOAE ('cochlear echo') and automated auditory brainstem response (AABR). These techniques require sophisticated equipment, but have been automated for screening purposes so that they can be conducted by trained lay staff.
- The first screen uses the AOAE technique and is usually done before the baby leaves hospital; babies who do not have a clear response in both ears (often due to fluid in the middle ear or a noisy environment) are re-tested. If there is still doubt, the next step is AABR.
- Both ears are tested, but although the main aim is to identify bilateral hearing loss of moderate or worse severity, unilateral hearing loss may also be identified. The policy for managing these babies is still evolving.
- Very few cases are 'missed' though some false positives are unavoidable. It is important to confirm that hearing is normal or to give the parents a definite diagnosis as soon as possible, in order to minimise anxiety. Staff need to understand their local protocols so that they can support parents whose baby needs more than one test.*
- Sedation is not needed in early infancy. It is expected that infants will undergo diagnostic audiological tests before 8 weeks of age when they can be carried out under natural sleep.
- Parents are given a leaflet after the newborn screen has been completed, explaining how they can identify any hearing problems that occur later on in infancy or early childhood.

---

* Helpful advice for parents, including a video, can be found at http://hearing.screening.nhs.uk/sitemap.php

How screening works
The screen is done in hospital before discharge, or in a community clinic (within 6 weeks) depending on local service provisions. There are different protocols for the well baby with no risks and those in intensive care. As for any screening test, parental consent is required. It is a safe, painless procedure that takes a few minutes. AOAEs use an ear probe, AABR uses three small sensors on the skin and an earphone, while the baby is quiet or during sleep. Screening may not be possible if the baby is restless or there is debris in the ear.

IDENTIFICATION OF VISION DEFECTS
Serious defects of vision
These can be defined as defects that affect the child's vision to the extent that he has difficulty in coping with normal schooling without some form of additional assistance. It corresponds very roughly to a corrected vision of 6/18 or worse (i.e. the best vision obtainable when wearing correct glasses). Other factors also determine the extent to which a particular defect causes a disability; for instance, field defects, photophobia and intelligence. Serious vision defects are uncommon; the incidence is around 4 children per 10 000. However, this figure does not include all the children with cortical vision defects (*see* page 185), which means it has been underestimated. The general practitioner may see only one new case of a congenital disabling vision defect in his professional lifetime, and a consultant ophthalmologist at a district general hospital may see only one or two cases per year.

Early diagnosis of serious vision defects is important for several reasons:

 ▶ some conditions need urgent investigation and treatment (e.g. retinoblastoma, cataract and glaucoma);
 ▶ eye defects are often accompanied by abnormalities in other organs and therefore early paediatric assessment is advisable;
 ▶ many eye diseases are genetic in origin and early counselling should be offered so that parents can make a choice and, if they wish, avoid the birth of a second affected child;
 ▶ severe visual defects affect all areas of development and may also result in secondary behavioural and emotional disturbances, which can often be prevented by appropriate management.

Minor vision problems
These are very common; between 5% and 10% of children have a squint, a refractive error, or both at some time in childhood. These terms are defined and explained in Box 9.3. Early diagnosis of minor vision problems is important because:

 ▶ A squint
   — may be a sign of serious ocular or neurological disease;
   — predisposes to the development of amblyopia.
 ▶ A refractive error
   — causes impaired visual acuity;
   — may predispose to the development of amblyopia.

BOX 9.3 Terminology used in vision screening

Definitions:

- **Partial sight**: some residual vision that can be used for education or work.
- **Blind**: the person can only use methods for education or work which do not require the use of any vision.
- An **ocular defect**: poor vision due to a defect of the eye itself or of the optic nerve.
- A **cortical defect**: the abnormality lies in the brain rather than in the eye. Cortical vision defects are often associated with other problems, such as cerebral palsy or learning difficulties (mental handicap).
- **Refractive error**: the eye is not functioning as a perfect optical system; the refracting structures of the eye, the lens and cornea, do not bring rays of light to a perfect focus on the retina. It is measured in terms of the correcting lens which must be placed in front of the eye in order to produce a sharp image on the retina.
- **Squint**: the visual axis of one eye is not directed to the same point as the visual axis of the other eye. A **pseudosquint** is the illusory appearance of a squint created by broad epicanthic folds. Pseudosquint and true squint can co-exist. A **manifest squint** is one which is constantly present. A **latent squint** is only evident under conditions of stress such as fatigue, illness or provocative testing. Manifest squints are cosmetically unattractive and predispose to the development of amblyopia, but latent squints are generally of less significance. An **alternating squint** is one in which the child fixates with either eye alternately. It is less likely to lead to amblyopia. **NB**: Some books on childcare still state that a squint can be normal up to the age of 6 months. This is misleading; some babies may have a transient loss of conjugate gaze when tracking a close moving object, but a **permanent squint in one eye is never normal.**
- **Ptosis**: drooping of the upper eyelid. It may be unilateral or bilateral. If it is severe enough to occlude the pupil it may cause amblyopia, otherwise its main significance is cosmetic and an occasional association with other paediatric disorders.
- **Visual acuity**: a measure of the subject's ability to discriminate visual stimuli. It normally requires some form of cooperation or behavioural response from the subject. The **Snellen letter charts** are the recognised method of ascertaining and recording visual acuity. The standard test is done at a distance of 6 metres between subject and chart. The result is given as a pseudo-fraction. Thus 6/6 means that the person can read at 6 metres the same as the average person; 6/12 means that the subject can read only at 6 metres the letters that the average person can read at 12 metres. Snellen charts should now be replaced by **LogMAR** charts, which, because of the design, are better at picking up visual impairment (0.2 on a LogMAR chart is roughly equivalent to 6/9 on a Snellen-based linear chart).When the subject is too young or disabled to cooperate, specialised techniques are needed to measure visual acuity.
- **Amblyopia**: a condition in which vision is impaired even when any refractive error has been corrected, in spite of there being no disease of the eye or visual pathways. It can be caused by any condition which prevents a clear image from reaching the retina; for instance, refractive error, particularly when there is a difference between the two eyes (anisometropia – *see* below), squint or severe ptosis. It occurs only during the period of brain maturation and is therefore only likely to develop in the

first 7 or 8 years of life. Amblyopia impairs the development of 3-D vision, which may cause a minor degree of disability in some sports. If it is severe, the person has effectively only one eye, and will be barred from some careers, such as the Armed Forces, and becomes seriously disabled if so unfortunate as to lose the other eye through disease or accident. A person who has good 3-D vision can be presumed to have no amblyopia and is unlikely to have a significant squint or refractive error.

- **Impaired colour vision**: much more common in boys than girls. Screening in the pre-school age group and among school entrants is not currently recommended (though its identification in older children may be useful as it can affect career choices).

Types of refractive error

- **Short and long sight** can be measured with a retinoscope. Most eyes have a slight degree of long- or short-sightedness, but the decision as to whether a person has a *significant* degree of refractive error depends on the *visual acuity* measurement.
- In **myopia** or short-sightedness, the subject has difficulty in seeing objects at a distance. Myopia is very uncommon in pre-school children, but the incidence rises steadily throughout the school years. Severe myopia is a disability both in sport and in classroom work, but there is little evidence that minor degrees of myopia cause any significant inconvenience.
- In **hypermetropia** or long-sightedness, distant objects are perceived clearly, but the subject has difficulty in seeing close objects. Children respond to this by increasing accommodation (i.e. the ability to converge the eyes and change the shape of the lens), but sometimes this results in a squint. A deficiency in near visual acuity is therefore unlikely to be the presenting feature of hypermetropia in young people. It is usually discovered when the child presents with a squint (with or without amblyopia).
- **Astigmatism** means that there is a different degree of refraction in the horizontal and vertical axes of the eye and results in a distorted image.
- **Anisometropia** is the situation in which there is a significant difference in the refractions of the two eyes.

Early detection of vision defects

The eyes of all newborn babies and infants of 6–8 weeks old should be observed for their morphology and to check for opacities (e.g. cataracts) by observing the red reflex using an ophthalmoscope. These are the only recognised screening procedures for children under 4 years old. Although various methods of screening infants and children under 4 for refractive error, squint and amblyopia have been studied (*see* Appendix 2), none has as yet been found to meet the national criteria for screening tests. The current recommendation in England is for a vision screening examination of all children, either conducted or supervised by an orthoptist, between the fourth and fifth birthdays. The tests used are summarised in Appendix 2.

Staff should be alert to clues and signs suggestive of visual impairment, at any age (*see* pages 247 and 289). If a serious vision defect is suspected at any age, an immediate referral for expert examination is essential and every effort should be made to obtain an urgent appointment. In some places, a telephone call to a paediatrician may be the fastest route to obtaining this, and also ensures that the child has a complete physical examination. This is important because (i) eye disorders are often associated with other congenital problems; and (ii) abnormal visual behaviour can be the presenting feature of serious disease, more generalised developmental delay or learning disability syndromes.

The organisation of ophthalmic services for children varies according to locality. The routes of referral should be defined and the point of entry may be a consultant-led children's eye clinic, a community orthoptist, or an optometrist, according to local policy.

DEVELOPMENTAL AND BEHAVIOURAL PROBLEMS

Many parents have anxieties about the behaviour and development of their young children, though it is difficult to obtain objective estimates of prevalence because some problems presenting in the under-5 age group are permanent and potentially disabling (Box 9.4), while others are transient, ill-defined and often difficult to identify in the first few years of life. Behavioural and emotional difficulties are extremely common in the first few years of life.

BOX 9.4 Prevalence estimates for developmental problems

Condition	Pre-school prevalence
Autism	4 per 1000
Other autism spectrum disorders	8 per 1000
ADHD	20–50 per 1000
Speech and language problems	30–100 per 1000
Permanent hearing impairment	1.9 per 1000
Visual impairment (other than cortical)	3–4 per 10 000
Cerebral palsy	2.5 per 1000
Severe learning disability	3.7 per 1000
Duchenne muscular dystrophy	1 per 3000 boys

Child development

An understanding of how children develop is used to:

- reassure worried parents that a child is normal;
- identify possibly atypical or abnormal development;
- assess, monitor and interpret development when there are risk factors, such as prematurity, or concern about a child's progress;
- recognise situations that are detrimental or beneficial to a child's development and, where necessary:
  - explain such situations to other professionals (social workers, magistrates, judges or adoption agencies);
  - use age- and stage-appropriate language and concepts to interview children, involve them in decisions and explain treatments or illnesses.

The models of child development traditionally used by health professionals focus on the emergence of skills, such as walking. Modern accounts of child development integrate genetic factors and an understanding of how the brain develops in the early years, with the family, educational and economic environments in which the child grows up. They incorporate aspects of development that are less easily measured, such as attachment, self-regulation, theory of mind and acquisition of a moral sense or prosocial development (a term that encompasses various positive interactions with other people including helping, sharing, cooperating and comforting).

Accounts of the more easily observed aspects of child development are an essential tool for health professionals. Examples are listed in Box 9.5, and the Denver Developmental Screening Test is shown in Figure 9.1. The clinician needs to know what most children are likely to achieve by a given age ('**milestones**'), and when to worry ('**red flags**'). A milestone is the achievement of a readily identified skill. The average or median ages for key milestones are useful but, as children are all different, it is also important to know the approximate age range within which most children achieve each milestone. *See* page 194 for further discussion of the role of developmental screening tests.

Red flags are of several kinds:

1 Failure to reach milestones by a certain time:[4]
   ▶ most full-term babies smile in response to social overtures by 6 weeks; so;
   ▶ no smile in a full-term baby by 8 weeks is worrying and no smile by 10 weeks is an indication for referral;
   ▶ not walking by 18 months;
   ▶ unable to walk up stairs (five or more treads) unaided at age 3;
   ▶ unable to produce an intelligible spontaneous sentence of four or more words at age 3.

2 Persistence of behaviours that are normally transient and disappear; for example:
   ▶ casting: repeated throwing of objects onto the floor, which usually reaches a peak soon after the first birthday, declines thereafter and usually stops by 16–18 months (persistence of repeated casting after this age is unusual);
   ▶ the same applies to persistent mouthing of objects.

3 Marked discrepancies between different areas of development; for example:
   ▶ inability to speak or understand and respond to speech in a 2.5-year-old child who shows advanced development in other fields.

4 Abnormal motor or movement patterns; for example:
   ▶ an infant who feels very stiff or very floppy on handling;
   ▶ an infant under 1 year of age with a strong hand preference.

5 Abnormal behaviour; for example:
   ▶ a toddler who shows no interest in people.

6 Regression in development:
   ▶ loss or deterioration of a previously acquired skill; it is common for young children to stop doing something that they appeared to have learned a few weeks earlier, but deterioration in a wide range of skills is more worrying.

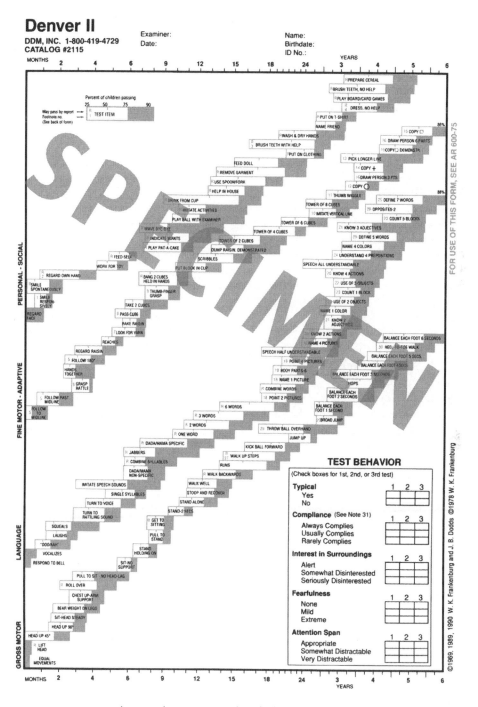

FIGURE 9.1 Denver Developmental Screening Test (DDST). The DDST provides a convenient summary of developmental progress and includes information about the *range* of ages at which abilities are usually acquired. It has been widely used and its strengths and weaknesses have been documented.[5] Reproduced by kind permission of Professor Frankenburg and Denver Developmental Materials Inc.

The early years educationists' viewpoint: competences, monitoring and teaching

Staff trained in health sciences often have a different view and understanding of early childhood problems from that of educationists. Health professionals use terms like 'delay' or 'deficit' in skill acquisition – terms that imply that the child's development may be abnormal. Educationists, in general, take for granted that rates and trajectories of development vary widely. They are less concerned about deficits and the categorisation or cause of disorders and are more interested in emerging competences and the ways in which these can be related to relevant teaching methods and the attainment of educational goals. They see these competences as being directly related to the kind of learning environment and activities offered both by parents and by early years educators.

In one important study[*] a cohort of children underwent developmental testing at 22 and 42 months and again at 10 years. Children who scored low on the tests at 22 and 42 months, but came from a high socio-economic background showed an improvement over time; whereas children whose early development was advanced, but came from a low socio-economic background experienced a decline over time. The gap widened so that by the age of 7 years the former group had overtaken the latter. These observations are probably partly explained by the greater learning opportunities experienced by the former group, with more exposure to language, books, and high-quality pre-school settings.

Day care settings (as defined on page 55), whether they are crèche facilities for babies, services for toddlers, or nursery school type facilities, need high-quality well-trained staff if they are to impact positively on child development. Leadership in day care will increasingly be provided by staff with the status of 'early years professional' (a graduate level qualification),[6] who can use developmental monitoring tools linked directly to the daily routine of activities and, because they use non-technical language and are based on daily observations, are readily shared with parents.

There are several aids to developmental monitoring; one popular example[7] builds on the 'Birth to Three' programme developed for Sure Start and the Early Years Foundation Stage and curriculum,[8] which set out goals for children up to age 5. These approaches recognise a hierarchy of competences that are acquired as the child gets older, so they provide invaluable guidance to early years educators and parents in their current format. However, they give little information that would help staff to identify the 'red flags' discussed in the previous section.

Early detection of developmental and behavioural problems

Some developmental and behavioural disorders are not obvious in the early years, so a proactive approach to early detection is desirable, aiming to ensure that special educational needs are identified before children start school. Autism spectrum disorders and speech and language disorders in particular can be difficult to identify (*see* pages 261–2). Although parents are often the first to suspect a problem, this is not always the case, for several reasons:

▶ In today's small nuclear families, many parents begin family life with little or

---

[*] *See* Feinstein L.: www.anzsog.edu.au/images/docs/forum/030000_How_early_can_we_predict_future_achievement_Feinstein.pdf

no experience of small children, nor do they always have such easy access to the wisdom of grandparents as their own parents would have done.

▶ Some are wary of professionals or find it hard to face the possibility of some serious problem.

▶ Parents' perceptions of normal development and acceptable behaviour – and therefore their use of child health services – vary widely according to their expectations of their children and of life in general. For example, parents living in deprived areas often do not recognise or worry about slow language development because they can only compare with the local population norm, which may be far below that of the population as a whole.[9]

▶ Parents who are under severe stress for any reason (*see* Chapter 5, page 86 onwards) have many other priorities and find it hard to focus on their child's development and learning.

▶ Both parents and professionals can be preoccupied with a child's behaviour and management problems, which sometimes make it more difficult to identify co-existing developmental delay.

For all these reasons, a universal child health programme – that is, one that is relevant to and accessible by all families – is important. There has been a long debate as to how such a service should be designed; should a modern child health service undertake a series of routine age-related contacts incorporating health, development and behaviour screening for every child under 5, as part of a child health programme?

There is widespread support for a universal service, but the emphasis, content and mode of delivery are changing, for two reasons: first, families do not all have the same needs; second, the evidence is growing that the development and behaviour patterns of all children – not just those with 'deficits' – benefit from optimal child rearing and early education opportunities and this calls for a shift of emphasis from screening (a 'deficit detection' model) to one with a greater emphasis on appropriate health promotion.

Parent–professional partnership: sharing and interpreting information

Responding promptly to parents' worries is an economic and effective method of early detection. Parents often sense that something is wrong with the child's development or health long before they can define exactly what it is. They watch their children playing at nursery and playgroup and discuss them with the staff; they talk to friends and neighbours; listen to grandparents; watch television programmes and read magazines (the media have done much to raise public awareness of disabilities in childhood). Developmental checklists often make use of parents' expertise about their own child[10] (*see* Box 9.5).

Many parents now like to monitor their child's progress themselves using information provided on the internet.* By the time parents bring a child to the doctor or health visitor with a concern about health, growth or development, they have thought about the suspected problem very carefully. It follows that if parents say something is wrong, you should assume that they are correct until proved otherwise. Parents should never be accused of being fussy, overanxious or neurotic!

Other people who deal with young children in the community are often the

---

* For example, www.babycentre.co.uk/. See also Williams N, Mughal S, Blair M. 'Is my child developing normally?' : a critical review of web-based resources for parents. *Dev Med Child Neurol.* 2008; **50**: 893–7.

first to raise concerns about a child, either with the parents or directly with health professionals, such as health visitors or community-based doctors, who visit their facilities. Playgroup leaders, foster parents, nursery staff and early years workers all acquire a substantial experience of what 'normal' children are like at different ages. This expertise can be enhanced by providing staff with appropriate further training, support and easy access to professional advice when they are in doubt, and with various aids and guides to normal development.

Parents should be encouraged to use health and early years professionals as a sounding board for vague anxieties and supporting them through their worries is important and useful. It is helpful to ask parents about any worries they may have, whenever the opportunity arises. One way of doing this is to use the 'Parents' Evaluation of Developmental Status' (PEDS)[11] which relies on asking the parents a series of questions (*see* Figure 9.2). PEDS should not be regarded as a screening test, but as a way of structuring conversations between parents, childcare staff and professionals about a child's development and progress.

Whatever method is used, there are some important caveats about discussing developmental and behavioural issues with parents:

▶ Open questions designed to elicit any worries are important, but should be followed by more precise questions; vague questions will produce vague answers.
▶ Parents are often objective and precise in their observations and rarely exaggerate, but they do *not* always understand the significance of what they see. For instance, they may describe the inability of a 3-year-old to understand simple instructions, but *not* realise that this is abnormal.
▶ When parents have difficulty in making or reporting their observations, it may be useful to ask them what the playgroup leader or nursery nurse thinks. People who spend their days working with a wide variety of children are often very astute in recognising atypical children as they can observe their development over a period of time.
▶ Parents are much better at telling you about **current** abilities than remembering past milestones, so you can ask when parents first became worried, but do not invest a lot of time in trying to establish exactly when a child first sat or walked. Ask the parents if they recorded milestones in the Personal Child Health Record.
▶ Some skills are easily described by parents or observed in the clinic; for example, walking, climbing steps or speaking. Some skills (e.g. verbal understanding) can be observed when the parent speaks to the child or the child is playing, but are harder for the layman to report accurately; and some skills can only be demonstrated by using a stimulus task, such as completing a puzzle, drawing or using building blocks. Check that the parent's description of what the child does is supported by observation. Watch the child and use what you see as a talking point with the parents.
▶ There are three important rules: (i) do not jump to conclusions on the basis of a single contact or brief observation period; (ii) do not over-interpret isolated delays in a developmental skill or 'failures' on a developmental task (look at the overall profile of development); and (iii) do not interpret reports, observations or data about development and behaviour without considering the various possible explanations, as summarised below.

PEDS RESPONSE FORM

Child's name: *Billy Morris*   Parent's Name: *Linda Morris*

Child's Birthday: 4/17/94   Child's Age: 3   Today's Date: 4/27/97

Please list any concerns about how your child's learning development and behaviour.

He's kind of quiet and doesn't say very much. Seems to prefer watching to interacting.

Do you have any concerns about how your child talks and makes speech sounds?

Circle one: No   Yes   (A little)   COMMENTS

As I said, I don't think he talks as well as he should for his age. Otherwise he's just loving, watches everything carefully. Figures things out quickly. Very bright.

Do you have any concerns about how your child understands what you say?

Circle one: (No)   Yes   A little   COMMENTS

Do you have any concerns about how your child uses his or her hands and fingers to do things?

Circle one: (No)   Yes   A little   COMMENTS

Do you have any concerns about how your child uses his or her arms and legs?

Circle one: (No)   Yes   A little   COMMENTS

Do you have any concerns about how your child behaves?

Circle one: (No)   Yes   A little   COMMENTS

Do you have any concerns about how your child gets along with others?

Circle one: (No)   Yes   A little   COMMENTS

Do you have any concerns about how your child is learning to do things for himself/herself?

Circle one: (No)   Yes   A little   COMMENTS

Do you have any concerns about how your child is learning pre-school or school skills?

Circle one: (No)   Yes   A little   COMMENTS

Please list any other concerns.

None.

FIGURE 9.2 The PEDS is a 10-question survey that relies on parent knowledge about their child. It offers a useful way of structuring interviews with parents. Data are available on sensitivity and specificity. Glascoe found that when parents have a single significant concern about their child's development (e.g. speech), or when there are difficulties in communication because of a language barrier, the use of a further screening test can help reduce unnecessary referrals. However, when parents have clear concerns in two or more areas of development (e.g. difficulty in understanding language *and* in social interaction), there is a higher probability of a significant problem that would merit more detailed assessment.[12] Reproduced with the permission of Frances Glascoe.

Developmental and behavioural screening

Developmental and behavioural screening tests and programmes do not satisfy the UK's strict criteria for a screening programme mentioned earlier in this chapter (*see* page 177). There is no evidence that they have delivered real improvements in outcomes for children and in the UK the routine use of developmental screening tests for all children is not currently considered an effective strategy. The reasons are discussed in depth elsewhere.[1] Reviews of a child's development form part of the Child Health Promotion Programme (*see* below); reviews may take several forms, but generally involve a professional who has the opportunity to observe and discuss the child's progress, developmental stages and needs. This is a more demanding task than working through a screening checklist and calls for a sound knowledge of child development.

When are developmental tests useful?

We do not recommend the routine use of tests *for screening* for the reasons outlined above, but the ability to use one or more standard tests for *assessment* should be part of the repertoire of child health professionals, as they are useful in several circumstances:

- to clarify concerns raised by parental comments or professional observations;
- to provide a quick source of information about the extent of normal variation and any delay (this is a useful feature of the Denver test);
- to help demonstrate the reason for your concerns to parents when they are not convinced that there is anything to worry about;
- to act as an aide-memoire and to help train staff who are not yet familiar with child development.

Tests and scales have several advantages: they have a structured approach, they use set tasks to examine skills that cannot easily be observed in spontaneous play, they offer information about what is expected at any given age (*see* Figure 9.1 for an example) and they categorise development to facilitate observations that are easy to make; for example:

- gross motor: sitting, standing, walking, running;
- fine motor and visuo-motor coordination: handling toys, stacking bricks, doing buttons;
- speech and language, including hearing;
- social behaviour.

Tests do not provide a medical diagnosis, they just tell you about current performance and function. For example, difficulties with fine motor coordination might be due to visual impairment or global delay, as well as conditions that specifically affect movement, such as cerebral palsy or muscle disease.

It is important to understand the *psychometric properties* of tests. This means that one needs information about how reliable they are, whether they measure what they claim to measure, how well they compare with other long-established tests used by psychologists and how well they predict future performance and problems. It is important to know their sensitivity and specificity; in other words, how many false positives (children who on subsequent investigation are found not to have any problem) and how many false negatives ('missed' cases) can be expected. Pre-school children cannot be expected to perform equally well in all circumstances, so we also need to know the reliability of the test when carried out on different days or by different people.

In the case of tests designed for screening, data are also needed on the skill level required to administer them, the time each test takes, the extent to which they can be generalised across social classes, cultures and language groups, and their acceptability to parents. Developmental screening tests vary widely in the quality and extent of the data on their psychometric properties; some are too insensitive and miss many cases, while others over-refer normal children.

Tests commonly used at primary care level in the UK are listed in Box 9.5.[13] Details of the most easily observed developmental skills and behaviours are described in the following chapters. Psychologists have access to a much wider range of tests that examine a variety of developmental functions, including measures of intelligence. Intelligence can be thought of as the ability to derive meaning from experience and apply it to solving problems. As a crude rule of thumb, curiosity is an indication of intelligence in the very young child; self-organisation in the older child. Motor milestones are a poor guide, creativity only a loose indicator, and memory is not very helpful. Speed of learning is virtually synonymous with intelligence. For older children, school performance provides useful information, though of course it is affected by many factors in addition to the child's innate ability.

Intelligence can be measured with reasonable accuracy, but there is danger in placing too much reliance upon IQ numbers without considering, for example, unusual circumstances, such as tiredness or recent testing, which might affect the child's performance. Tests only sample a child's problem-solving behaviour; they cannot indicate potential in some magical way. Furthermore, a child's IQ can change significantly during maturation so that absolute stability over time is not expected.

BOX 9.5 Tests and scales used by community health staff in the UK

- The Denver Developmental Screening Test – reproduced in Figure 9.1. Available for purchase from www.denverii.com
- Sheridan's guide to child development: Sheridan MD, Sharma A, Cockerill H. *From Birth to Five Years: Children's Developmental Progress*. 3rd ed. London: Routledge; 2007. A structured developmental examination package, the *Schedule of Growing Skills*, based on Sheridan's work, is only available to registered users at: www. onestopeducation.co.uk/icat/4064004main
- Language: the Sure Start Language Measure is currently the most accessible for UK primary care staff and is available at: www.surestart.gov.uk/research/keyresearch/ earlylanguagedevelopment/surestartlanguagemeasure/. For other options see review by Pickstone, *et al.*[13]
- Screening tests for autism are described on page 262.
- Behavioural screens or checklists: *The Strengths and Difficulties Questionnaire* (SDQ) is the best validated and most widely used behaviour screening test (for current problems; it does not predict future disorder). There are versions for two different age ranges (3-4 years and 4-16 years); and for teacher, parent. There is also a self-completion version for adolescents (11-16 years). Available at: www.sdqinfo.com/
- The *Ages and Stages Questionnaire* (ASQ) and the *Child Development Inventory* (CDI) are popular in the USA, and the ASQ has recently been used in the UK. Available at: www.brookespublishing.com/store/books/bricker-asq/index.htm

CHILD MENTAL HEALTH SURVEILLANCE

There is no hard and fast line to be drawn between a child's developmental progress, physical health and mental health. Emotional and behavioural difficulties are extremely common in young children. During routine healthcare consultations, opportunities often arise for the appraisal of psychological development and prognostic signs by asking a series of simple questions. If a formal checklist of behavioural problems is required, the Strengths and Difficulties Questionnaire (Box 9.5) is often used, though whole-population screening for these problems is not currently recommended. Chapter 14 describes in more detail an approach to child mental health surveillance and the management of the more common emotional and psychological problems.

UK POLICY FOR CHILD HEALTH PROGRAMMES

The content and structure of preventive child health programmes has been modified in the light of the evidence discussed above. The current policy is to provide a universal or core programme for all families and targeted approaches for those with additional needs. The preferred term is now Child Health Promotion Programme (CHPP) to reflect the greater emphasis on promoting health as opposed to the 'defect and problem' detection model implied in the term 'surveillance'. In order to ensure that all children receive essential services of proven value, a core programme of contacts and actions was set out in the National Service Framework (NSF)* (Box 9.6). A revised CHPP was published by the England Department of Health in 2008.[14] It lays clear responsibility on the health visitor to oversee the programme for individual children, but recognises that there will often be other people involved in delivering it. The content of the CHPP programme can be summarised as follows:

- establishing contact and a relationship with the family;
- providing information, advice and support;
- offering and arranging contacts with other individuals or organisations who may be helpful to the parent(s);
- identifying children at risk because of developmental or health problems or possible neglect or abuse;
- recognising mental health and lifestyle problems in the family;
- carrying out standard screening procedures;
- ensuring that preventive health measures and information are made available to all parents.

The NSF recommended that all children should receive the basic programme of care and that by 1 year of age there should be an agreed plan setting out what further input the parents want and the child needs, from the primary care and community child health team(s). In addition, the new CHPP (2008) recommends a review at 2 to 2.5 years. There should also be a targeted programme that addresses specific identified needs and issues; this may be short-, medium- or long-term according to need and should be linked to whatever early educational and social care interventions are required.

---

* This refers to the NSF for England; the other three countries of the UK (Scotland, Northern Ireland and Wales) have published their own approaches to community child health.

BOX 9.6 Summary of the Child Health Promotion Programme (2008)

Age/Stage	Intervention
Pregnancy up to 28 weeks	Promotion of health and well-being, including physical care and screening, signposting to resources and needs assessment. Preparation for parenthood
Pregnancy after 28 weeks	As for above, but details are different
Birth to 1 week	Infant feeding, health promotion, maintaining infant health, reviewing pregnancy and delivery, promoting sensitive parenting, screening (including physical examination, hearing and blood spot tests listed in Box 9.1), immunisations if indicated (hepatitis B and BCG), SIDS prevention, vitamin K
1–6 weeks	Infant feeding, promoting sensitive parenting, promoting development, assessing maternal mental health, immunisations (hepatitis B and BCG) if indicated, SIDS prevention, safety, maintaining infant health
6 weeks to 6 months	Nutrition, health review at 6–8 weeks (including physical examination), immunisations (8, 12 and 16 weeks), maintaining infant health, promoting development, keeping safe
6 months to 1 year	Distribution of Bookstart pack, health review by 1 year, dental health, immunisations (Hib/Men C at 12 months), maintaining infant health, promoting development, keeping safe
1–3 years	MMR and PCV at 13 months
	Health review at 2–2.5 years; development, behaviour, advice on nutrition and activity, dental health, check immunisations are up to date, respond to concerns, signpost resources, keeping safe
3–5 years	Immunisations at 3 years 4 months (MMR and pre-school booster), support of parenting and promotion of development with emphasis on healthy lifestyles
School entry	School entry review. Health visitor handover to school nurse. Measure/plot height and weight. BMI, Foundation Stage Profile by teacher. Hearing screening test
Throughout primary and secondary school	Open access to school nurse. Some nursing care. Input to PSE. Advice in general and about specific children. Yr 6 – BMI
Secondary school	HPV immunisation for girls in year 8 (and catch-up programme) and school leavers' booster to all at 13–18 years old

BCG = Bacillus Calmette-Guérin; **BMI** = body mass index; **Hib** = *Haemophilus influenza* type b; **HPV** = human papilloma virus HV; **Men C** = meningococcal C; **MMR** = mumps, measles and rubella; **PCV** = pneumococcal conjugate vaccine; **PKU** = phenylketonuria; **PSE** = personal and social education; **SIDS** = sudden infant death syndrome.

PRIMARY CARE DECISIONS

After ensuring that a child and family has received all the appropriate advice about primary prevention, professionals working in child health promotion programmes may find it helpful to ask themselves three key questions:

1 Is there any significant abnormality in this child's development, health, growth, behaviour or experiences; and if so, what aspects are affected?

2 Are there any underlying factors that need further evaluation or that could be altered or improved?

If the answer to either question is YES, a more detailed assessment may be required. You must then decide:

3 Should you refer the child onwards for more detailed assessment and if so, to whom? Or should you manage the problem within the primary care team? This depends on the level of skill available and on ease of access to specialist services. Many community staff are competent to deal with common management problems and many more can acquire the necessary skills if appropriate training is provided.

Assessment

Assessment is distinct from screening and surveillance. It is a process involving several stages:

▶ recognition that a child has or may have a problem, disorder or disability;
▶ gathering information about the child and family from a variety of sources;
▶ integrating that information;
▶ formulating a view about the situation, its causes, prognosis and the scope for intervention;
▶ sharing and discussing that view with the family;
▶ initiating whatever interventions may be indicated.

In the context of early child development, assessment is usually regarded as a specialist activity; that is, it is secondary or tertiary level care rather than primary care. This does not necessarily mean that staff employed in primary care settings must refer all children needing assessment to another service; many community-based staff have specialist skills.

Difficult cases

Developmental cases are often complex and emotionally loaded. In many cases, input from a wide variety of health service disciplines and other agencies may be required. For pre-school children, the requisite multi-disciplinary and multi-agency services are often coordinated under the umbrella of a child development centre or team. A close working relationship with education services is crucial (*see* page 347). If you have any doubts, discuss and debate the case with colleagues.

It will often be useful to consult CAMHS (Child and Adolescent Mental Health Service) professionals who are attached to many schools and GP surgeries, who may be able to provide useful information about the child. Often these cases do not have a single correct answer, but for primary care staff a useful rule of thumb is to refer the child for more intensive assessment if there is no improvement after two or three visits. More rapid referral is often justified in cases with worrying prognostic features (*see* page 306).

When contemplating a referral to CAMHS, spend time discussing this with the parents, otherwise there is a high risk that they will not attend the appointment(s). They need to know how long the waiting list is and should be advised that it may involve several hours of interview and talk, sometimes spread over more than 1 day; it may include various games; and the team may wish to see not only the child and the parents, but sometimes other members of the family.

REFERENCES

1 Hall D, Elliman D, editors. *Health for All Children*. 4th ed. revised. Oxford: OUP; 2006. *See* also Regalado M, Halfon N. Primary care services promoting optimal child development from birth to three years. *Arch Ped Adolesc Med.* 2001; **155**: 1311–22.

2 *See* the web site of the National Screening Committee: www.nsc.nhs.uk/

3 http://hearing.screening.nhs.uk/

4 Silva PA. Predictive validity of a simple two item developmental screening test for three year olds. *New Zeal Med J.* 1981; **93**: 39–41.

5 www.denverii.com/ (lists references to studies using the DDST; test materials may be ordered through this web site) (accessed 31 December 2008).

6 www.cwdcouncil.org.uk/eyps

7 Mortimer H. *Trackers 0–5: Tracking children's progress through the Early Years Foundation Stage*. Stafford: QEd publications; 2008. Available from: www.qed.uk.com/nurseries_and_early_years.htm

8 www.standards.dcsf.gov.uk/eyfs/site/resource/index.htm (accessed 31 December 2008).

9 Pachter LM, Dworkin PH. Maternal expectations about normal child development in 4 cultural groups. *Arch Ped Adolesc Med.* 1997; **151**(11): 1144–50.

10 Rydz D, Srour M, Oskoui M, *et al.* Screening for developmental delay in the setting of a community pediatric clinic: a prospective assessment of parent-report questionnaires. *Pediatrics.* 2006; **118**(4): e1178–86. Available at: http://pediatrics.aappublications.org/cgi/content/abstract/118/4/e1178 (accessed 31 December 2008).

11 Available at: http://shop.healthforallchildren.co.uk/pro.epl?SHOP=HFAC4&DO=USERPAGE&PAGE=peds06

12 www.pedstest.com/ – this web site gives detailed information about the design, validation and use of PEDS.

13 Pickstone C, Hannon P, Fox L. Surveying and screening preschool language development. *Child Care Health Dev.* 2002; **28**: 251–64.

14 Department of Health. *Child Health Promotion Programme*. London: DH; 2008. Available at: www.dh.gov.uk/en/Publicationsandstatistics/Publications/DH_083645 (accessed 31 December 2008).

CHAPTER 10

Birth to 6 months

CHAPTER CONTENTS

The routine examination of the newborn and subsequent contacts between parents and health professionals offer opportunities not only to assess the infant's health and identify any abnormalities, but also to support and advise the parents in a variety of ways. This and the next three chapters discuss the common health concerns in children under five and outline key aspects of development.[1]

CARE AND ASSESSMENT OF INFANTS: AN OVERVIEW

Most parents appreciate professional advice and support in the first few weeks of their baby's life, particularly if it is their first child. Although the focus is often on examining the baby and identifying any problems, it is equally important to use each contact as an opportunity to discuss aspects of childcare and family life with the parents. Parents who have experienced routine newborn care delivered by doctors and by nurses sometimes seem to prefer the latter, not because nurses examine the baby with greater expertise, but because parents appreciate their more holistic approach.[2]

The following topics and questions may be relevant in the newborn period or at some point in the early weeks of life for most babies:

▸ Ask open questions: how is the baby? How are you feeling? How are you coping? (Enquire about both parents!) Are you getting adequate sleep?
▸ Review any pregnancy problems and do a 'de-brief' about the labour and birth as this may provide an opportunity to explain and often lay to rest any lingering anxieties. Do the parents have any worries about the pregnancy (e.g. equivocal scan results) or the birth (e.g. abnormal fetal heart tracings)? Were any problems noted in antenatal or labour records and if so, is any postnatal investigation or imaging needed?
▸ Check and, if necessary, ask about any mental health problems. Listen

sympathetically and if appropriate create opportunities to discuss issues such as depression, substance abuse, domestic violence, other risk factors for child neglect and abuse (*see* Box 10.1 and page 59).

▶ Ask about any worries regarding the baby's general health, weight gain, responsiveness, vision or hearing. Have a discussion about baby care: feeding (particularly breastfeeding), crying, skin care, sleep patterns and management of any medical problems.

▶ Advise on managing a baby who was premature (*see* Chapter 15).

▶ Demonstrate infant behavioural responses[3] (many parents find this fascinating).

▶ Explain any anomalies or abnormalities found on examination.

▶ Consider whether the baby is in a high-risk category for vision defects, hearing defects or any other congenital disorder.

▶ Check whether the baby needs vitamin K, according to local policy (*see* page 103)

▶ Check whether the newborn screening tests have been done (*see* Chapter 9) and how will the parents receive (and interpret) the results?

▶ Check whether the parents are familiar with – and implementing – the advice on reducing the risk of sudden infant death (*see* page 229)

▶ Clarify that the parents understand and accept the immunisation schedule (including hepatitis B and BCG if relevant – *see* Chapter 9).

▶ Discuss other health promotion topics; e.g. home safety.

▶ Agree what arrangements for the type and frequency of further professional support (home visiting, clinic attendance, etc.) are most appropriate for the family.

▶ Assess whether the mother needs the MMR vaccine (if sero-negative).

▶ Do the parent(s) need contraceptive advice?

▶ Ensure that parents understand the role and use of the Personal Child Health Record.

See also Chapter 15 for specific issues such as sudden infant death, asphyxia, prematurity, sick babies, etc.

BOX 10.1 Assessing the risk of child abuse and neglect

Early risk factors for child neglect and abuse:

- Very young parent(s).
- Lack of social support network.
- History of deprivation or abuse in parent's own childhood.
- Parent(s) attended special school.
- Handling problems: baby held at arm's length, lack of eye contact, no evidence of pleasure in the baby, rough or careless handling.
- Disparaging remarks about baby's appearance, behaviour, responsiveness or sex.
- Failure to thrive.
- Failure to seek medical advice when appropriate.
- Abnormal baby: prematurity, handicap, chronic illness, etc.
- Baby with difficult temperament.
- History of previous unexplained infant death in suspicious circumstances.
- Arrival in household of new partner who is not the baby's natural parent.

- Substance abuse.
- Family history of violence.
- Parents lacking basic knowledge of child development.

Family factors – look for:

- evidence of additional stress on the family: bad housing, financial problems, relationship under strain;
- maternal depression, which is *very* common (*see* page 44). Ask the mother what she is feeling, how are her spirits, is she enjoying the baby?

Parents' worries:

- Parents who *express* a fear of hurting the baby should be taken seriously, but do not create a sense of panic or overreact! Discuss the reasons and what support they have and need, and help them plan what to do when they feel under stress.

NORMAL DEVELOPMENT IN THE FIRST 6 MONTHS
Parents' relationship with their baby

The parent(s)' attitude to their baby, their circumstances and their mental state impact in many ways on the infant's development. The infant is an active participant in these interactions and even in infancy differences in temperament can be recognised. These topics are discussed in detail in Chapter 3. When the parent–infant relationship is disturbed or abnormal, it is important to consider if there are risk factors for child neglect and abuse and to take any steps necessary to protect the baby (*see* Box 10.1)

Social behaviours: imitation, turn-taking and smiling

Infants sometimes imitate adult gestures, such as tongue protrusion or opening the mouth. The phenomenon of 'turn-taking' can be observed within the first few hours or days of life and normally involves both vision and hearing. The infant looks intently at the parent and this gaze is returned. When the parent makes sounds to the baby, he stills and listens and when the sounds stop, the baby vocalises and increases his bodily movements. As the baby gets older, he may look puzzled, become distressed and even burst into tears if the parent does not give the expected response.

Occasionally a parent may suspect that something is wrong before it is obvious to any professional, because they sense that the infant's responses and behavioural patterns are not normal. Conversely, parents who are very well informed about child development may over-interpret such behaviour patterns and suspect problems that do not exist. Some young, inexperienced parents fail to appreciate the importance of talking and playing with infants. 'Difficult' babies may just be trying to elicit social interactions with their parents.

In the first few weeks of life babies may 'smile' in response to being well-fed, or during REM sleep. By 4 weeks, a dramatic sight, such as a colourful moving toy, may produce a smile. The true social smile in response to the human face, often accompanied by cooing, appears between 6 and 10 weeks.

Habituation

Infants are 'programmed' to seek novelty. They are bored by repetition of identical stimuli (habituation) and respond to a new stimulus with an increase in alertness, respiratory and heart rates, and sucking (recovery). These responses can be used to assess what infants perceive as a new stimulus and therefore how discriminating they are. Habituation and recovery are quite good predictors of later intelligence.

Taste and smell

Infants can distinguish between the smell of formula and that of breast milk and between their own and an unfamiliar lactating mother. They initially prefer sweet tastes to sour, but by 4 months they begin to like more salty tastes. However, they can adapt to whatever food alleviates hunger. Infants who are given a special feed in the first 6 months of life, because of some gastrointestinal or metabolic disorder, may subsequently reject ordinary milk. Offering a wide variety of flavours in the first 6 months may make it easier, subsequently, to introduce a range of foods. One advantage of breastfeeding may be that the flavours of the foods in the mother's diet are transmitted to the baby.

Vision

Visual acuity is limited in newborns and they do not focus very well. They prefer colour stimuli to grey tones, but cannot readily discriminate between hues. Focusing and eye movement control mature rapidly over the first 3 months and by 6 months the visual acuity and colour sensitivity are approaching adult levels. As the baby learns to sit and then to crawl, his perception of depth and distance also improve. Newborns look at face-like patterns; between 1 and 2 months they begin to distinguish between the face of their mother and an unfamiliar woman and by 3 months can make quite fine distinctions. Over the same timescale they also learn that an object's shape and properties are stable even if viewed from different angles or partially concealed.

Learning social skills and routines

As early as 14 weeks, the baby may stare with obvious fascination at an unfamiliar person and by 6 months it is usually obvious even to the casual observer that he regards his familiar caregivers as different from other people. His laughter at his own reflection in a mirror suggests that he has some sense of himself as a person although true self-recognition is thought to occur only in the second year.

At this stage he has not yet acquired a deep suspicion of strangers and it is usually quite easy to 'make friends' with a baby of this age. The formation of strong **attachments** is a natural part of the infant's development (*see* page 46) but these may be formed with either one or several people and indeed there may be advantages in a child having several attachment figures. Some parents recognise this and actively plan ways to achieve it, though it is also important to realise that some babies cope with being handled and cared for by several different people much better than others. The strength of attachment is related more to the quality of interaction between the baby and the caregiver than to the actual amount of physical care. This point is important for parents who feel guilty about making use of a child-minder while they are at work (*see* also page 190).

In the first 6 months of life, the infant **learns** about daily rituals such as bath time, feeding, changing, etc. He reveals this knowledge by showing **anticipation** when he sees or hears the preparations for these events. He also enjoys games where anticipation is needed and he may begin to develop '**procedures**' to encourage their performance. For instance, he may rock back and forth with excitement or may vocalise loudly.

Hearing, listening and communicating

Newborns can tell the difference between random noise and certain sound patterns, such as a series of tones, a wide range of speech syllables and speech with emotional overtones of anger or sadness. They respond differently to the voice of their mother to that of other women and to their own language as opposed to a foreign language. They orientate towards sound within the first few days of life and can reach towards a sound source in darkness by 4 months.

'Cooing' is followed at around 3–4 months by babbling (the repetitive use of single syllables such as 'gaga' and 'ah-goo', followed by 'da', 'ma', 'ka', 'der') and blowing raspberries. This behaviour seems to be innate as it also occurs in deaf babies and deaf babies whose parents use sign language 'babble' with their hands; however, they do not begin to incorporate the wider range of sounds peculiar to the child's native language as hearing babies do, at around 7 months.

Parents follow their baby's direction of gaze and at around 4 months babies begin to follow the direction of the adult's gaze. This ability to engage in 'joint attention' allows adults to comment on what the baby is seeing and this is an important element of early language development. Adults also begin to 'teach' the baby about turn-taking games such as peek-a-boo; the baby is at first puzzled and then an amused observer, but gradually begins to anticipate and then to enjoy these games.

Adults use 'child-directed speech' to engage and keep infants' attention. They use short sentences, a high-pitched exaggerated intonation, and clear-cut pauses. As the baby gets older, words are repeated in different ways and in varying grammatical settings, with stress on the key word that is being 'taught'. (Adults do the same when talking to foreign adults!) Infants prefer this kind of conversation to ordinary adult intonation. Alert parents fine-tune their speech to the baby by observing his responses.

Some parents enjoy using signs to communicate with their baby and this is increasingly popular in many nurseries. Early concerns that this might inhibit speech development have not been confirmed and the opposite seems to be the case.*

Motor development

Motor development (*see* illustrations on pages 205-12) is the easiest aspect of development to observe and assess and for this reason sometimes receives dispro-portionate attention. The sequence of motor development is fairly uniform, although some infants do follow atypical pathways (*see*, for example, page 265). The rate of development varies widely, as illustrated in the Denver chart (*see* Chapter 9). Some of the variability is genetic, but cultural practices also have some influence; for example, infants reared in cots in an orphanage do not become mobile till after 2 years of age; some cultures discourage mobility for safety reasons; others deliberately bounce and exercise babies and believe that this accelerates motor competence. There is no

---

* Advice on how to sign is available on several web sites, for example www.netmums.com

evidence that baby walkers enhance motor development and some people think that they are both harmful and dangerous.

Reaching for objects is attempted by newborns, but they lack the necessary coordination to make reliable contact. This stage is called 'pre-reaching'. This usually disappears by about 7 weeks and is replaced by true reaching at around 3 months, which gradually improves in accuracy.

Observations in the first weeks of life

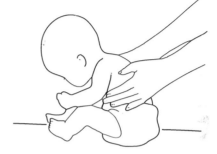

- The newborn infant presents with a mixture of floppiness of the head and neck and strong flexion of the limbs and trunk.
- When handled he requires support to his head and remains curled up in a bundle.
- He may be very insecure lying on his back, tending to startle easily.
- The baby may be happier laid prone or on his side.

Supine:

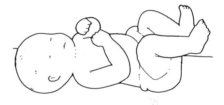

- Posture symmetrical.
- Flexion of all limbs and trunk.
- Unable to stretch his limbs.

Prone:

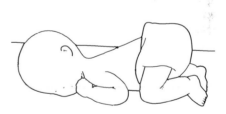

- Flexed posture.
- Head turns to one side.
- Knees tucked under abdomen.
- Unable to raise head.

Reflex reactions:

- *Grasp reflex.* If palm of hand stroked or traction applied to fingers, the infant will close his fingers tightly around the object;
- *Moro* (startle response). In response to a sudden stimulus of noise or movement, the infant will fling his arms and legs wide and then draw them back into flexion.
- *Reflex walking.* If the infant's feet are placed against a firm surface he will move his legs as if walking.
- *Positive supporting response.* Reflex standing.
- *Sucking reflex.* If infant's mouth is stroked he will suck rhythmically.
- *Rooting reflex.* If the cheek is stroked near the mouth, the infant will turn his head to suckle.

These reflexes are prominent in the early weeks of life. They disappear gradually and at a variable rate. The ease with which they can be elicited depends to some extent on the baby's state of arousal. It is not necessary to insist on demonstrating these reflexes as part of a routine examination. Although neurological and developmental disorders affect them in various ways, there are always other and more reliable signs.

Grasp:

▶ Hands held strongly fisted.

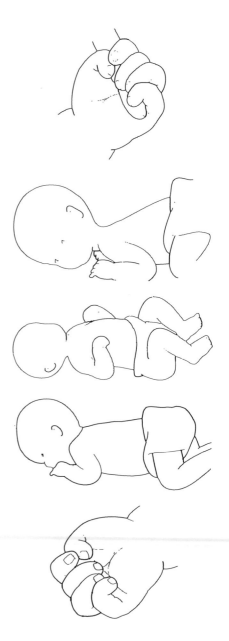

Age 1 month

▶ By 1 month the infant's limbs are more supple and movements more fluent.
▶ He is more tolerant of being handled and moved. He has a little movement of his head under voluntary control.

Supine:

▶ Head usually turned to one side.
▶ Flexion in limbs still marked.
▶ Tendency to roll off back onto either side.
▶ Can partly extend arms and legs.

Prone:

▶ Pelvis lies flatter.
▶ Legs more extended.
▶ Raises head briefly.
▶ Makes small movements with arms.

Grasp:

▶ Hands less fisted.
▶ Finger movements seen.

Head control:

- Held in sitting position; balances head briefly.
- Head-lag when pulled to sitting position.
- In lying position turns head through arc to follow dangling object.

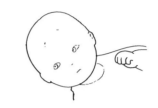

Age 2 months

- By 2 months the infant shows more spontaneous active movement.
- He is becoming happier in supine position.
- His postures are rarely symmetrical and he lies with his head turned to one side or the other.

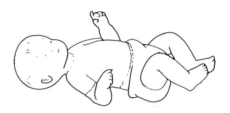

Supine:

- Lies flat on the supporting surface with pelvis and shoulders supported.
- Head adopts mid-position for only brief periods.
- Flexion of limbs decreasing; they rest in semi-flexion and can nearly extend fully actively.

Prone:

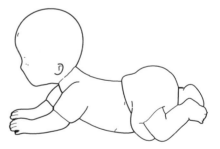

- Raises head to 45 degrees and holds this posture for up to half a minute.
- Watches and follows toy placed about 22 cm from face.
- Follows this toy through small arc.
- Kicks with both legs alternately.
- Takes small amount of weight on forearms.

Grasp:

- Hands open most of time.
- No longer grasps finger automatically.
- Hands may accidentally contact a toy in line of movement. This knocking action may be repeated if rewarded by sound or movement.

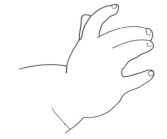

Being moved:

- When held in mother's arms posture is more symmetrical.
- Shows a degree of head balance. This is not sustained or reliable.
- When dangled on his tummy (ventral suspension) his head does not flop but is held in line with body.
- Arms extend and abduct a little.
- Hips remain slightly flexed.

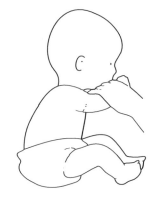

Standing:

- Bounces gently on flexed knees.

Age 3 months

- By 3 months the infant has developed a remarkable degree of voluntary control of his movements.
- Most of his waking time is spent moving arms and legs.
- He is able to maintain his head in a mid-position and is free to watch, follow and reach towards moving objects.
- He has more defined periods of wakefulness.

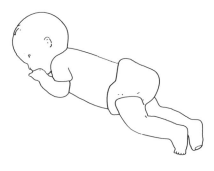

Supine:

- Maintains head in mid-position.
- Moves head freely to watch dangling object, side to side and up and down.
- Stares at hands.
- Kicks legs into flexion and extension – mostly reciprocally (i.e. one leg up, one down) as in cycling.

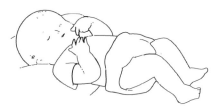

Prone:

- Raises head to 60 degrees and holds this position for minutes at a time.
- Weight is taken firmly on forearms.
- Pelvis rests flat on supporting surface.
- Hips extend and knees rotate outwards.
- Kicks with one or both legs, either reciprocally or symmetrically.

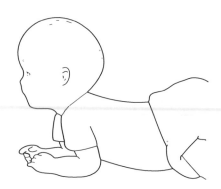

Sitting:

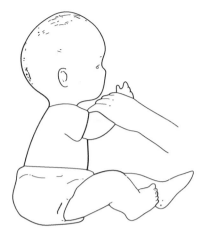

- Placed in sitting position, balances head and has a little control of upper trunk.
- Head control is adequate to allow turning and following of a moving object.
- No balance of trunk.

Standing:

- Takes some weight.
- Head remains balanced in line with trunk.
- No reflex stepping.

Grasp:

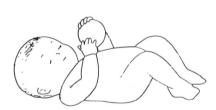

- Grasps object if placed in hand.
- Uses total fisted grasp described as 'contact grasp'. This grasp is partly involuntary.
- Will loosen grasp (not release) after a few seconds.
- Unable to reach and grasp.
- Unable to move hand with object in it.

Age 4 months

- By 4 months symmetry is becoming established.
- The infant lies with head in mid-position and hands engaged in mid-line, typically with fingers in mouth.
- Legs flexed and abducted.

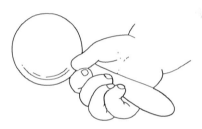

Supine:

- Head mostly in mid-line.
- Hands engage in mid-line.
- Plays with fingers.
- Legs rest in flexed abducted posture.
- Kicks legs into full extension.
- Places feet on surface and hitches bottom for 1–2 seconds.
- May place one foot on opposite knee.
- May roll from back to side and side to back.
- Patterns of movement are extremely varied (i.e. not stereotyped).

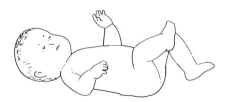

Prone:

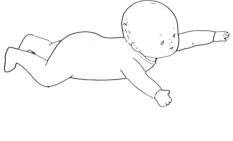

- Head firmly raised to 90 degrees.
- Alternately takes weight firmly on elbows or extends arms and legs into aeroplane or swimming posture.
- Elbows starting to be placed forwards for weight bearing (no longer tucked under chest).
- Kicks legs in a variety of movement combinations using either or both legs.

Sitting:

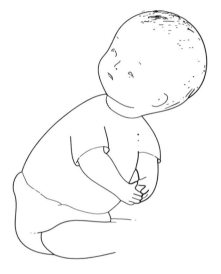

- Placed in sitting position supports head and trunk firmly.
- Lower back still needs support.
- Held firmly in sitting position, he is able to control arm movements.
- May reach and touch toys placed just in front of his feet.
- May either collapse forwards or brace shoulders into retraction to gain stability.

Standing:

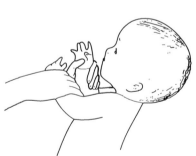

- Extends legs rhythmically and supports most of weight.
- Rises up onto toes.
- Grasps with toes.

Being moved:

- Pulled up to the sitting position, has only a slight head lag.
- Dangled on tummy (ventral suspension) shows intermittent extension of all limbs. Even when relaxed does not collapse into full flexion.
- When carried does not require support to head and shoulders.
- Makes small adjustments to changes of position on lap.

Grasp:

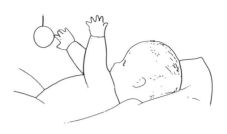

- Primitive clutch.
- Starts to finger toys.
- Plucks at clothes and blankets.
- Plays with own hands.
- Grasps at attractive objects, but may not hit the target!
- Takes all objects to mouth.
- Maintains rattle in hand for few minutes.

Age 5 months

- By 5 months the infant is physically very active.
- He spontaneously changes his position from lying flat on his stomach to pushing up onto extended arms.
- He reaches and grasps toys and has some ability to roll.

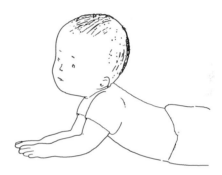

Supine:

- Very active in this position.
- Grasps toys and brings them to mouth.
- Flexes legs and pelvis and plays with toes. Often places toes in mouth and sucks them.
- Places feet on mattress and lifts pelvis (bridging).
- Rolls from back to side with ease and almost to prone.
- May stay on side and play with toys or toes.

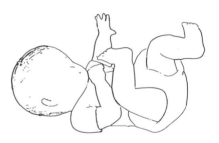

Prone:

- Increasing variety of movement.
- Adopts aeroplane-position: arms and legs raised off floor and spread into abduction.
- Pushes up from forearms to extended arms.
- Transfers weight onto one arm and frees the other arm to reach for a toy.

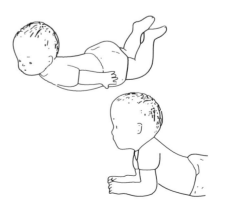

211

- May start to move round in a circle
  – pivoting or pushing backwards on
  extended arms – pre-creeping.
- Rolls to supine.

Sitting:

- Needs only a little support to lower
  trunk.
- Head held firmly.
- Back held straight.
- Makes small adjustments to balance of
  trunk when tilted side to side.
- Early weight-bearing on hands to side-
  propping.

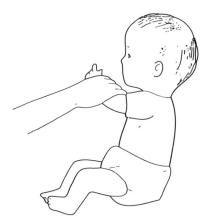

Being moved:

- Pulled to the sitting position, baby
  actively assists by bracing his shoulders
  and raising his head.
- Independent mobility is starting
  through rolling, pivoting and pre-
  creeping.

Standing:

- Takes weight firmly.
- Makes pedalling movements with legs.

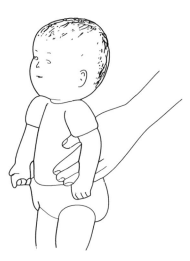

Grasp:

- Use of hands is best seen in supine or
  sitting with support. Hand function
  will otherwise be masked by the need
  to use hands to maintain balance.
- Reaches towards objects on table
  surface or dangled on a string.
- Grasps with palm and outer three
  fingers only, thumb and index finger
  not involved.
- Reaches, grasps and takes toy to
  mouth.
- Bangs toy.
- Release of toys is accidental and visual
  pursuit of a lost toy rare.

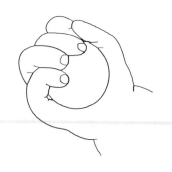

COMMON TOPICS: BIRTH TO 6 MONTHS
Neonatal behavioural assessment

The normal newborn is equipped with a variety of capacities that support survival, elicit caregiving and encourage social attachment to the parent(s). These abilities can be assessed in various ways, but the best-known is the Brazelton Neonatal Behavioural Assessment Scale (NBAS).[3] This examines the baby's state of arousal and a range of motor and social behaviours and responses. A single NBAS score is less useful in predicting future development than the changes in scores over the early weeks of life; however, the greatest benefit of demonstrating infant behaviour using the NBAS is that it gives parents exciting new insights into their baby's needs and behaviour patterns and this translates into more responsive parenting.

Behavioural states

Normal newborns move in and out of six states of arousal: (i) regular or non-REM (rapid eye movement) sleep; (ii) irregular or REM sleep; (iii) drowsiness; (iv) quiet alertness (a state when the infant is relaxed and attentive); (v) waking, often accompanied by irregular breathing and uncoordinated activity; and (vi) crying. Disturbed organisation of sleep and arousal states may occur. These may be associated with a variety of neonatal problems though innate differences in temperament may also be responsible (*see* page 42).

Crying

Babies sometimes cry in response to physical needs, or because of pain. Prolonged inconsolable crying is often attributed to 'colic' although there is very little evidence that this is due to any gastrointestinal disorder (*see* the advice in Box 10.2). Parents may think that they can distinguish different cries for different causes, but this is doubtful. Often there is no obvious reason for the crying, but in most cultures it peaks at about 6–8 weeks and then reduces, partly because the baby matures and learns to regulate his own emotional state more effectively and perhaps also because the parents become more confident at comforting and settling him. Some babies cry more than others and in most cases this is probably due more to their innate temperament rather than anything the parents do or fail to do.

Cross-cultural comparisons stimulate debate (but do not produce much evidence) as to whether it is better to respond quickly whenever a baby cries (on the grounds that this makes the baby feel safe and secure) or to wait for a while (so that the baby does not grow into a whiny, demanding child). No single manoeuvre can be guaranteed to stop a baby crying, but these procedures may help: holding the baby to the shoulder and walking around or rocking; taking the baby out in a car or buggy; swaddling (this may be useful for brain-injured infants); using a pacifier (dummy); making soothing rhythmic sounds; giving the baby a massage.

BOX 10.2 Colic

Features of colic

'Colic' is common in the first few months of life. A useful definition is 'paroxysms of irritability, fussing or crying lasting for a total of more than 3 hours day and occurring on more than 3 days in any one week'. These paroxysms are unexplained and difficult or impossible to soothe. 'Three-month colic' starts typically at about 3 weeks and persists until 14 weeks of age. Colic is no longer regarded as a sign of gastro-intestinal dysfunction. 'Colicky' crying, sometimes accompanied by clenched fists and flexed knees, indicates high levels of arousal or distress, but is not qualitatively very different from crying that indicates hunger and is terminated by feeding. Colic is now thought to be related to difficulties in self-regulation and to temperamental styles.

Consider: Gastro-oesophageal reflux and intolerance to cow's milk (but many breastfed babies are colicky). Altering the size of the hole in the teat has little or no effect. True colic is not relieved by a burp. Colic in a screaming baby who cries and screams intensely for long periods, draws his knees right up and looks pale could also be due to:

- pain from an acute infection (ears, urine infection, abdomen, balanitis);
- intussusception;
- skin problems (napkin rash, eczema);
- anal fissure;
- injuries, fractures.

If the baby flexes the **entire** trunk and lets out a brief cry this may signify a sinister form of epilepsy called salaam attacks, which are infantile seizures that may result in the child appearing to draw up his knees during a jack-knife spasm. Immediate referral is mandatory.

Colic is not caused by anxious parents and varying parental and cultural styles of child rearing do not have much effect on its prevalence; but parents who are unable to soothe a screaming infant develop feelings of ineffectiveness and helplessness, anxiety and depression. Bad-tempered handling, rows between tired, desperate parents and shouting at the baby will exacerbate the baby's distress. There may even be a risk of child abuse.*

Management

Medications should not be used. The following steps are sensible.

- Examine the baby, asking the parents what they fear might be wrong, and commenting on the physical signs of the conditions listed above that you are seeking, but very seldom find.
- Explain that the problem is colic, which is common and short-lived.
- The explanation of 'gut spasm', though probably wrong, will already have been suggested. Without necessarily debunking it, you can add that babies vary in their temperament – some have a very 'strong' personality even as infants.
- Emphasise that it is not caused by poor feeding or handling; make sure this message gets through to the father and the rest of the family.
- Say that there is no known definite cure, but that it will pass by 14 weeks (or 16 weeks to be absolutely sure).
- Consider offering to give them a printed summary that explains about colic, or if the

mother is under great pressure to 'solve' the problem, even put all this in a letter to them so that they can show it to in-laws and neighbours.

Remind them that it is a parent's first duty to survive and they should:

- Take turns in attempting to soothe the baby, out of earshot of the other if possible, by rhythmic rocking, massaging the tummy, giving gripe-water, rides in the pram, etc. A small baby can be carried prone over and along a horizontal forearm and have his back rubbed while being carried around.
- Put a calendar on the wall with the 16-week deadline marked, and cross off each day as it passes.
- Ensure that the mother gets some sleep during the day so that she is not exhausted by the evening. She can sleep while her baby sleeps.

Offer follow-up within a week or two.

* For useful parent guidance, *see* http://dontshake.ca/information/information.php?id=70&type=5

Sleeping in the parents' bed

There is also a debate about the benefits and hazards of having the baby sleep in the parents' bed ('co-sleeping'). Some argue that this practice is normal and desirable and may result in less night time disturbance; others worry about the risks of overlying and the difficulty they will face in the future when they want the child to sleep in his own bed.

Co-sleeping may increase the risk of 'cot death' (*see* page 229), particularly if either or both parents are under the influence of alcohol or drugs, or are very tired. There are differences in crying and in feeding frequency between babies who experience prompt responses to their crying and who sleep in the parents' bed, compared to those who do not, but it is not possible to say that one policy is superior to another in terms of medium- or long-term outcome. Babies and parents should never sleep together on a sofa.

Constipation

Breastfed babies may only pass a stool once or twice a week; straining, accompanied by going red in the face, or 'colic' that appears to be relieved by the passage of a stool, can mislead parents into thinking that their baby is constipated, so it is important to get a description of the stool. Serious causes of constipation in infancy include Hirschsprung's disease, anal abnormalities and hypothyroidism. Other clues to these diagnoses are usually present: delay in the passage of meconium, vomiting, distended abdomen or failure to thrive. Hirschsprung's disease is unlikely if the constipation began after early infancy, but should be suspected if a gentle rectal examination with the fifth finger releases flatus and loose stool. If any specific diagnosis is suspected, specialist referral is necessary. If stools are hard and dry, but there are no other concerns, lactulose 2.5 mL twice daily can be tried.

Sleep difficulties

It is helpful to consider sleep behaviour and sleep problems separately for babies under 6 months of age, infants between 6 and 24 months (*see* Chapters 11 and 12) and children over the age of 2 (*see* Chapter 13).

About two-thirds of babies sleep at night for at least 5 hours by 12 weeks of age (*see* Table 10.1). Babies who have very frequent feeds in the first few weeks are less likely to sleep through the night. Parents need to understand that it is normal for babies to wake several times at night and it is best if they 'learn' to go to sleep by themselves rather than relying on parents' providing comfort. Crying, when put down to sleep after a feed, is often due to tiredness rather than pain or distress.

TABLE 10.1 Sleep cycle of newborns and 3-month-old babies

	Sleep per day	Cycle	Longest sleep
Newborn	16–17 hours	A 90-minute rest-activity cycle	4 hours
3-month old	14–15 hours	Longer cycles, often in the night	8–10 hours

A behavioural programme initiated in the first 12 weeks of life is reported to have some benefits both immediately and in reducing the risk of disturbed sleep patterns later on. Several components may play a part in helping the infant to develop good sleep patterns.[4] Parents are advised to:

▶ maximise the difference between day and night, by minimising light intensity and social interaction at night;
▶ develop a daytime routine for stimulating activities such as bath time and feeding;
▶ learn to recognise signs of tiredness such as yawning and grizzling;
▶ observe how infants can calm themselves (allow some time for this to happen and only intervene if the infant clearly is not going to settle);
▶ be aware that infants sometimes seem to wake, but may fall asleep again *if* they are not stimulated;
▶ feed or change the infant at night, if necessary, quietly, in dim light and with minimal stimulation;
▶ have a consistent time, place and plan for bed time each night;
▶ try to put the infant down to sleep while still awake; settle a sleepy baby in a cot or similar place, and avoid feeding or cuddling to sleep at night time, so that the baby learns to go to sleep on his own;
▶ providing the baby is healthy and gaining weight, introduce a delay, for example by changing the nappy, before giving a feed, so that the baby does not associate waking with feeding.

Massage

Infant massage has beneficial effects on mother–infant interaction, sleeping and crying, and on hormones influencing stress levels, both in low birth weight infants and in normal full-term babies. The research is not conclusive regarding any effect on growth and weight gain. Massage, both at home and in groups with other parents, is popular with mothers; babies seem to enjoy it and there is no evidence that it does any harm.[5]

Kangaroo mother care

This approach to caring for low birth weight and premature infants is discussed on page 343.

Pain

Infants are sensitive to pain; painful procedures elicit a stressed cry, sweating and rises in heart rate, respiratory rate and blood pressure. Sucking a nipple that delivers a sugar solution while being cuddled lessens the infant's perception of pain when a painful procedure is being undertaken.

PHYSICAL EXAMINATION: NEWBORN AND 6–8 WEEKS OLD

Every infant should be examined soon after birth. A study in Germany found that up to 15% of newborn babies have minor anomalies or injuries.[6] Although the neonatal examination is usually performed by paediatric staff, sometimes midwives, nurses or GPs undertake this important check. There is a trend towards early discharge from postnatal wards (sometimes as early as 6 hours); however, if the newborn examination is done on day 1 there is an increased risk of missing some cardiac defects and low bowel obstruction. A further examination is recommended between 6 and 8 weeks of age. These two routine examinations together produce a higher yield of abnormalities than at any other age.

Begin by asking the parents if they have any worries or questions about the pregnancy, the birth or the baby's current status. Explain to parents what you are doing and why. Ensure that they have received all relevant health education information; in particular, make sure that they know about the programmes of universal newborn hearing screening and the neonatal blood spot programme.

This section focuses on the examination of the newborn, but the procedures are similar for neonatal and 6- or 8-week examinations. It is described in three parts:
1 General examination, including check for dysmorphic features.
2 Examination of individual systems.
3 Developmental examination. (Whenever a baby is examined, it is important to check for developmental and behavioural abnormalities as well as physical disorders.)

General examination

If the baby is quiet or asleep, do not ask the mother to undress him until you have listened to his heart and chest; this can usually be done by loosening the top clothing. While the baby is being undressed, look at his general state of health, nutrition and care. The baby should be weighed while undressed. Observe colour (unusually pale, cyanosed); breathing; alertness and activity. Note the pulse rate – normally it should be 100–160 per minute.

Check for **jaundice**. Be familiar with local protocols. Visible jaundice is very common in the first week of life and in most cases is benign or 'physiological'; however, with the trend to early discharge, there is a risk that serious conditions leading to rapidly rising levels of bilirubin may be overlooked. GPs, midwives and health visitors must be prepared to urgently refer any baby whose jaundice is deepening. If this is not done promptly there is a risk of **kernicterus**, leading to permanent brain injury.[7]

Dysmorphic features

It is good practice to ask yourself if there are any dysmorphic features whenever you examine a child at any age, but this is particularly important in the newborn examination. The term 'dysmorphic features' includes any anomaly of structure that results in an abnormal appearance of any part of the body. They may result from chromosome or single gene defects, adverse intrauterine influences, such as alcohol, or from a wide variety of as yet unspecified causes. Some dysmorphic features are regarded as minor and are of little significance, for example clinodactyly (incurved little finger).

With a little practice, it is possible to carry out a systematic examination for dysmorphic features in a very short time, and you should not be put off by the long list of abnormalities given below. Experience is required to know whether a particular dysmorphic feature is likely to be significant and, if so, what diagnoses need to be considered. More than one dysmorphic feature is more likely to be of significance than just a single item. Always check whether the feature is a family characteristic, but also remember that the characteristic may be a marker of an as yet undiagnosed familial condition. If in doubt, ask a paediatrician for advice.

A number of features should be checked during the examination.

Begin your inspection by looking at the baby's **overall appearance**. If you feel that the child does look dysmorphic, different or 'odd', try to decide what specific features give that impression.

Examine the **face** carefully. The **ears** may be regarded as low set if all of the pinna is below the level of the angle of the orbit. They may be underdeveloped, of an abnormal shape, or protruding excessively ('bat ears'). Make sure that the **auditory canal** is patent, but there is no need to spend time trying to visualise the eardrums unless the baby is ill. The **nose** may be uptilted so that the nostrils face forwards; this may be significant if combined with other dysmorphic features. A swelling at the root of the **nose** may look like an innocent cyst, but it could be an encephalocoel and merits a neurosurgical opinion. The presence of **teeth** at birth may denote one of several dysmorphic syndromes. **Cleft lip** is obvious, but **cleft palate** is easily missed. Palpation with a finger in the mouth is not reliable and ideally the palate should be inspected visually. If the diagnosis is missed, it may present with milk regurgitation through the nose. Clefts should be referred promptly to the plastic surgeon and cleft palate team. **Tongue tie** is a possible cause of breastfeeding problems and is discussed on page 101.

Look at the **shape of the head** and check the **fontanelles**. The posterior is often very small and may be hardly palpable by 6 weeks; the anterior usually closes by 18 months. The fontanelles vary considerably in size, and the variations are rarely significant unless the head is of abnormal size or shape. A long, thin head is characteristic of very premature babies, but otherwise may suggest premature fusion of the sagittal suture. A tower shaped head may occur with premature fusion of the coronal suture. Parents worry about asymmetric head shape (*see* Figure 10.1).[8]

BOX 10.3 Head shapes

Premature babies often have a rather long narrow head. **Plagiocephaly** (lop-sided or skewed head shape) is a common finding and is usually associated with positional deformity and pressure rather than early closure of the lambdoid suture (which is rare).

Central flattening of the occiput (**brachycephaly**) similarly worries parents. These head shapes are probably more common in premature infants and in those with low muscle tone or slow development. They have been seen more frequently since parents were advised to put babies to sleep on their backs to reduce the risk of cot death. Parents have sometimes wrongly interpreted the 'Back to Sleep' campaign as a ban on prone positioning at any time; in the UK, the message is now 'Sleep on the Back, Play on the Front' not only to stress the importance of the Back to Sleep campaign, but also to promote head-repositioning manoeuvres and 'tummy time'; infants should spend more time prone when awake.

Flattening of the occiput is more common on the right. There may be other related features such as torticollis and asymmetric motor function (*see* page 265). The natural history of positional skull asymmetry is to become more obvious in the first few months of life followed by gradual improvement by the age of 2. In the vast majority of infants, any residual asymmetry of the skull is of no practical or cosmetic significance.

Advice to parents. Parents who are concerned about the shape of their baby's head should first be reassured and then shown simple positioning manoeuvres – they should lay the child's head on the opposite side to that which is flattened when lying down. This can be facilitated by placing objects of interest on that side of the cot to encourage head movement in that direction. Some authors advocate assisting positioning with foam wedges to ensure that the head is held in the required orientation. A more drastic (and very expensive) approach is to 'correct' the head shape using a helmet that applies pressure to the head. It is uncertain how effective this is, what harm might result and how the benefits, if any, of the usually modest change in head shape should be measured. Very few UK paediatricians or neurosurgeons recommend this approach.

When to worry. Other peculiarities of head shape are more likely to be important, particularly if present from birth, and may be a sign of premature closure of one or more of the sutures: **craniosynostosis**. Feel for a prominent ridge along the sagittal and coronal suture lines and see if the anterior fontanel has closed earlier than expected (the fontanel usually closes between 6 and 18 months). If in doubt, don't delay: ask an expert.

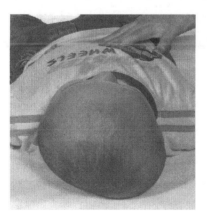

FIGURE 10.1 Vertex view of plagiocephaly without synostosis. Parallelogram due to compensatory bulge of frontal bone on ipsilateral side. Reproduced from Saeed, *et al.*[9] with the permission of BMJ Publishing Group.

Check the eyes and vision (*see* Box 10.4). Ophthalmic terminology is summarised on page 185, vision screening policy on page 184 and the care of children with visual impairment on page 344. Persistent **downward deviation** of the eyes is often called the 'sunset sign' because the white rim of sclera above the pupil gives the appearance of the sun going down behind the horizon. It may be a sign of raised intracranial pressure (e.g. in hydrocephalus), and if combined with other signs, is an indication for urgent referral. However, transient 'sun-setting' may be seen in normal babies.

BOX 10.4 Detection of serious vision defects in infancy

Ask the parents whether they have any concerns about the child's eyes or vision. Enquire about family history of eye disorders. Consider other risk factors, in particular prematurity and dysmorphic syndromes.

Observe visual behaviour. Does the baby look at the parent's face and follow it as she moves from side to side in his field of vision?

Inspect the eyes carefully. (Ask the parent to hold the baby upright if he is reluctant to open his eyes; do not try to force them open.) Are they the same size? If one eye is smaller than the other, the smaller one may have poor vision. A slight asymmetry in the size of the pupils is normal. Look for opacities, cloudiness of the cornea, defects in the iris. Note any photophobia.

Use the ophthalmoscope set on plus 3, held at 10–12 inches, to look for the red reflex, to exclude cataracts. This is not easy, especially in Afro-Caribbean babies whose retina is more heavily pigmented. Do not try to see the fundi; it is very difficult to get an adequate view in the infant without using drops to dilate the pupils and this is not justified as a routine procedure.

Findings suggestive of serious vision defect and needing immediate referral:

- abnormal appearance (white mass, cataracts, etc.);
- eye unusually small or large;
- lack of fixation or following movements of the eyes;
- wandering or roving eye movements;
- nystagmus;
- photophobia;
- lack of pigment in the eyes (appear pink in certain light);
- abnormal reflection of light in a photograph taken with a flash.

Refer the following babies for expert examination:

- premature infants (birth weight <1250 g) who have required oxygen therapy, if they have not already been examined in the neonatal unit (cases of retinopathy of prematurity are still missed in units where there is not a strict policy);
- infants with a positive family history for heritable eye disease;
- children known to have other disabling conditions;
- a permanent squint in one eye is never normal; prompt referral is necessary to exclude cataract and retinoblastoma.

An unduly **short neck**, with or without webbing, may be found in Turner's or Klippel-Feil syndrome. An **underdeveloped lower jaw** is found in Pierre-Robin syndrome (respiratory and feeding difficulties). A sternomastoid 'tumour'* is a swelling in the muscle, associated with some restriction of movement. Gentle stretching exercises may be helpful and can be demonstrated by a physiotherapist.

Look at the **limbs**. Unusually short limbs occur in various skeletal dysplasias. **Asymmetry** in the size of the limbs, or indeed between the entire left and right sides of the body, is found in a number of syndromes.

Examine the **hands**. Accessory digits, single palmar creases and clinodactyly are generally of no significance on their own, but may offer a clue to the presence of a dysmorphic syndrome if associated with other findings.

Look at the **lower limbs**. Under-development or wasting of one leg or calf may be the result of spinal dysraphism (*see* below). Deformities of the **feet** are common in the neonate. The most common is positional talipes, in which the abnormal position of the foot can be corrected passively. Any other abnormality of the feet requires orthopaedic advice. Unexplained non-pitting **oedema** of the **feet** in the neonate can be a sign of Turner's syndrome.

Examine the **skin**. Stork Bite birthmarks, pink capillary naevi on the **forehead** or back of the neck and erythema toxicum are common and generally of no significance. However, a naevus distributed in the territory of the trigeminal nerve suggests the Sturge-Weber syndrome; it may be small or extensive. Excessive **laxity** of the skin, so that it can be picked up in folds, suggests a congenital connective tissue disorder.

Strawberry naevi, which are invisible or tiny at birth and grow rapidly in infancy, are the cause of considerable alarm and distress to parents, but are nevertheless benign and should usually be left alone. One exception to this rule is when the strawberry naevus occurs on the eyelid or margin of the orbit as it may then obscure vision and cause amblyopia.

Look for evidence of **occult spinal dysraphism** (spina bifida occulta). A tiny dimple whose floor is easily visible is commonly found in the cleft between the buttocks and is of no importance. However, there are a number of other cutaneous findings over the mid-line of the spine, particularly in the **lumbosacral region**, which, though apparently trivial in themselves, may indicate the presence of a potentially serious anomaly of the spinal cord. Look carefully for a discrete tuft of hair that may look like a pony-tail; a deep sinus or pits whose floor is not visible; a capillary naevus; a lipoma or dermoid; a Z-shaped deviation in the buttock cleft. If any of these are present the child should be referred promptly to a paediatrician or paediatric neurosurgeon.

Inspect the **genitalia**. In *boys*, note and record whether both **testes** are fully descended into the scrotal sac. If they are, they are unlikely to ascend subsequently, but there is emerging evidence that this does happen on occasion.[10] Make sure it is the testis that you are feeling; the gubernaculum to which the testicle is attached can be mistaken for the testis. If both testes are undescended at birth, the infant should be seen by a paediatrician to exclude any endocrine or intersex disorder.

If there is *any* doubt about the baby's gender or whether the genitalia are normal, refer the baby at once to a paediatrician. The urgency is for two reasons: first, the

---

* Explain to the mother that the word 'tumour' is old-fashioned, but still used. The lump is actually a fibrous scar and is *not* malignant or serious.

psychological impact on the family of uncertainty about the gender of their baby is devastating; second, some causes of intersex, notably congenital adrenal hyperplasia, are life-threatening and need urgent investigation.

If either or both testes are not *completely* descended by 8 weeks, the baby should be reviewed at 5–6 months and if still undescended, the infant should be referred to a paediatric surgeon before the first birthday. Check for **hypospadias**. You may be asked about circumcision (*see* Box 10.5). In *girls*, check for fusion of the labia and any anatomical abnormality of the external genitalia.

BOX 10.5 Circumcision[11]

Circumcision may be recommended for a variety of reasons.

Religious: circumcision of infant boys is required in Judaism and Islam. Generally circumcision for religious reasons is not available on the NHS.

Public health: possible reduction in risks of cancer of the penis (uncertain), cancer of the cervix in sexual partners, transmission of HIV and possibly other STDs.

Reducing the risk of urinary tract infection (UTI): In the UK this is not considered sufficient reason for routine circumcision but it may be worthwhile in boys with recurrent UTIs, particularly if they have anomalies of the urinary tract. Proteus infection is said to be a strong indication for circumcision (after investigation of the urinary tract).

Non-retractile foreskin is *not* an indication for circumcision. At birth, 4% of babies have non-retractile foreskin. With age, the foreskin becomes retractile without medical help. In boys who have had no medical or surgical intervention, at age 5, 90% have non-retractile foreskins; at age 17 this has reduced to only 1%.

Pushing the foreskin towards the baby shows an orifice whose small size may alarm the parent; but if the foreskin is pulled towards the observer, the orifice is demonstrated to be adequate.

Ballooning of the foreskin on micturition is *not* an indication for circumcision, unless it is causing urinary dribbling.

Preputial adhesions usually resolve without treatment. They may be *caused* by misguided attempts to retract the foreskin.

In 3- to 5-year-olds, a tight rim proximal to the meatal orifice can often be loosened by application of 0.5% hydrocortisone cream twice daily for a few days.

Recurrent balanoposthitis may be an indication for circumcision but one attack is not. Chronic balanitis, true phimosis (with scarring of the foreskin) and meatal stenosis need specialist attention.

Doctors who undertake or advocate circumcision are required by the UK's General Medical Council to keep up to date with the indications, techniques and complications and allow a religious adviser to be present for the procedure. Those who disagree with ritual circumcision should refer the family to a colleague who is willing to undertake the task.

Parents need to know that (i) circumcision may reduce the sensitivity of the penis in the adult; and (ii) it has a morbidity and mortality, although these are very low.

Examination of individual systems

Examine the **cardiovascular system**. The most important features of serious congenital heart disease in the first few weeks of life are **increased respiratory rate (tachypnoea), cyanosis, tiredness with feeding and failure to thrive**. The respiratory rate varies quite widely according to whether the infant is calm, restless or asleep, so it is not helpful to specify an upper limit of normal; however, cardiac or lung disease are likely to result in *sustained* rapid breathing with less variability in relation to the infant's activity. Serious heart disease can be present even when there is no audible murmur. Check the quality and rate of the radial or brachial pulse, palpate the femorals or the dorsalis pedis pulse, feel for right and left ventricular enlargement and thrills. Auscultate for murmurs. If you hear a murmur, listen over the back as well as the front of the chest; some murmurs are louder posteriorly (e.g. patent ductus).

Even the most expert examiner will be unable to detect all cases of heart disease in the newborn, so it is important to consider the possibility in any unwell infant. If you suspect congenital heart disease in the first few weeks of life, consider the urgency of the referral. It is **urgent** (same day) if the baby is cyanosed or tachypnoeic, because deterioration can be rapid and catastrophic. Symptomatic infants with congenital heart lesions can deteriorate very rapidly. If the only finding is a murmur, it may be less urgent, though from the parents' perspective *any* worry about heart disease is urgent.

Routine oxygen saturation measurement by pulse oximetry would facilitate detection of some cardiac defects, but would also increase the false positive rate. The costs, benefits and disadvantages of this procedure are currently under investigation.

Examine the chest. Look for asymmetry, **tachypnoea** and recession. Some babies who are slightly wheezy do have some tachypnoea, but are otherwise obviously well. A **persistent cough in early infancy** is unusual and may indicate some serious problem such as cystic fibrosis.

Examine the abdomen. In the neonate, check whether there are one or two umbilical arteries. A single artery without other abnormalities is usually of no significance, but it should be recorded.

Small umbilical **granulomas** are common. Most will resolve on their own. Applying salt or wiping the granuloma with alcohol wipes may help. If the granuloma persists in spite of this, the traditional treatment is to touch it with a silver nitrate stick, having first protected the surrounding skin with Vaseline. Warn the mother not to leave the baby in wet nappies for long periods as an unpleasant skin reaction may result.

Confirm that the **anus** is patent. Meconium is usually passed within the first 48 hours. Parents may ask about the normal frequency of bowel movements. The most usual pattern is every day in the first 2 weeks of life; by 6 weeks, the range is from three motions per day to one every 3 days.

Check for enlargement of the **liver, spleen** and **kidneys**. The liver edge may be felt up to 2 cm below the costal margin. The tip of the spleen can sometimes be palpated in infancy and childhood and this is seldom of any significance.

Developmental dysplasia of the hip (DDH)

Dysplasia of the hip (DDH; previously known as congenital dysplasia of the hip) includes congenital hip dislocation (hip is dislocated but may be reducible), congenital dislocatable hip (hip dislocates fully when stressed), subluxable hip (the hip feels unstable), acetabular dysplasia (the acetabulum is shallow). The incidence of all types of dysplasia is 4 per 1000 births. It is five times more common in girls.

Screening for DDH by clinical examination in the newborn cannot detect all cases at birth, but experts can identify around 80%; inexperienced examiners may only detect half as many. Training and practice are more important than professional background. As no screening programme finds all cases, vigilance must be maintained until the child is seen to be walking normally. *Make sure parents understand this.*

Ultrasound screening can detect hip disorders, but it has a high false positive rate, so is not recommended for the screening of all babies. Current policy in the UK is for high-risk babies to be examined by ultrasound. It is important to ensure that this is done as failure to do so would probably be considered negligent in the event of a missed case. The current screening procedure has three elements.

1 *Identify the following high risk groups*, examine them with particular care and refer for ultrasound. Check for a **relevant family history**, which is defined as a positive reply to the following question: 'Is there anyone in the family who has had a hip problem that started when they were a baby or young child?' Was the baby a **breech presentation**? This is defined as breech presentation at delivery *or* clinically diagnosed in pregnancy *or* history of intervention for breech during pregnancy (e.g. external cephalic version), irrespective of gestational age at delivery or mode of delivery.

2 *Inspect for classical signs of dislocation.* These are sometimes detected at birth but become more common thereafter (*see* page 265).

3 *Examine to detect hip instability.* **The modified Ortolani and Barlow manoeuvres** should be used from birth up to the age of 3 months. There is an increased false positive rate if the test is done within the first 48 hours, but in practice it is often necessary to do it on the first day before the baby is discharged. It is recommended that this should be repeated at the 6- to 8-week examination. The tests must be performed gently, with warm hands and the baby relaxed (*see* Figure 10.2). It may sometimes be easier to examine the hips at the same time as checking the baby's motor development (*see* below). The procedure is described for examination of the left hip:

> ▸ the infant lies supine with the hips partially abducted and fully flexed, and the knees fully flexed;
> ▸ the examiner steadies the pelvis between the thumb of the left hand on the symphysis pubis and the fingers under the sacrum;
> ▸ the upper thigh of the left leg is grasped by the examiner's right hand with the middle finger over the greater trochanter, with the flexed leg held in the palm and with the thumb on the inner side of the thigh opposite the lesser trochanter.

The manoeuvre has two stages:

1 *Ortolani test for dislocation.* The hip is gently abducted; simultaneously the middle finger presses on the greater trochanter in an attempt to relocate the head of the femur (which dislocates posteriorly) into the acetabulum. If dislocation is present the head will relocate with a movement of up to 5 mm and a definite clunk.

2 *Barlow test for subluxable hip.* With the thumb on the inner side of the thigh, backward pressure is applied to the head of the femur. If the latter is felt to move backwards over the fibro-cartilaginous rim of the acetabulum, again with a

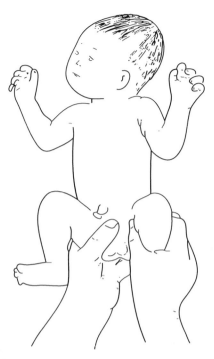

FIGURE 10.2 Modified Ortolani/Barlow manoeuvre.

movement of up to 5 mm and a clunk, the hip is subluxable or dislocatable. If this happens, the hip is gently abducted and will relocate. When the hip is adducted again, it will remain located.

Ligamentous clicks without any movement of the head of the femur are generally thought to be of no significance.

If you do detect a case, do not encourage all your colleagues to come and manipulate the hip in and out of the acetabulum! Urgent referral to an orthopaedic surgeon is mandatory. Results are said to be better if treatment begins before 8 weeks.

A plastic training simulator ('Baby Hippy') which demonstrates the feel of a dislocation and relocation is a useful training aid.[*]

NB: All children with cerebral palsy and other severe disorders of the motor system should be considered at risk for dislocation of the hip and associated spinal deformity **throughout childhood**.

Developmental examination

A developmental examination needs to cover a number of areas.

Look first at social behaviour. Observe the eye contact between baby and parent. Note whether he **visually tracks** the parent's face if they move in front of him. This can usually be demonstrated well before 8 weeks, but it cannot always be observed as it depends to some extent on the baby's state of arousal.

---

[*] Available from Laerdal and Co.: www.laerdal.co.uk/document.asp?docid=1013530

Ask if the baby is **smiling**; this is usually observed by 6 weeks of age or very soon afterwards. Delay of more than a few weeks in this milestone is worrying.

Ask the parents about the baby's **hearing and vision**. Do not attempt any formal hearing test, but check for risk factors; make sure that the baby has had the newborn hearing test and that parents know about access to advice if they have any concerns. Examine the eyes and observe visual behaviour.

Look at **motor development**. Observe the resting posture while the baby is in the parent's arms. **Hold the child yourself** in order to assess the muscle tone and then place him supine on the couch. Note the amount, symmetry and pattern of spontaneous movements. Hold the baby's hands and gently **pull** him to the **sitting** position, then lower him to supine again, noting the tone of the muscles and the amount of **head control**.

Place the baby in the **prone** position and observe the posture of the head and any attempt to lift the head and shoulders clear of the couch.

Do not try to demonstrate the Moro response unless you already suspect asymmetry of arm movement, which can usually be observed just as accurately by watching spontaneous activity.

Do not worry about the other primitive reflexes; they are only unequivocally abnormal when other easier signs of developmental problems are also present. Do not routinely test the tendon reflexes or look for ankle clonus.

Paperwork

Complete the records including any anomalies and details of advice to parents and plot the weight, head circumference and length (if measured) on the chart (*see* page 137 for further discussion on how to interpret the charts).

NB: Examination of the **hips** and measurement of the **head circumference** and **length** are often left till last as they upset some babies. Length is not measured routinely but must be checked and recorded for low birth weight babies and those with any significant anomaly or suspicion of a dysmorphic syndrome.

Interpretation of developmental observations

Delays in smiling, social behaviour and visual tracking are encountered not only in babies with vision defects, but also in those with more generalised developmental backwardness and learning disability (previously called mental handicap). **Severe floppiness** or **hypotonia** may be due to illness, learning disability (mental handicap) syndromes (central hypotonia) or disorders of peripheral nerve or muscle (neuromuscular causes). Of these, the best known is **spinal muscular atrophy** of severe type **(Werdnig-Hoffman disease)**. These babies present in infancy (sometimes with a quite acute onset) with floppiness of profound degree, but a bright alert appearance. Floppiness of sufficient degree to be detected on routine examination or noted by the parent is an indication for prompt referral.

After discharge

Primary care staff normally visit newly discharged mothers and babies on several occasions in the first few weeks. Common concerns include feeding and weight gain, parental mental health problems, and understanding the blood spot screening test.

Care of the umbilical cord

The cord stump will normally fall off between 10 and 21 days after birth. Cord care is outlined on page 223.

Congenital heart disease

Congenital heart disease may present in the first few weeks after the baby goes home. (*See* page 222 for warning signs.)

Jaundice

Jaundice is said to be **prolonged** if it is still visible at 14 days (21 days in premature infants). About 10% of breastfed babies are still visibly jaundiced at 28 days and in many it persists for several more weeks.[12] Breast milk-related jaundice is benign; the baby is entirely well and, as the National Screening Committee does not currently advise screening for prolonged jaundice, many of these babies never come to the attention of health professionals. The cause is unknown, though genetic differences in how the liver metabolises bilirubin probably contribute.

Prolonged jaundice can be due to liver disease, urinary tract infection, haemolysis or other serious conditions. Prompt referral to a paediatrician is mandatory for:

- any *formula-fed* baby with prolonged jaundice;
- any *breastfed* baby with prolonged jaundice who is unwell or has *any* of the following features: not thriving; unexplained bruising (which can be an early sign of liver disease); pale, creamy or clay coloured stools; urine which is yellow or orange rather than the almost colourless urine normally seen in babies; clinical suspicion of anaemia; itching (very rare).

A stool and urine colour chart can be downloaded from the Children's Liver Disease Foundation.* This helps staff and parents to recognise abnormalities at an earlier stage.

If there is any doubt about the cause of the jaundice in a breastfed baby, a blood split bilirubin estimation should be requested – this measures both conjugated and unconjugated bilirubin. In breast-milk related jaundice, there is an increase only in the unconjugated fraction; if the conjugated fraction is elevated, the baby should be referred to a paediatrician.

Missed hearing screening

Any babies born in private hospitals who have not had a private hearing screen, any babies born at home, new immigrants and babies missed for other reasons must be referred immediately to the children's audiology team who will decide on the degree of urgency and make the appropriate arrangements.

Summary of the 8-week examination

This examination is very similar to that described for the newborn infant.

Check records. Are they up to date? Are there any particular issues that need review? Are the newborn screening test results (blood and hearing) in the record and have they been explained to parents?

---

* Children's Liver Disease Foundation: www.childliverdisease.org/uploaded/File/CLDF%20Stool%20Chart%20Bookmark.pdf OR www.childliverdisease.org/uploaded/File/Jaundice_Prot_07.pdf.

Review progress: It is important to do this with the parent(s) and health visitor.

First impression: How are the parent(s)? Any evidence of maternal (or paternal) depression? Other psychosocial problems? Is the baby well? Does he look healthy? Is he growing?

Consider risk factors: For example, consider risk factors for vision and hearing defects and other congenital or inherited conditions. Note that the newborn hearing screen does not detect or exclude progressive hearing loss. It is important for parents and professionals to remain vigilant after neonatal screening. Even if the child has passed the screen, they should still be referred for audiological assessment if there are concerns **at any age**. No attempt should be made to test the infant's hearing in primary care settings as no behavioural test is reliable at this age.

Inspection: Look for:

▶ jaundice;
▶ anaemia;
▶ dysmorphic features – systematic inspection of head, face, neck, trunk, limbs, back;
▶ tachypnoea and cyanosis;
▶ genital abnormalities, especially undescended testes;
▶ listen to the heart.

Development:

▶ social and visual responsiveness;
▶ smiling;
▶ muscle tone and movements – handle the baby, lay him prone and supine.

Leave till last:

▶ checking the hips;
▶ measuring and recording the head circumference, and length (if indicated);
▶ checking for cataract with ophthalmoscope.

Complete the records including the Personal Child Health Record.

HEALTH EDUCATION TOPICS: THE FIRST 8 WEEKS

Key health topics should be discussed in the first 8 weeks, including injury prevention, which is summarised in Box 10.6. Ensure parents are familiar with measures to reduce the risk of sudden infant death ('cot death') (*see* Box 10.7). Explain the immunisation programme to the parents, deal with any queries and give the first dose, if appropriate. Other topics include:

▶ **feeding and nutrition**: establishing and maintaining breastfeeding, preparation of formula feeds, age of weaning (*see* page 111);
▶ **parental smoking habits**: exposure to cigarette smoke increases risk of sudden infant death syndrome (SIDS), respiratory tract infections, meningitis and middle ear disease;

◗ **crying and 'colic'**;
◗ **symptoms of illness** in young babies;
◗ **early infant development;**
◗ **parents' needs**: sleep, return to work, etc.;
◗ **problems with siblings** (*see* page 275);
◗ **how to cope** with stress, sleep disturbance, frustration, etc.

BOX 10.6 Injury prevention

Provide, or advise parents to obtain, the publication *Keep Your Baby Safe*.[*] This gives details of standards for equipment such as pushchairs, cradles, etc., and summarises the common hazards for young babies.

- **Fire risks**: every household should have a working fire alarm and an escape plan.
- **Carbon monoxide**: low cost detectors are now available. Blocked or partially blocked flues or chimneys and appliances that are old or have not been regularly serviced are the main risks but even newly installed systems can be faulty.[†]
- **Car journeys** – Safe transport in the car (*see* the CAPT factsheet – 'In-car Safety').
- **Falls** – do not leave unattended unless safely positioned. Small babies wriggle!
- **Scalds** – Check temperature of bath water carefully.
- **Microwave ovens** make fluids deceptively hot – great care needed if used to heat feeding bottles.
- **Inhalation** – Beware of small toys, furry toys, etc. – ingestion and suffocation risks. Long strings on dummies have been known to strangle babies.
- **Dogs** – do not leave a dog alone with a young child.

BOX 10.7 Sudden Infant Death Syndrome (SIDS)

Approximately 300–400 babies die each year in the UK from SIDS (this can be defined as a death between 1 week and 1 year of age that is unexplained by autopsy, laboratory tests or scene of death investigations). The magnitude of the risk of SIDS is related to the following factors:

- social class;
- smoking;
- age of mother;
- short interval between births;
- infection in pregnancy;
- maternal drug addiction;
- sex of infant – risk is higher for males;
- feeding intention (breast or bottle);
- maternal depression;
- premature or low birth weight;

---

[*] www.capt.org.uk (CAPT – The Child Accident Prevention Trust: Telephone 0207 608 3828).

[†] For information on carbon monoxide poisoning, *see*: *Recognising Carbon Monoxide Poisoning: 'Think CO'.* PL/CMO/2008/8, PL/CNO/2008/8 13 November 2008. Available at: www.dh.gov.uk/en/Publicationsand statistics/Lettersandcirculars/Professionalletters/Chiefmedicalofficerletters/DH_090128

- multiple births;
- congenital defects;
- infant sleeping position;
- previous sudden infant death in the family.

The Confidential Enquiry into Stillbirths and Deaths in Infancy (CESDI) study emphasised three main risk factors: smoking; mother with more than one child *and* aged under 27; no employment income in the family. Families with *no* risk factors had approximately a 1 in 8000 risk of losing a baby from SIDS; families with *all three* risk factors had a 1 in 200 risk; that is, 40 times higher.

Advice on how to reduce the risk of SIDS is provided and regularly updated by the Foundation for the Study of Infant Deaths:[13]

- Place your baby on its back to sleep (there is an eight-fold increase in risk with sleeping prone).
- Your baby can safely play in the prone position (*see* Box 10.3).
- If your baby has been nursed prone in intensive care, s/he should start to sleep supine before discharge.
- The safest place for the baby to sleep is in a cot in the parents' room for the first 6 months.
- Parents should never sleep on a sofa or armchair with their baby.
- If parents choose to share a bed with their baby, there is an increased risk of sudden infant death if either parent: is a smoker; has recently drunk any alcohol; has taken medication or drugs that make them sleep more heavily; or is very tired.
- Breastfeeding is a protective factor.
- Preferably give up smoking. If unable to do so, cut smoking in pregnancy – fathers too! Do not let anyone smoke in the rooms where your baby sleeps or spends the day. Do not smoke when travelling with the baby in the car.
- If your baby is unwell, seek medical advice promptly.
- Do not let your baby get too hot or too cold (the ideal temperature is 16–20°C. Parents cannot easily estimate temperature of a room, so a thermometer is useful.) Do not let your baby sleep next to a radiator or in direct sunlight. If the baby has to be put down to sleep in a warm room, use fewer blankets until the room is cooler.
- Keep baby's head uncovered. Place your baby in the 'feet to foot' position to prevent from wriggling down under the covers; hands should be allowed movement (i.e. no swaddling). Ill babies do not need extra clothing.
- Quilts and baby nests increase the risk of over-heating. No more than 10–12 tog units of insulation are needed under normal circumstances; less in summer.
- Use of a pacifier (dummy) may reduce the risk of cot death; do not use it in the first month if breastfeeding and do not stop using it suddenly.
- There is *no* evidence that toxic gases from mattresses play a part. The mattress should be firm, not sag and show no sign of deterioration. Keep it well-aired and clean. Mattresses with a PVC surface or a removable, washable cover are easiest to keep clean. Ventilated mattresses (with holes) are not necessary.
- Never put your baby to sleep on a pillow, cushion, bean bag or water bed.

Standard tog values:

Vest 0.2	Babygro 1
Pyjamas 2	Jumper, trousers 2
Cardigan 2	Disposable nappy 1
Sleeping suit 4	Baby nest 4
Sheet 0.2	Old blanket 1.5
New blanket 2	Quilt (variable) 3–9

For management of a family who have lost a baby to cot death (or other causes), *see* Chapter 15.

HEALTHCARE FROM 8 WEEKS TO 6 MONTHS

There are no routine examinations or health checks during this period, but there are many incidental opportunities to examine babies, both during consultations for minor ailments and also when the baby attends for immunisation. Problems that may present in this age group are more often related to general health or management issues than to developmental problems; for instance, colic, crying at night, feeding difficulties, poor weight gain, constipation. Health education topics include the prevention of accidents and injuries (*see* page 232), as well as infant feeding practice and dental care.

The procedure depends on the reason for the consultation, but the following observations take little time and help to reassure you and the parent:

▶ Observe the baby's **social behaviour** in response to the parents and to you or other strangers in the room. Vocalisation, smiling and other facial expressions in response to the parent's voice should be more readily observed now than at 8 weeks. Vocalisation at 3 months still consists of vowel sounds only, but the baby is beginning to gain some control over the voice and modulate the sounds as he coos in response to the parent.

▶ Ask about the baby's **response to sound**. At 4 months, he may orientate towards a sound, particularly when in the supine position. Parents often expect more rapid and precise localisation than is realistic at this age, and this can result in unnecessary referrals to the audiology clinic.

▶ **Visual following** is now present through 180 degrees and the baby can turn his head to follow an object at the extreme of lateral gaze.

▶ At around 3 months, the infant becomes **fascinated by his hands** and looks at them with intense interest. When an object is placed in the baby's hand, it is grasped on contact, but he cannot voluntarily release it. He is unlikely to reach for the object or to move it around, but if it is held close to him – but not near enough to grasp it – he may reveal, by excited activity, that the desire to obtain it is greater than the actual level of motor competence.

▶ When placed in the **sitting position**, the trunk and head control can be observed; safe independent sitting is unlikely to be achieved before 5 or 6 months, but the baby is progressing towards this goal.

Interpretation

Defects of vision and hearing may sometimes first be suspected by parents during this period. Low muscle tone, lack of responsiveness, excessive stiffness and irritability, and being 'too good', can be early warning signs of developmental problems.

BOX 10.8 Danger advice

Parents should be thinking about the next stage in development: the child will soon be mobile!* Precautions need to be taken against some possible incidents.

- **Falls**: do not leave the baby unattended in baby walker (better still, do not use a baby walker at all as they are associated with a high risk of accidents e.g. falls, scalds and poisonings due to increased reach; furthermore, they do not result in an earlier age of walking).
- **Toppling down stairs**: check access to stairs – is a gate needed?
- **Scalds/burns**: do not leave hot food or drinks within reach. Do not make or drink hot beverages while holding the child. Guard all fires and radiators.
- **Inhalation**: keep small objects (peanuts, ballpoint pen-tops, small toys, etc.) out of reach.
- **Sunburn**: The SunSmart campaign run by Cancer Research UK advises that infants under 6 months should not be exposed to the sun, nor should sun cream be used on them.
- **Overheating**: Warn parents about the dangers of heaters left on by mistake in warm weather; baby left to sleep in the car during summer months.

Reinforce the advice given previously, including infant feeding practice, dental care, sugar intake and weaning.

REFERENCES

1 Berk LE. *Child Development*. New York: Pearson Education; 2005. (This gives an excellent introduction to the science of child development.)
2 Hall DMB, Wilkinson A. The Ashington experiment. *Arch Dis Child Fetal Neonatal Ed.* 2005; **90**: F195–200.
3 www.brazelton-institute.com/intro.html
4 France KG, Blampiedw NM, Henderson JMT. Infant sleep disturbance. *Cur Paediatr.* 2003; **13**: 241–6.
5 http://iaim.it2003.co.uk/index.htm. *See* also www.bliss.org and www.netmums.com
6 Green K, Oddie S. The value of the postnatal examination in improving child health. *Arch Dis Child Fetal Neonatal Ed.* 2008; **93**: F389–93.
7 Manning D, Todd P, Maxwell M, *et al.* Prospective surveillance study of severe hyperbilirubinaemia in the newborn in the United Kingdom and Ireland. *Arch Dis Child Fetal Neonatal Ed.* 2007; **92**: F342–6.
8 Gill D, Walsh J. Plagiocephaly, brachycephaly and cranial orthotic devices: misshapen heads and helmets. *Arch Dis Child.* 2008; **93**: 805–7. *See* also Singh A, Wacogne I. What is the role of helmet therapy in positional plagiocephaly? *Arch Dis Child.* 2008; **93**: 807–10. *See* also Stellwagen L, Hubbard E, Chambers C, *et al.* Torticollis, facial asymmetry and plagiocephaly in normal newborns. *Arch Dis Child.* 2008; **93**: 827–31.

---

* *See: Now I Can Crawl, I Can . . .* (www.capt.org.uk).

9 Saeed NR, Wall SA, Dhariwal DK. Management of positional plagiocephaly. *Arch Dis Child.* 2008; **93**: 82–4.
10 Sijstermans K. *Different aspects of undescended testis.* van de Vrije Universiteit, De Boelelaan 1005, Amsterdam; 2005.
11 American Academy of Pediatrics: Policy Statement on Circumcision (1999). Available at: www.cirp.org/library/statements/aap1999/ (accessed 1 January 2009).
12 Crofts DJ, Michel JM, Rigby AS, *et al.* Assessment of stool colour in community management of prolonged jaundice in infancy. *Acta Paediatr.* 1999; **88**: 969–74.
13 Foundation for the Study of Infant Deaths: www.fsid.org.uk (accessed 1 January 2009).

CHAPTER 11

6–12 months old

CHAPTER CONTENTS

NORMAL DEVELOPMENT: 6–12 MONTHS[1]

Learning and communication

During the second half of the first year, the infant's attachment to his main caregiver(s) becomes increasingly strong. The significance of attachment behaviours is discussed in detail in Chapter 3. The baby's understanding and use of **speech sounds** matures rapidly during the second 6 months of life. He listens carefully to speech, distinguishes between familiar and unfamiliar words and clearly prefers chunks of speech with intonation and natural pauses. He enjoys looking at books with an adult and listening to the adult reading (*see* 'Bookstart', page 248). He pays attention to the structure of words and sentences long before he can understand their meaning. Parents make increasing use of 'joint attention' (*see* Figure 11.1) in promoting language development. As the infant's gaze falls on an object or person, the parent names it and talks about it. In this way, the relationship between the object and its word label gradually becomes established.

By 7 months he coughs or vocalises to get attention. His own vocalisations now include a wider variety of sounds, with a growing number of consonants, and by 9 or 10 months he begins to imitate sounds. The average age for first words is around 12 months but the 'normal' range is very wide, from 8 months to at least 18 months. Some babies use the same sound to indicate a particular object before it could be recognised as a word and to some extent the variability may reflect differing parental interpretations of what is a word.

There is always a time gap between understanding and speech production. For example, on average, a baby understands 50 words at 13 months and uses 50 at around 18 months – a 5-month lag.

At around 12 months a baby starts to use new gestures to influence the behaviour of other people. Proto-declarative gestures involve touching or pointing to an object and then looking at the adult to make sure they are paying attention. Proto-imperative gestures involve reaching, pointing or making sounds to get the adult

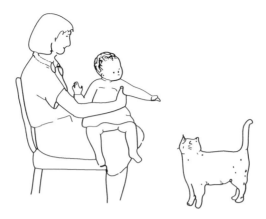

FIGURE 11.1 Joint attention. The child looks at the cat; the mother follows his line of gaze and says 'Yes, that's a cat.'

to do something. These gestures gradually become more explicit in their meaning. The ability to engage in various modes of social communication and exchange may be impaired in children with autism spectrum disorder (*see* page 262), though it is unusual to recognise this in the first year of life.

The ability to **localise the source of sound** also improves so that by 7–9 months the baby can locate sounds to either side and behind him quite accurately, though he may still have difficulty localising sounds made directly above or below him. The 'auditory world' also expands and the infant becomes aware of sound stimuli at an increasing distance from him.

Visual behaviour

Visual acuity is approaching adult levels by 9 months, and binocular vision, depth perception and a sense of parallax are established. The visual world expands and the baby now shows an ability to look at and follow objects or people some distance away; for instance, on the far side of a room. Objects in the far distance are less likely to attract visual attention at this stage. Very tiny objects can capture the baby's attention; for example, tiny bits of fluff on a carpet, or biscuit crumbs. As with hearing, a reduced visual awareness of small objects and apparent lack of interest in visual stimuli at a distance of more than a few feet may sometimes be a sign of general slowness in development rather than of a vision defect.

Learning concepts and skills

Between 6 and 9 months, the baby discovers an important principle: that objects have a continued existence of their own, even when out of sight. This concept is known as object permanence (*see* Figure 11.2). By 7 months, the baby will search briefly for an object that has been dropped. By 9 months he will make a more determined and prolonged search. At first, covering an object seems to make it disappear from the infant's awareness; however, by 9 or 10 months – and certainly by the end of the first year – the infant should quickly be able to locate an object covered by a cloth. The task can be made more complex as the baby gets older. For instance, he can be confused deliberately by the parent hiding the object under one of several cloths. By

15 months, the well-developed sense of object permanence is shown by the child's ability to locate lost toys and to know where prized possessions are kept.

Object permanence develops in parallel with **person permanence**. The baby begins to realise that his parent exists even when not in the same room. The establishment of a mental image of familiar people is a necessary pre-requisite for eventual separation and independence from the parent. These concepts are closely linked to the understanding of how attachment behaviours develop.

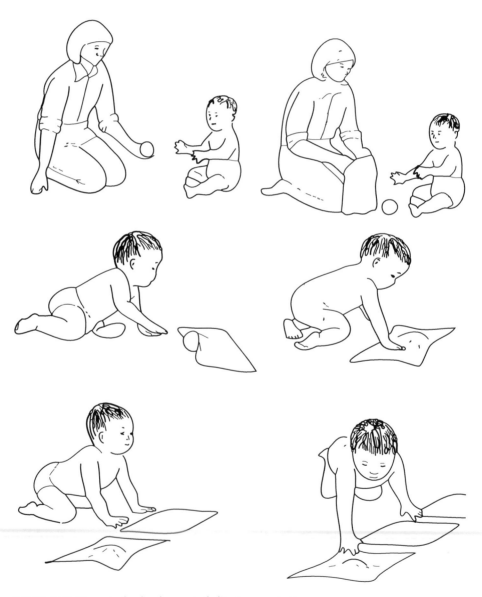

FIGURE 11.2 Stages in the development of object permanence.

Memory

Memory is difficult to assess in infants. Babies aged 3 months can be taught to activate a mobile toy and remember how to do this a week later; the retention span increases to several weeks in babies aged 6 months. At 9–12 months, infants can watch a peer open a container, and then remember how to do it themselves a day later. Memory in babies is highly context dependent: they are much more likely to remember something in the same setting where they first learnt it. This becomes steadily less important in the second year. The ability to predict what a person or toy will do is probably related to memory as infants prefer toys and companions who allow them some predictable control, rather than subjecting them to uncontrollable surprises.

Play

Other areas of learning can be observed by watching the baby play. He experiments with the effects of pulling, shaking and dropping objects; he discovers the mechanism of cause and effect; he examines the size, shape and weight of objects and their relationship to each other. By 1 year of age he can concentrate for surprisingly long periods on a single task.

MOTOR DEVELOPMENT

Summary of motor development in the first year

A more detailed description of motor development in the first year is outlined below. In brief, the baby rolls prone to supine (at 16 weeks); sits unaided (at 5–7 months); rolls supine to prone (24 weeks); can adopt a creeping position (at 36 weeks) followed by crawling (at 44 weeks) – though it should be noted that some babies shuffle instead (*see* page 265); walks (at 10–11 months, with the median around 13 months; and 97% by age 18 months).

Age 6–7 months

▶ By 6 months the baby is developing the ability to initiate changes of position and make his desires clearly known in respect of whether he will sit up, lie down, etc.
▶ He is no longer happy to stay in one position and rolls from prone to supine and back again.
▶ He is starting to move in the horizontal plane in several directions and may even pursue a discarded toy.

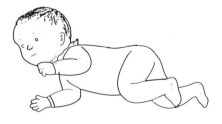

Supine:

▶ Does not stay in this position for long – rolls to prone.
▶ Raises head from floor in an invitation to be sat up!

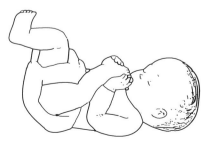

237

▶ Pulls up on adult's fingers to sitting position.
▶ Plays with fingers and toes.
▶ Still places foot on opposite knee.

Prone:

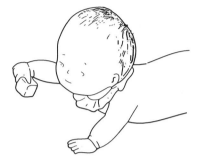

▶ Active!
▶ Pushes up onto arms.
▶ Moves round in circles.
▶ Pushes backwards.
▶ Starting to heave self forwards either using both arms together or alternate arms.
▶ Legs may only assist minimally at this stage.

Sitting:

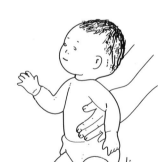

▶ Sits without support for increasing periods.
▶ Needs cushions around him to protect from heavy falls to sides or backwards.
▶ Has good control forwards.

Standing:

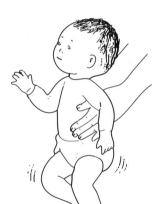

▶ Bounces on feet.
▶ Flexible.
▶ Rarely takes all of weight.

Moving:

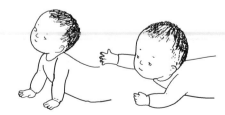

▶ Starting to move alone flat on belly using Commando creeping or pivoting.

Grasp:

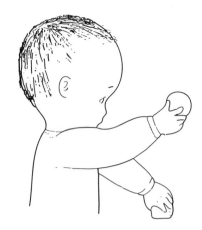

- Grasp remains crude (described as a palmar or scoop grasp).
- The functional area of the hand is moving across and the thumb is minimally involved.
- Considerable variation of manipulation.
- Picks up objects of differing sizes, shapes and weights.
- Transfers objects hand to hand and hand to mouth.
- Manipulates with either hand or both together.
- Can modify grasp effort from banging a toy hard on the table to gentle flicking of a rattle or patting a mirror.

Age 8–9 months

By 8 months the baby has increasing fluency between movements.

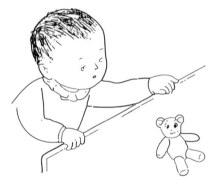

- He can move between positions (e.g. sitting to crawling to sitting), and change from the horizontal, lying, to the upright, sitting.
- Attention span is increasing and individual objects are investigated for long periods.
- The baby has started to gain control of movement of his own body in his environment and control of objects that he encounters.

Supine:

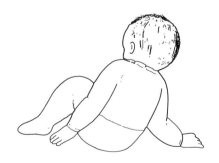

- Does not like this position – feels stranded and vulnerable.
- Either sits up or rolls over to escape from supine.

Prone/moving:

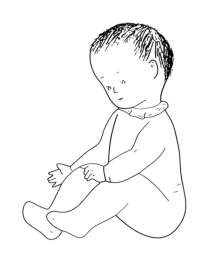

- Freely adopts this position from supine or sitting.
- May continue to creep, or have developed an all-fours position (i.e. prone kneeling).
- May rock on all fours or start to crawl backwards initially.
- Moves between sitting and crawling and crawling and sitting.
- Moves around in sitting, twisting and shuffling to pursue a toy.
- Some babies develop this ability to move in sitting position to a greater degree and become 'bottom shufflers' (*see* page 265).

Sitting:

- Sits for longer periods from 1 minute upwards; can get into and out of this position.
- Saving and propping on hands is well-developed forwards and emerges sideways by around 9 months.
- Sitting no longer a static position, but a dynamic posture.

Standing:

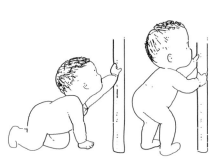

- Pulls up to standing on furniture, in cot as well as on adults.
- Leans trunk against support and takes weight firmly on soles of feet.
- Toes may claw intermittently especially on effort (e.g. rising to standing).
- Toes intermittently relax and wriggle.
- Weight is no longer taken symmetrically at all times and is shifted slightly from one leg to the other.
- Rises to standing with ease but has great difficulty in getting down.

Grasp:

- Pincer grasp emerging.
- Thumb touches side of index finger.
- Grasp has shifted from the outer side of the hand across to the inner.
- The index finger is active in poking and prodding toys.
- Release of objects is starting. May still need a little nudge on the floor or from an adult's hand to completely release.
- Baby tosses toys for a short distance and then retrieves them.
- He watches the effect intently and pursues them even when they go out of sight.

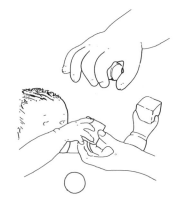

Reflex reactions:

These also give useful evidence that there is no asymmetry between the right and left arms.

- Balance reactions developing in sitting.
- Saving reactions developing forwards and sideways in sitting.

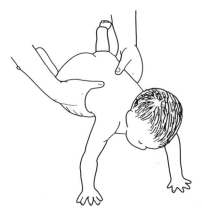

Downward parachute reaction.

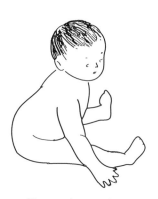

Forwards reaction.

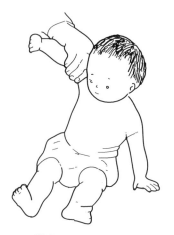

Sideways reaction.

Age 10–11 months

- By 10 months the baby has developed a new dimension to his control of his body in space – he can move fluently from flat (prone or supine) to standing through kneeling or sitting, or either.
- He can travel from place to place either by crawling, 'cruising' or more unusually, by bottom shuffling.
- By 11 months he moves sideways along furniture or cot: 'cruises'.
- Still uses three points of balance: two feet and chest; two feet and one arm; two hands and one foot.
- Gradually over these 2 months these points of balance move more distally (i.e. away from leaning on a chair or low table with trunk to standing well back from the table using only hands or finger tips for support).
- Starting to drop from standing to sitting with control.
- Pushes stable wheeled toys (e.g. brick truck).
- Walks with adult if two hands held.

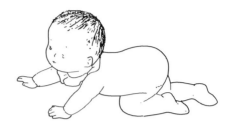

Supine:

- More tolerant of this position, but still rarely stays in it.

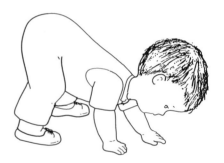

Prone/moving:

- Increasing variations of creeping and crawling.
- Moves forwards using any or all of a variety of methods: four-point crawling using alternate hands and knees; two hands, one knee and one foot; two hands and soles of feet: 'bear walking'.
- Pulls up to standing on furniture.
- Transfers weight from foot to foot.

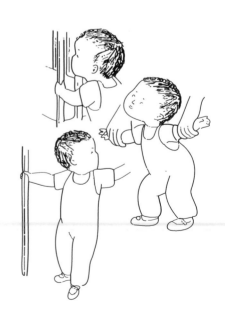

Grasp:

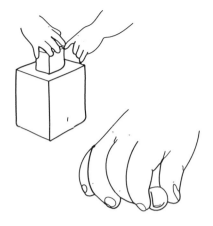

- Places objects into and out of container.
- Release of objects becoming more controlled.
- Teases adult by offering toy, but not releasing.
- Alternately drops object for adult to retrieve!
- Pincer grasp emerging involving thumb and tip of index finger.
- Uses index finger to point and poke.
- Grasp now more economical; only opens fingers enough for the task in hand.
- Starting to estimate size and weight of objects.

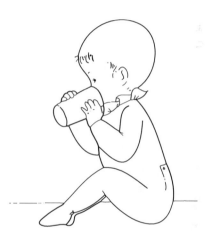

Reflex reactions:

- Balance reactions emerging in standing.
- Saving reactions in sitting: well-developed forwards and sideways; emerging backwards.
- Saving reactions in standing becoming more effective.

SUMMARY OF TOPICS TO CONSIDER BETWEEN 6 AND 12 MONTHS

No specific screening tests or procedures are recommended between 6 and 12 months, but for some parents it is helpful and reassuring to review their baby's progress and to discuss health and development concerns with professionals. They may value some guidance on the next stages of development and the implications for learning. A review with the parents by the time the infant reaches 1 year old is recommended in the 2008 Child Health Promotion Programme (CHPP).[2] Depending on the issues raised, the following may be relevant.

- **Discussion with the parents**: make use of their extensive store of knowledge about their baby's temperament, behaviour and development. Talk to the parents while allowing the baby a few minutes to settle and become used to the presence of a stranger. He should be seated on the floor or on his parent's lap, with a few simple toys within reach.
- **Ask open questions.** Are there any worries about growth, health, appetite or development? How are the parents coping and how do they feel?

243

▶ **Watch the baby's response to you and to his parents.** Suspicion and wariness are normal at this age. Take your time; do not alarm the baby by making friendly advances too soon. Move slowly, speak gently and retreat if he becomes restive and anxious. Offer a small toy as a gesture of friendly intent.

▶ **While establishing rapport with the baby, ask the parents** about his ability to distinguish between them and familiar adults, such as grandparents. At this age most babies know their familiar family figures and respond differently to them compared with strangers.

▶ **Ask the parents about vocalisations.** Does he modulate his cooing sounds (eee-ahah), chatter with a range of consonant sounds? Does he enjoy sound games – for example copying raspberry noises or imitating a cough?

▶ **Does he begin to understand voice** (though not the actual meaning of words)? Ask the parents to call him and observe the response. Does he listen when they talk to him and does he try to have a conversation?

▶ **Enquire about his other methods of communication.** Does he convey his excitement at mealtimes or bath time? Does he insist on attention by shouting or indicate by other means that he wants a particular object? Can he play anticipation games such as 'peep-bo'?

▶ **Motor development**: consider hand and finger movements, sitting balance on the parent's lap and on the floor; check the balance reactions and the response to vertical suspension. Sit him on the floor or couch.

▶ A **physical examination** including length, weight and head circumference is indicated *if* some problem has been raised by the parents or has been suggested by an appraisal of the child's health or developmental progress.

Hip problems

Most significant hip problems should be identified in the first 2 months of life. The features of hip dislocation that have escaped early diagnosis are variable and difficult to detect. They can be missed even by expert examiners. For this reason, the UK National Screening Committee[3] advises that examining the hips after the age of 2 months should not be regarded as a screening test; and the decision not to provide a universal screening programme for hip problems after 2 months of age does not constitute negligence, nor does a 'missed' case. However, failure to act on expressed parental concerns or on physical signs that might point to a dislocated hip could be regarded as negligent.

Parent reports suggest that a dislocated hip in the first year of life may be suspected initially for a number of reasons: the leg 'looks funny'; the hip feels tight or different when the baby is washed or sat on the parent's lap; nappy changing is difficult. Any of these concerns may be sufficient to justify referral for a specialist opinion or an ultrasound or x-ray, according to the age of the baby and local guidelines. It is much easier to detect the signs of unilateral dislocation because of the resulting asymmetry (*see* Box 11.1). Because of the effect on the gait, bilateral dislocation has sometimes been mistaken for muscular dystrophy and vice versa (*see* page 265).

BOX 11.1 Hip dislocation

There are a number of signs of hip dislocation in non-ambulant babies:

- The thigh on the abnormal side lies in partial lateral rotation, flexion and abduction.
- Above-knee shortening is seen by comparing the level of the knees with the hip flexed.
- There may be asymmetry of the thigh and groin creases (although on its own this is not a very reliable sign).
- The buttock on the affected side may appear flattened when the baby is prone.
- Reduced range of abduction is detected by placing the infant on his back with the hips flexed to 90 degrees and gently abducting the thighs simultaneously. The range of normal is wide, but the average is 75 degrees. Abduction may also be reduced in irritable hypertonic babies.
- The resistance to abduction may give way with a clunk as the head of the femur relocates. This sign becomes less common as the infant gets older, but may persist until the second year.
- With bilateral dislocation there may be a perineal gap between the thighs.

PROBLEMS AND CONCERNS
Concerns about motor development

Developmental examination at 6–9 months is very dependent on the infant's ability to give **motor** responses to stimuli. It may therefore be difficult to decide if an infant who is late in achieving motor milestones has purely a movement problem or whether this is simply a reflection of more general backwardness. Conversely, gross motor development may be normal or even advanced in spite of quite severe intellectual backwardness.

Some babies have rather low muscle tone, dislike the prone position and later, will shuffle on their bottoms or sit on one buttock and hitch themselves along with a hand on the floor.[4] These 'shufflers' are often late to walk (*see* also page 265). Also, there is often a family history of late walking.

Two common developmental concerns at this age are:

1 **Delay in reaching gross motor milestones.** There is no precise age at which one can say that delay in reaching a milestone, such as sitting, is pathological. As a rough guide, most babies can sit unsupported by 10 months, and almost all by 12 months. Most babies can stand by 13–14 months and walk by 18 months.

  'Generalised' or 'global slow development' (also called 'learning disability' or 'mental handicap') is an important cause of delayed gross motor development. There are likely to be corresponding deficits in fine motor skills and social behaviour. Responses to hearing and vision assessment may also be poor or immature (*see* page 235). Muscle tone is usually normal or reduced, but profound floppiness is rare and there is usually a reasonable range of spontaneous movement. Babies who present in this way may have one of many disorders and will need a detailed paediatric assessment.

  Cerebral palsy can usually be diagnosed by the age of 9 months. With this condition there is delay in motor milestones; a reduced range, speed and accuracy of movement (particularly of the hands); the muscle tone can be increased or decreased and often varies with position and handling. The baby does not *feel* right and his movements do not *look* right. Do not be misled by the absence of an abnormal birth history; many cerebral palsy cases are of unknown origin and cannot be explained on the basis of perinatal asphyxia or prematurity.

2 **Asymmetry of motor function.** This is usually first observed in the hand rather than the leg. Failure to use a hand, or apparent strong hand preference in the first year, is sufficient indication for referral. The baby may have congenital spastic hemiplegia or a brachial plexus lesion (Erb's palsy). There is also a benign developmental asymmetry called 'preferred head turning'. These babies always turn more to one side, have a strong hand preference and walk 'crabwise' (some of them also have an asymmetric head shape;[5] *see* page 265).

Clues to possible hearing impairment

At any time when a parent is worried about their child's hearing, there should be easy access to expert testing. In some clinics, self-referral is accepted and therefore delay is kept to a minimum. **When parents suspect a hearing loss, there is a high probability that *something* is wrong, though the diagnosis sometimes turns out to be a developmental problem rather than a hearing impairment.** Unfortunately, parents' conviction that their child has **normal** hearing is not so reliable, though their observations can be made more accurate by providing written information about normal hearing behaviour in the Personal Child Health Record. Ask the parent these questions:

▶ What do *you* think about his hearing?
▶ Do you have any worries at all about your child's hearing?
▶ *Why* do you think he can/cannot hear? Ask for examples:
  — listens and turns to voices;
  — wakes when bedroom door opens;
  — hears dog bark, parent's key in lock, etc.;
  — hears rustling of sweet or biscuit paper;
  — responds to name.
▶ Can he tell where a sound is coming from?
▶ Does he respond better if you raise your voice?
▶ Does his hearing seem to vary from day to day?

Consider if there are any high risk factors for **sensorineural deafness** in the past or family history. Babies with no risk factors who were not screened in the neonatal period should have a **hearing assessment at 7–9 months**. Concerns raised by parents, or any of the risk factors listed on page 181, are indications for referral to the audiology clinic at *any* age if neonatal testing has not been done.

Are there any pointers in the baby's history that suggest an increased risk of **secretory otitis media** (otitis with effusion, glue ear)? (*See* box on page 287.)

The infant distraction test

Screening for hearing loss using the distraction test, which used to be conducted by health visitors when the baby was 7–8 months old has been replaced by newborn screening and enhanced surveillance. The distraction test was found to be unreliable when used for whole population screening.[6] The procedure is described in Appendix 1, because distraction testing is still used for diagnostic purposes by trained audiology personnel.

Detection of vision defects

The terminology used to describe vision defects is summarised on page 185.

History

To ascertain the possibility of vision defects, ask the parents these questions:

- Have you any worries about his vision?
- Does he look at you and follow with his eyes?
- Does he look at his hands?
- Does he look at objects or pictures?
- Does he recognise you when he sees you?
- Does he look at tiny objects (e.g. crumbs on the floor)?
- Have you ever noticed a squint/cast/wandering or turning eye?
- Do both eyes look red in flash photos? (Several cases of retinoblastoma – tumour in the eye – have been discovered when parents reported that one eye looked grey or white rather than red in a photo.)
- Is there a family history of vision defects?

Squints tend to be more common in some families. If there is a sibling or parent with a squint, local guidelines may suggest that the child should have an orthoptic examination and refraction. Squint is most often noticed first by the parents or other family members, but they do not always regard it as important and may not mention it unless specifically asked. In some cases, refractive error may also be familial. It is unnecessary to refer infants solely on the grounds of a family history of myopia appearing later in childhood or in adult life. However, severe hypermetropia or astigmatism in a first degree relative may justify referral.

Observe the child's visual behaviour. Does he look at you, his parent, or around the room? Notice how he looks at toys or objects. There is rarely any doubt about a normal child's ability to see.

Inspect the eyes carefully. Look at the eye movements. Wandering or jerking movements are abnormal and are often a sign of poor vision. Nystagmus may be an isolated and often familial condition, or a feature of any disorder causing impaired visual fixation. It is not present at birth, but becomes evident within the first few months. Nystagmus in one eye only suggests poor vision in that eye. If one eye is smaller than the other it may have reduced vision.

Detection of squint. The most efficient way of detecting squint in infancy is to **ask the parents**. When parents report a squint they are usually correct, although they do experience the same difficulty as professionals in distinguishing between squint and pseudosquint.

Visual acuity. The measurement of visual acuity is very difficult in children too young to cooperate. Normal visual behaviour and conjugate gaze are the best indicators of satisfactory vision at this age. The ability to detect very small objects can be used to demonstrate visual behaviour. These tests are known as measures of 'minimum observable vision'. They do not assess the ability to separate adjacent visual stimuli and therefore are not capable of detecting minor degrees of refractive error. Their value is in exploring and recording impaired visual behaviour in infants, which is more often related to general developmental backwardness rather than primary vision disorders.

Infants show an obvious interest in objects of 1 or 2 mm diameter by 6 months of age, although they may not be able to grasp them. Tiny cake decorations (e.g. hundreds and thousands) are often used to test this. They should be placed on a dark, flat surface, and if the infant does not immediately show an interest they should be rolled around. (Note, however, that a visually impaired baby may appear to see a moving object, but be unable to fixate his gaze on it when it is stationary.) There may be an attempt to poke at the sweets with a finger tip. If you can only retain the child's attention with larger objects, consider whether this reflects developmental immaturity rather than a vision problem.

This procedure may be carried out with each eye patched in turn. If the baby objects violently to one eye being covered, but not the other, or there is an obvious difference between the two eyes in the ability to fixate, a unilateral defect should be suspected.

Formal examination of the eyes for refractive error and squint

Appendix 2 summarises the observations and procedures most commonly used by orthoptists and ophthalmologists to examine the eyes of infants and young children. Other staff should not use these methods unless they have been taught how to use the equipment and correctly interpret the results. The orthoptist spends 3 years learning these skills and they cannot be mastered in half an hour!

Research on automated methods of assessing vision in infants suggests that these might reduce the risk of squint and amblyopia, but as yet none of these approaches has been introduced for population screening.[7]

HEALTH EDUCATION TOPICS

When talking with parents about the development of their child at 6–12 months old, some or all of the topics listed below may be covered.

Immunisations. Are these up to date?

Developmental progress. Discuss the need for play and language stimulation and what parents can do to help by applying what is known about language development. Advise about **day care** if parents are concerned.

Introduce books and the idea of reading to babies. For example, the Bookstart scheme is a good introduction.[8] Parents are offered a pack of books, usually by the health visitor, when the baby is 7–9 months old, and parents are encouraged to join the local library. Early years librarians are often very helpful in suggesting suitable books for each age group. Babies enjoy looking at books with an adult; they listen to the sound of the adult voice and learn to be interested in books from an early age.

Sufficient stimulation. Contemporary middle class parents worry as to whether they are providing sufficient stimulation for their child's intellectual development. There is a risk that they will try too hard and put the child under unreasonable pressure or bombard him with stimulation that goes right over his head. Stimulation should be at the child's level of understanding; be relevant to his interests (must engage him); and allow for his participation in it as far as possible (be interactive).

Television can be appropriate when it is providing information, but less useful when it is just producing escapist entertainment.

Nutrition and diet. Discuss weaning; how to introduce a wide range of foods and flavours and to reduce the risk of obesity; dealing with eating problems.

Teeth. Careful and regular tooth brushing once teeth appear is essential. Parents need to be aware of the risks of sweet energy-dense drinks, both for dental disease and obesity.

Dentist. The child should be registered with a dentist and should attend at least once annually for a dental check-up and health advice.

Accident prevention. This is covered in Box 11.2.

BOX 11.2 Advice for accident prevention

From the crawling stage, infants can encounter all manner of dangers, which all too often are accidents just waiting to happen. Some ways to avoid these dangers are listed here.

Scalds: safety flexes should be coiled and dangling kettle flexes should be out of reach. Cups of tea are a common cause of scalds. Where and when do you have your cup of tea?

Falls: make sure the child is properly restrained in buggies and highchairs. Put a gate across stairs – top and/or bottom – depending where the infant is. Take care with baby-walkers, but preferably, don't use them as they are potentially dangerous (*see* page 205).

Car seat: is the car seat safe, secure and correctly fitted? Is the child always strapped in? Some parents are reluctant to be firm about this – with tragic consequences if they are involved in an accident. Do not put a baby in a car seat on a surface such as a table, unless supervised, as infants can fall off and suffer severe injuries.

Poisoning: keep medicines and household products out of reach (including dishwasher powder).

Cuts: beware of sharp edges on furniture and toys.

Choking: keep small objects out of reach.[*]

Severe sunburn: there is an increased risk of skin tumours in later life after severe sunburn in early childhood. Children with fair hair, pale skin and freckles are particularly at risk. The SunSmart campaign run by Cancer Research UK advises:

- Stay in the shade from 11 to 3.
- Make sure you never burn.
- Always cover up – wear a t-shirt, hat and wraparound sunglasses.
- Remember, children burn more easily.
- Then use factor 15+ sunscreen.

Use shades and umbrellas; wear long sleeves and hats when in the sun – it makes no difference how hot it is.[†]

---

[*] *See* factsheet: *Choking Accidents* www.capt.org.uk

[†] *See* http://info.cancerresearchuk.org/healthyliving/sunsmart/

REFERENCES

1 Berk LE. *Child Development*. New York: Pearson Educational; 2005.
2 Department of Health. *Child Health Promotion Programme*. London: DH; 2008. Available at: www.dh.gov.uk/en/Publicationsandstatistics/Publications/DH_083645 (accessed 2 January 2009).
3 National Screening Committee: www.nsc.nhs.uk
4 Robson P. Shuffling, hitching, scooting or sliding: some observations in 30 otherwise normal children. *Dev Med Child Neurol*. 1970; **12**(5): 608–17.
5 Robson P. Persisting head turning in the early months: some effects in the early years. *Dev Med Child Neurol*. 1968; **10**(1): 82–92.
6 Russ SA, Poulakis Z, Wake M, *et al*. The distraction test: the last word? *J Paediatr Child Health*. 2005; **41**(4): 197–200.
7 Atkinson J, Braddick O, Nardini M, *et al*. Infant hyperopia: detection, distribution, changes and correlates-outcomes from the Cambridge infant screening programs. *Optom Vis Sci*. 2007; **84**(2): 84–96.
8 www.bookstart.org.uk

1–2 years

NORMAL DEVELOPMENT: 12–24 MONTHS[1]

Language acquisition

The pace of language acquisition varies enormously. Nearly all 18-month-olds can understand some words and many can respond to simple commands; for example, 'put the car on the table'. The normal 18-month-old child may have no words or as many as 200. Some will start to join words at or before this age. By the age of two, the vocabulary may be many hundreds of words, but some normal children will have few or none. Most will be joining two or even three words to make short sentences.

Books

In the first 18 months of life, behaviour with books is influenced to some extent by how much parents or childcare staff use books with the child. The responses the child gives depend on whether he is shown his own familiar books or one that he has never seen before.[2]

Before the child is 15 months old, a book is usually treated like any other attractive object. From 15–18 months, the child shows active interest in the pictures; he may turn pages though often several at a time. By the age of 2, most children can turn pages singly.

Play

Between 12 and 15 months, play and experimentation with objects occupy the infant for long periods. He learns about the relationships between objects, putting things in and out of containers or dropping them on the floor. He begins to demonstrate by appropriate use that he understands the function of common objects, such as a hairbrush or a cup and spoon (*see* Figure 12.1).

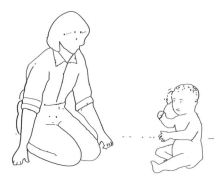

FIGURE 12.1 Definition by use.

By 18 months, the toddler is exploring actively, opening cupboards, climbing on furniture and so on. He understands daily routines and tries to imitate housework and other adult activities. The relationships between shapes and the properties of liquids and solid objects are investigated. He plays with miniature toys; for example dolls or cars, but the activities performed with them are still fragmentary and it is a few more months before he will act out detailed sequences with them.

It is normal for a child to pass through a phase of putting objects in the mouth and throwing them away ('casting') but this does not last for long and does not usually persist beyond 18 months (apart from dummies or pacifiers). If casting (other than in a temper tantrum) or persistent indiscriminate mouthing of objects continues beyond the age of 2, this is a worrying sign suggestive of some developmental problem.[3]

Attention control

The infant's attention is very focused and, once immersed in an interesting activity, he has great difficulty in absorbing spoken instructions or suggestions offered by demonstration. The ability to handle several streams of information simultaneously is a more sophisticated skill that emerges between 18 and 36 months. This is also a period of increasing social poise, self-confidence and independence.

Attachment and security

Very strong attachments are shown to his caregivers and the child may still be wary of strangers, although this varies considerably as some toddlers make friends very easily. The process of development can be facilitated by the continued involvement of the caregiver who can offer encouragement and security. There is a gap between the problem-solving that the child can manage independently and the level that he can achieve with guidance. Within this area (called the 'zone of proximal development' by the Russian psychologist Vygotsky) adults can facilitate active learning by interventions at appropriate moments, while still allowing the child to make his own discoveries whenever possible.[1]

Atypical patterns of development

A child can have severe delay in language development yet understand the rules of social behaviour and show advanced ideas in the way he plays. The clearest example of this is seen in the late-diagnosed, partially hearing child and such a pattern of development should always raise a suspicion of hearing loss. However, more commonly, one finds that the child who has slow language development is also immature in the development of attention control, the acquisition of social skills and the emergence of imaginative play. Impaired social and communicative skills may offer early clues to a diagnosis of autism spectrum disorder.

Friendship

Infants show an interest in each other even in the first year of life, and in the second year they begin to initiate games that involve imitation; for example jumping or banging a toy. Gradually they develop more joint understanding and by the second birthday may be starting to use words to influence each other's behaviour. Some children as young as 18 months can form quite firm friendships and show real distress if these are disrupted; for example, if there is a change of playgroup or if the family moves house.[4]

Motor development
Age 12–14 months

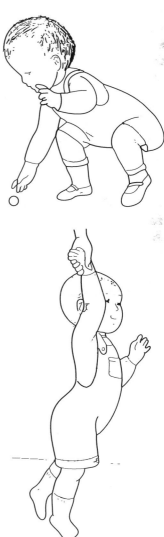

- The precise stage at which a toddler walks alone varies with his personality and physical make-up. This is usually between 12 and 15 months, but may vary by several months earlier or later.
- Independent mobility is more important to the child than the method used.
- For many children, crawling remains their chosen method of mobility for a prolonged period. Walking is no more important to the toddler than any other skill which gives him control over his world (e.g. manipulation, communication or socialisation).

Mobility:

- The toddler has the ability to crawl, pull up to standing, cruise, return to the floor, push a chair or a truck and an infinite variation or combination of these.
- He will cruise along the furniture, drop to crawling to bridge a gap and rise to standing again at the next piece of furniture.
- He will walk with one hand held.
- He may rise to standing in free space without the support of furniture, but his balance is hazardous!

▶ He may drop from standing to sitting or crawling in free space.

▶ He adopts numerous varieties of sitting positions thus allowing himself to get close to his toys (e.g. side-sitting with legs wind-swept to one side or sitting on heels bunny style).

▶ He bends down from standing to retrieve a fallen toy.

▶ He hitches along the floor on his bottom.

▶ He can move from place to place while hoarding objects in his hands (e.g. crawls around with a brick in each hand).

▶ He experiments with his body in relation to objects: crawls under chairs and tables, sits up and bumps his head, climbs up into chairs and onto tables.

Grasp and manipulation:

▶ Can grasp with almost adult precision, but release is still not fully developed.

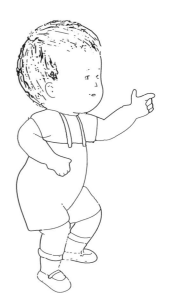

▶ Can now release an object in an intended direction, but it takes time and effort.

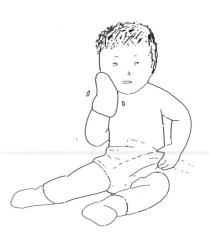

- Plays with objects and containers.
- Enjoys fitting things together.
- Places round shapes into posting box.
- Attempts to build cube tower: places brick on top of brick, but fails to release with precision.
- By 13 months can grasp two cubes in one hand simultaneously.

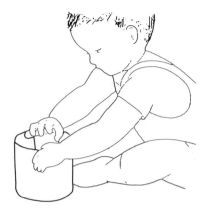

Age 15–18 months

- The toddler has adopted walking as his most usual means of mobility.
- He uses a wide-based gait to increase his stability and will retain this for several months, returning to it when attempting demanding physical tasks.
- Release of objects has become sophisticated, enabling him to engage in building, throwing and posting games.

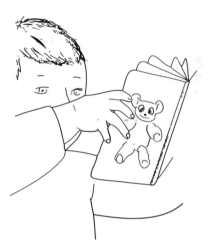

Mobility:

- Walks alone on a wide-based gait.
- Rarely falls.
- Attempts to run, but knees remain stiff and feet flat on the floor.
- Climbs stairs on all fours or walks up with one hand held and the other on rail or stair.
- Descends stairs by hitching on bottom or sliding down on stomach.
- Kneels upright unaided.
- Moves with increasing fluency between standing and squatting, and squatting and standing.

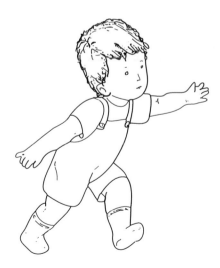

Grasp and manipulation:

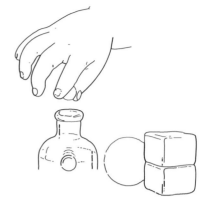

- Balance now adequate to free hands for manipulation.
- Release of objects is well developed.
- Places rings over a post.
- Builds tower of two cubes.
- Manoeuvres cubes into post box.
- Throws ball to adult.
- Carries toys for most of day, tucked under arm.
- Turns pages of books.
- Scribbles spontaneously, mostly circular, but some vertical strokes.

Age 18–24 months

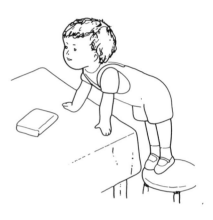

- By 2 years the toddler has become a physically confident, ambulant child.
- He has an increasing repertoire of mobility and dexterity with which to explore his world.
- The physical skills which he acquired in the first 18 months of life form the basis of all his future refinement of movement.

Mobility:

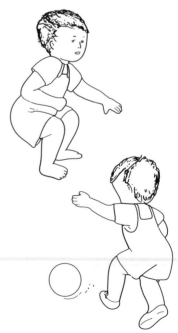

- Climbs up stairs with two feet on each step, hand on rail much of the time (he is returning to three points of balance because the task is risky).
- Runs fast and with flexibility of knees and ankles.
- Changes direction.
- Kicks a ball without falling over. Jumps with both feet together.
- Can bend to retrieve a toy and play for long periods in either squatting or semi-squatting position (half way between standing and squatting).
- Sits in long-sitting (with legs straight out in front) for long periods looking at a book or playing with a doll on lap.
- Sits astride a tricycle and paddles it along, but takes little interest in the pedals.

Grasp and manipulation:

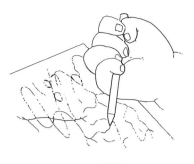

- Increased movement of wrists and rotation of forearms.
- Now opens and shuts doors, twisting handle.
- Puts on socks.
- Builds tower of six cubes.
- Turns individual pages of book.
- Starts to join large Lego type bricks.
- Places objects in precise positions constructing neat rows and lines.
- Draws vertical and horizontal strokes.
- Places and manoeuvres simple jigsaw pieces.
- Uses non-dominant hand to steady objects.
- Starts to manoeuvre objects within hand – no longer puts them down to turn them around – may use body to assist.
- Emerging use of individual fingers to assist in manipulation.

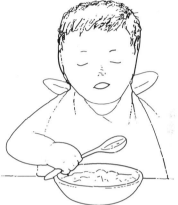

IMPORTANT TOPICS BETWEEN 12 AND 24 MONTHS
Reviewing the 12- to 24-month-old child

Children in this age group are particularly difficult to evaluate in a clinic or consulting room and if either parents or professionals have any concerns it is often better to make a home visit. There are no formal screening tests in the second year of life, but developmental guidance, information on playgroups or nurseries, and help with behavioural and eating problems, are often appreciated.

Whether or not children are seen for routine review is largely a matter of policy and resource allocation. In some cases, an agreement can be made with parents during the child's first year that no further routine reviews are needed and they can be invited to contact their GP or health visitor if there are any concerns. Other parents may welcome continuing support and guidance in managing their child. The content of any consultation depends on the reason for the review and may include any or all of the following:

- A **physical examination** is *not* included as a routine at this age but, depending on the reason for the consultation, it may be important to examine the child and to measure the **weight** and the **height** or **length** (page 131).
- Observe if the child is **walking** and whether the **gait is normal**. By 18 months, 97% of children are walking.
- No attempt should be made to screen for vision or hearing defects except by simple observation and by asking the parents appropriate questions. Refer any

child if you or the parents have worries about hearing problems, or squint or vision defects.

▶ Review **language development**. Although most children are beginning to produce some words and to show more definite evidence of understanding language, the variation is too wide and evaluation is too difficult to recommend formal whole-population screening for language delays and disorders.[5] Ask the parents about the child's **use of words** and **understanding of instructions**. Observe how the child responds to any comments or remarks made to him by the parent, and to any extraneous noises in the room.

▶ Discuss ways in which children can be helped to develop their language and play abilities.

▶ Watch how the child **plays with toys**. Note persistence of **mouthing** and **casting**; this usually indicates that the child does not understand their function or symbolic meaning and by the second birthday this behaviour should have disappeared or at most be only occasional and brief.

▶ Ascertain the child's **social skills** by asking the parents, supported by observation as necessary. By the age of 2, most children can use a spoon and a cup adequately without spilling, can remove several items of clothing, try to put on their shoes, appreciate the functions of a book so that pages are turned singly, and play for a short time alone.

▶ Often the main concerns at this age are to do with **management issues**, such as tantrums, sleep disturbances, food fads or poor appetite, toilet training battles and so on. Some parents value advice on how to deal with these; others may simply want reassurance that their approach is sensible. These common problems are discussed elsewhere in this book.

▶ **Iron deficiency** is quite common at this age, particularly in children who are fussy eaters or have small appetites. This may be a cause of irritability, developmental and behavioural problems as well as anaemia.[6]

▶ **Developmental needs.** Discuss the importance of mixing with other children, learning to play with them and to share possessions; playgroups and nurseries; language stimulation.

▶ **Behavioural difficulties.** Disturbance of sleep, eating battles, toilet training, tantrums are all *very* common.

▶ It is normal for the 2-year-old to be **aggressive** in defence of his possessions and to play alongside rather than *with* other children. (*See* page 326 for more information about aggression.)

COMMON ISSUES AND CONCERNS
Speech and language acquisition

By 21 months, 75% of children can point to a named body part and **follow a single instruction**. The parent may be able to give equivalent examples (e.g. 'Where's your nose?', 'Take the shoes to Daddy'). Between 80% and 90% of children aged 2 can understand at least one such request. The more advanced child will be able to identify pictures, and be able to point to pictures that indicate actions such as running, jumping or crying (e.g. 'Which girl is running?')

Strategies that support language development

Many factors affect the rate of language development. One of these is the interaction between parent and child[7] and it is possible to teach parents to interact more effectively. Box 12.1 summarises some of the strategies that can be used.

BOX 12.1 Interaction between parent and child

Child oriented strategies
Encourage parents to:

- follow the child's lead by talking about the topic and activity that is holding his attention;
- wait for the child to respond;
- use a pace of language that allows the child time to process it.

Responses that promote interaction

- Looking at and reading books together: parents should be encouraged to join their local library and to meet the early years librarian.
- Engaging the child in conversation.
- Using open questions (i.e. questions that cannot be answered solely by 'Yes' or 'No').
- Encourage the parent to take turns with the child in conversation.
- Encourage the use of comments rather than mainly questions.
- Viewing TV and DVDs: unrestricted, unsupervised viewing is undesirable, but can be helpful if appropriate material is chosen. The parent sits with the child while viewing and uses the programme as a basis for conversation (as with books).

Modelling of language
Encourage parents to:

- provide good models of language for the child to imitate, including labelling, and the use of varying grammatical forms (verbs, adjectives, adverbs, etc.);
- repeat, expand and paraphrase what the child says;
- focus on content of what the child is trying to say rather than pronunciation or factual accuracy.

Recognising language delay

The problem for the health professional is that between 10% and 20% of children are quite slow in language development and this figure may be substantially higher in areas of poverty or deprivation. The challenge is two-fold: (i) to distinguish between those children who, in spite of a normal family background, are slow in starting to talk and who have a good prognosis, from those whose environment offers insufficient opportunities for language acquisition; and (ii) to identify the minority who have a more serious and potentially disabling problem underlying their difficulties with language.

It is also important to ensure that spurious explanations are dismissed and not used as an excuse for inaction. Conversely, parents often complain that professionals have offered them spurious reassurance instead of arranging an expert assessment. Some parents may wait until the child is in his third year before taking action, hoping that he will improve. So when they do finally seek advice, one can be reasonably sure that there is a problem and their concerns, or those of any professional who knows the child, must be taken seriously.

Spurious explanations

The following are often put forward as 'explanations' for delay in speech and language development:

- exposure to more than one language is holding him back;
- boys are always slower than girls;
- second children are slower than first;
- twins have a secret language;
- he is lazy;
- his mother doesn't talk to him.

Differences between boys and girls, birth order effects and the 'secret' language of twins may play a small part in some cases, but in general such 'explanations' should be rejected, at least until other causes have been excluded. Deprivation, parental depression, poverty and neglect are sometimes significant contributors to language delay, but the relationship between them is rarely simple.

Bilingual families

Research on language acquisition shows that the infant's brain can respond to any speech sound, but this ability disappears by the first birthday and he can no longer readily distinguish sounds not heard in his own language. For example, distinguishing 'r' and 'l' is difficult for those who grew up exposed only to Asian languages where these sounds are interchangeable. The child who listens to and learns two languages from infancy has all their language activity in the same part of the brain; whereas if the child learns the second language later in childhood there will be two different areas of language activity. Thus it seems that the process of learning two languages simultaneously in very early childhood is different from the acquisition of a second language later in childhood.

Bilingualism has positive benefits for the child.[*] Children in bilingual families learn both languages almost as fast as monoglot children, but they can quickly lose one of the languages if they do not use it. This may occur as a result of family relocation, separation, or school entry. When two languages are learned together in early childhood, the vocabulary size in each language may initially be somewhat smaller than in the monolingual child, but the gap is soon closed. Children learning a second language at school age may take much longer than pre-schoolers to become fluent. A second language may present more difficulty when a young child arrives in a new country; for example as a refugee, and has to stop using his native language, as yet incompletely mastered, and learn a new one (*see* page 88).

Bilingualism may cause more problems for a child who, for genetic or neurological

---

[*] *See* 'Supporting Children Learning English as an Additional Language', Department for Education and Skills (now Department for Children, Schools and Families): 2007. Available at: www.standards.dfes.gov.uk/primary/publications/foundation_stage/eal_eyfs/eal_eyfs

reasons, has a major developmental deficit in language skills, though this is uncertain. Therapists and teachers working with young children whose first language is not English often have difficulties in assessing and treating those with suspected language difficulties.

Gesture and sign
When parents use both gesture and speech together to communicate with their child before the child learns to talk, word learning can probably be helped (and there is no evidence that it is impaired). The parents often feel that their interaction with their child becomes closer.*

Deaf parents
Children with normal hearing who are living with deaf parents can acquire normal speech, if they have 5–10 hours of exposure to fluent speakers each week.

Twins
Twins often acquire speech slightly slower than singletons. This is likely because of the reduced quantity and increased complexity of parent-twins verbal interactions.[7]

Recognising the child with a serious language development problem
Although 80–90% of 18-month-old children can say at least a few words, delay in beginning to speak is of less concern at this age *provided that* there is evidence that the child understands when the parent(s) talk to him (i.e. comprehension of speech). A child who uses less than six words at age 2 is at the slow end of the range, but although understandably worrying to parents, this is not necessarily abnormal. The parents may recognise the child's frustration at being unable to communicate his ideas or wants, often expressed as tantrums. This problem reaches its peak incidence early in the third year.

Sometimes it may help to use a structured instrument, such as the Sure Start Language Measure (*see* page 195), to get a clearer idea of the child's abilities, particularly if it is anticipated that obtaining an expert assessment will be delayed. However, perhaps the best solution is a speech and language service that offers a triage clinic; this should be run by experienced therapists who can see children quickly and make a decision as to whether further follow-up, assessment and intervention are needed and whether a hearing assessment is also required.

There is more likely to be a **serious problem** if:

▶ the child is very silent: he does not vocalise or make any sounds that seem like attempts to say words;
▶ there is persistent or continuous dribbling;
▶ the child has significant problems with chewing and swallowing;
▶ there is other evidence of a movement disorder, such as floppiness or clumsiness, which might suggest a more widespread problem;
▶ the child does not show any desire to communicate by any means (*see* next section on autism);
▶ a child of 18 months with little or no **understanding** of simple familiar words

---

* For example, *see* www.babysigns.com

and phrases spoken by the parent, or a 2-year-old unable to show, for example by pointing, that he can identify some toys or objects correctly when they are named, should be regarded with concern;

▶ sometimes, the child whose speech and comprehension are delayed in this age group is also somewhat immature in other respects, notably in play, concentration and attention control; the child who cannot maintain his attention on any task is at increased risk of having persistent developmental and behavioural difficulties.

If you see a child with substantial difficulty in comprehension, but who has well-developed play and normal social interactions, the diagnosis is **hearing loss** until proved otherwise. Any child in this age range who does present with concern regarding poor *understanding* of speech *must* have a **hearing test** before any conclusions can be drawn about the cause of the delay in comprehension. There is no screening test suitable for routine clinic use in this age group. Any doubt about hearing is an indication for referral to the second-tier audiology clinic. This remains true even if the child passed a newborn screening test as not all deafness is present at birth.

Early recognition of autism spectrum disorder

Autism spectrum disorders (ASDs) are diagnosed on the basis of abnormalities in social, communicative and imaginative behaviours, and the presence of repetitive and stereotyped patterns of interests and activities.[8] The degree of abnormality in each of these dimensions can vary widely, hence the considerable variability in the clinical features[9] (*see* Box 12.2) and the confusing variety of terms used to describe the observed patterns: autism, autistic spectrum disorder, Asperger's syndrome and pervasive developmental disorder.

It used to be thought that autism was rare, but we now know that at least 4 in every 1000 children have autism and another 8 have other autism spectrum conditions, but the true figure may be even higher. This apparent increase is probably due to greater recognition and willingness to use the label, particularly in children with normal intelligence who are coping in mainstream settings; in these children, the diagnosis is often delayed.

Some children with ASDs show atypical behavioural patterns even in infancy; whereas others seem normal to start with and then 'become' autistic. Between one-fifth and one-half of children with autism show regression after apparently normal early development (although studies of videos made when the baby was thought to be normal sometimes show that they were less likely to look at others, point to objects or respond to their name). Spurious explanations for apparent regression are common (e.g. moving house), but the most recent explanation among some people is the concern that autism might be caused by the MMR vaccine. This concern still persists among some parents in spite of overwhelming evidence that there is really no connection (*see* Chapter 8).

As public awareness of autism and ASDs has increased, parents are more often the first to suspect autism; indeed, the proliferation of checklists on the internet may lead to over-diagnosis by parents. However, early features may be subtle and it can be hard to recognise social impairment in toddlers, though this may become more obvious when the child starts a playgroup. Slightly older children with autism ignore people, like to be alone and lack eye contact, gestures or expression. Social uncommunicative impairment is probably the best indicator. Reports of unusually rapid growth in head circumference in infancy are of theoretical interest, but are not useful as a means of early identification.

BOX 12.2 The range of behaviours seen in children with autism spectrum disorder[9]

A child's problems with *friendships* are on the continuum from:

- friendships break down; to
- wants friends but can't make them; to
- doesn't see the need for special friends; to
- no interest in others.

The level of a child's problems with *imaginative play* ranges from:

- shows imaginative play alone, but not with others; to
- scripted or late developing imaginative play; to
- no imaginative play.

Language problems range from:

- subtle language difficulties; to
- disordered, difficult to understand language; to
- single words or babble; to
- no language.

The severity of *repetitive behaviours* ranges from trivial to overwhelming:

- has routines;
- increased flapping;
- upset when routines disturbed;
- rigid;
- severely restricted interests;
- continuous self-harm.

Several screening procedures for ASDs are being developed, but as yet none is ideal for population screening. The CHAT (Checklist for Autism in Toddlers) is the best-known screening procedure in the UK.[8] It was designed to help professionals to identify autism in children 18 months old. This age was chosen because it is a good time to identify key behaviours that would be present in most normally developing children. The CHAT assesses simple pretend play (appropriate use of a tea set, doll play, object substitution) and the joint attentional behaviours, pointing for interest (in combination with eye contact) and following gaze, by parental report and by professional observation and direct testing (*see* Box 12.3 for details). The CHAT has not been introduced as a general screening test for two main reasons: first, it is important to administer it fairly close to the age of 18 months for which it was designed, otherwise it is less effective (and this presents practical problems); second, it does not adequately fulfil the UK criteria for a screening test (*see* Chapter 9).

The Modified Checklist for Autism in Toddlers (M-CHAT)[10] has not been widely adopted in the UK so far.

For primary care staff, the challenge is to recognise the early features and to respond to parental anxieties. When an ASD is suspected, a checklist such as the Social Communication Questionnaire or the M-CHAT can be used to decide if expert assessment is needed, but these should only be used by those who have received appropriate training and as part of an agreed local referral pathway. The investigation, diagnosis and management of ASDs is largely the province of child development teams and in many districts suspected cases will be referred direct to a team with particular expertise in this area. They will have access to formal diagnostic methods and their assessment is often crucial in obtaining the best available intervention for the child.

Parents value early recognition and intervention although it is not yet clear how much this alters the long-term outcome for the child. For children with major social communication problems, long-term interventions can produce significant behavioural gains, especially when they are very intensive. However, the benefits fade away after the intensive input ends, and no current intervention can be regarded as a 'cure' for ASDs. Programmes may involve speech and language therapy, medication, one-to-one help in school, specialist behaviour management (provided by schools and Child and Adolescent Mental Health Services (CAMHS)), specialist education in mainstream schools, and special or residential schools. As ASDs vary widely in severity, no single intervention is likely to suit every child.[11]

BOX 12.3 The five key items on the CHAT screen

Ask the parent:

1 Does your child ever PRETEND, for example, to make a cup of tea using a toy cup and teapot, or pretend other things?
2 Does your child ever use his/her index finger to point, to indicate INTEREST in something?

Health practitioner observation:

3 Get child's attention, then point across the room at an interesting object and say 'Oh look! There's a (name of toy)!' Watch the child's face. Does the child look across to see what you are pointing at?
4 Get the child's attention, then give the child a miniature toy cup and teapot and say 'Can you make a cup of tea?' Does the child pretend to pour out tea, drink it, etc.?
5 Say to the child 'Where's the light?', or 'Show me the light'. Does the child POINT with his/her index finger at the light? To record YES on this item the child must have looked up at your face around the time of pointing.

Based on Baird, et al.[8] with permission from BMJ Publishing Group.

Common movement problems

It is surprisingly rare in the UK that late walking is the presenting complaint in this 12- to 24-month age group. There are two likely reasons for this: either the child has already been diagnosed as having some neurological or developmental disorder, or the parents decide not to seek referral because they have a family history of late walking. Nevertheless, it is wise to look carefully at any child who is not walking at 18 months.

Unilateral dislocation of the hip

Unilateral dislocation of the hip will give rise to a limp and is unlikely to be overlooked. Delay in walking may occur, but is unusual. However, many children with late presenting unilateral hip dislocation have other features whose significance is easily overlooked. For example, the parents report that the child: is walking on tiptoe; has a short leg; can only place one foot on the ground in the baby-walker; has difficulty in crawling; has a 'funny walk'; is dragging one leg; has an inability to sit astride a bicycle or adult's knee; falls to one side; has pain on walking; and grating or clicking sensations are felt by the adult when holding the child. Parents and professionals often assume that a dislocated hip must be very painful, but this is not usually the case in children with congenital dislocation.[12]

Bilateral dislocation of the hips

Bilateral dislocation of the hips is associated with a delay in walking in some children, but the majority walk at the normal time. The gait is waddling and there is a marked lumbar lordosis. Observe the gait carefully. Any boy who has an **abnormal gait**, evidence of weakness on stairs or steps, or does not learn to run within a few months of starting to walk, or who has difficulty in stooping and recovering the upright position, should be referred for a blood CPK test to exclude Duchenne muscular dystrophy. Note that the signs of muscular dystrophy are occasionally mistaken for those of hip disorders and vice versa! *See* page 244 for further details.

Bottom shufflers

Babies who are bottom shufflers are rather floppy, slow to sit, dislike being placed in a prone position, tend to stick their legs out in front of them when held vertically, instead of placing their feet down and taking weight, and shuffle on their bottoms instead of walking. They walk late, sometimes as late as 30 months. There is often a positive family history of shuffling. If you do not know about it, you may wrongly suspect cerebral palsy or muscle disease. But babies with these disorders may also shuffle![13]

Tiptoe walking

Tiptoe walking is an unusual pattern of development. In most cases it is intermittent and the feet can be placed flat on the floor. The balance is often remarkably good – it has to be to permit the ballerina gait characteristic of these toddlers. Occasionally the heel-cords are very tight and although spontaneous resolution by the age of 3 is the rule, a physiotherapy assessment is reassuring to both doctor and parent. If there is any additional feature, such as weakness or a family history of any neuromuscular disorder, full paediatric evaluation is essential.[14] Children with other developmental problems, such as autism, may occasionally walk on tip toe.

Hand preference

Right or left handedness is not usually established during the first year. Hand preference may be detected by the first birthday in about 10% of children. By the second birthday, most children show hand preference, but it is not well established until age 3–5. Strong hand preference in infants suggests some abnormality in the non-preferred limb.

Common minor orthopaedic anomalies: frequent falls and funny feet [15]

Two common and often related complaints in children who have just begun to walk are that the child falls too often and that the feet 'do not look right'. The most common problems are **in-toeing, out-toeing, metatarsus adductus** (banana-shaped feet), **knock knees, bow legs** and **flat feet**. Correct diagnosis of these usually benign problems and adequate explanation and reassurance for the parents depend on an understanding of normal growth patterns in the lower limbs. The femur and tibia spiral as they grow and therefore, during growth, the feet may not point the same way as the legs. They may point inward (**in-toeing**), so that each can catch on the other leg as the child runs. If they point outwards (**out-toeing**), they may catch on obstacles, again leading to more falls than expected. Consider the following points in conjunction with Figure 12.2:

▶ Establish if there is a family history of bone or joint disease or any evidence of progressive deterioration in gait. In most cases neither is present and the parents can confirm that although the child falls frequently, he is walking, running and climbing and becoming progressively more expert at these skills. If there is any doubt about these points, consider the possibility of **muscular dystrophy** or **cerebral palsy**.

▶ Watch the child walking and running. If there is any limp or asymmetry of gait or any hint of weakness, specialist referral is advisable.

▶ Even if the child has been screened previously, congenital dislocation of the hips can be missed, particularly if the condition is bilateral. This results in a waddling gait with protruding buttocks. With the child supine, flex the hips and look for limitation of abduction. Obtain an x-ray if there is any doubt.

▶ Always look at the base of the spine for abnormalities characteristic of **occult spinal dysraphism**.

Once any serious problems have been excluded, take a more careful look at the child's feet and legs.

In-toeing

This can be associated with one or more of the following:

▶ **Femoral neck anteversion.** In infancy, the angle between the femoral neck and head, and the femoral shaft is different from that observed in the older child and adult. Instead of pointing inwards, the head and neck point forwards. As the child grows, the femur spirals until the adult position is reached. If the child starts to walk while the femoral heads are still pointing forwards, the child rotates the leg inwards as he walks, in order to maintain the position of the femoral head firmly in the acetabulum. The child therefore walks with the knee-caps facing each other and the feet pointing inwards. This can be demonstrated to the parents by placing the child prone and showing that the legs can be rotated inwards often to 90 degrees, whereas the outward or external rotation is greatly reduced (Figures 12.2a, 12.2b). This apparently alarming 'deformity' almost always resolves with growth, usually by age 8 or 9 years, and no treatment should be given or suggested.

▶ **Tibial torsion.** The tibia spirals as it grows in the same way as the femur. If the growth and rotation of the tibia is out of step with that of the femur, the foot may be either inwardly or outwardly rotated. Inward rotation of the foot is associated with internal tibial torsion and leads to in-toeing. It is usually associated with outward curving of the tibia, giving an apparent bow-leg appearance. Clinical assessment is rather more difficult than in the case of the thigh. It is necessary to assess the thigh-foot angle as shown in Figure 12.2c.

▶ **Metatarsus adductus (varus).** Some children have feet with an inward curve between the heel and the toes, giving the foot the appearance of a banana. The condition is distinguished from clubfoot by the normal position and appearance of the heel. In most cases the deformity is minor and corrects spontaneously. The child need only be referred if the deformity is severe (Figures 12.2d, 12.2e).

Out-toeing

Parents often become alarmed when they observe that as the child stands and begins to walk, the feet turn out, sometimes to nearly 90 degrees. Examination shows that the hips are externally rotated and internal rotation is much reduced (the opposite situation to that shown in Figure 12.2a). Spontaneous correction occurs in most cases and no treatment is needed.

Knock knees and bow legs

A mild degree of bow legs (genu varus) is commonly seen up to the age of 2 (Figure 12.2f) and between 2 and 4 years old, knock knees (genu valgus) is a normal finding (Figure 12.2 g). The degree of rotation of the hips should be checked because internal rotation of the hips leads to the appearance of knock knees. The extent of the deformity is easily determined. For bow legs, the ankles are brought together until they just touch and the distance between the knees is measured. To assess the degree of knock knees, the knees are brought together until the inside of the knees just touch and the feet are pointing straight forward. The distance between the malleoli of the ankles is measured and recorded. Up to 6 or 7 cm is generally accepted as normal in each case. However, *progressive* genu varus is an indication for referral as it may be caused by Blount's disease.

Rickets is only rarely the cause of knock knees or bow legs, and other diseases causing these deformities are even less common, but if the child is unwell or miserable in any way, or has a poor diet (*see* Chapter 6) he should be referred for paediatric assessment.

Other foot problems

Parents may become anxious about **flat feet**, particularly if they had supposedly 'suffered' from flat feet in childhood themselves. The child should be asked to stand on tiptoe. If the arch is seen to form normally when he does this the foot is normal and no treatment is required (Figure 12.2 h).

High arched or 'cavus' feet, and **clawing of the toes**, are more likely to be abnormal and may have a neurological cause; such children should be referred. Over-riding of the fifth toe over the fourth is common and though not serious can be a troublesome problem to treat. Attractive simple solutions such as strapping do not help, but if necessary, the toe can be straightened by surgery.

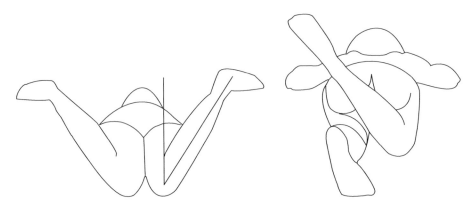

FIG 12.2A (assessing medial rotation) and **B** (assessing lateral rotation). How to assess hip rotation: the child should be lying prone on the examination couch. Flex the knees to 90°. Hold the feet and move them outwards so that the thighs rotate inwards (medially). With femoral neck anteversion, rotation may be to 90°. Then move each leg in turn so that the thigh rotates outwards (laterally). With femoral neck anteversion, this will be much reduced compared to the medial rotation.

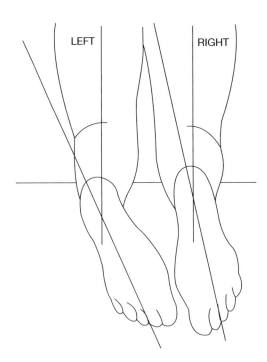

FIGURE 12.2C How to assess thigh-foot angle. The child should be lying prone on the examination couch. Flex the knees to 90°. Hold the ankles and look down on the feet. Draw an imaginary line through the axis of the foot – from the middle toe to the heel. Then draw an imaginary line through the axis of the thigh. The angle between the two axes is the thigh-foot angle. The 'normal' value is around 10° of out-toeing, i.e. the foot points slightly outwards relative to the thigh. In the figure, the right foot shows slight (normal) outward rotation relative to the thigh while the left shows inward rotation associated with internal tibial torsion. A difference between the two legs is common.

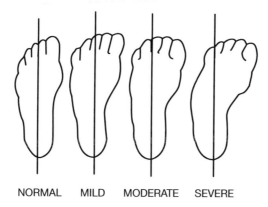

NORMAL   MILD   MODERATE   SEVERE

FIGURE 12.2D Metatarsus adductus (banana shaped feet).

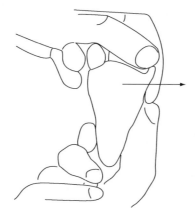

FIGURE 12.2E Check that the adducted foot is flexible by stabilising the heel and gently abducting the forefoot.

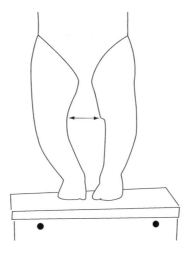

FIGURE 12.2F Bow legs (genu varus) – measure the inter-condylar distance to assess severity.

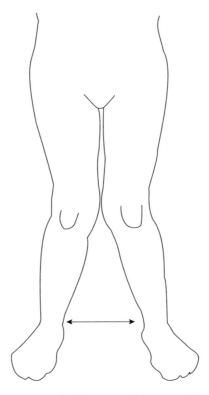

FIGURE 12.2G Knock knees – (genu valgus). Measure the distance between the malleoli to assess severity.

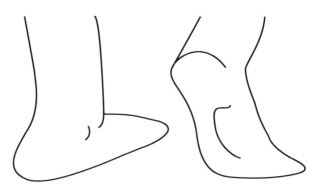

FIGURE 12.2H Flat feet. Young children's feet often look flat but if the arch forms normally when the child stands on tiptoe, the foot is normal.

Referral

The child should be referred if any deformity appears to be asymmetrical, deteriorating, or unusually severe. Often parental concern will only be eliminated by a specialist opinion, even if the primary care staff are confident that the child's physical findings are within the normal range.

COMMON MANAGEMENT PROBLEMS
Breath-holding

There are two sorts of breath-holding spells: blue and white.

Blue (cyanotic) spells are seen in babies and toddlers and are not uncommon, affecting perhaps 5% of all children and they appear to run in families. A typical spell is precipitated by frustration and rage; furious crying halts at the end of expiration after a few yells. The glottis is then held closed, blocking inspiration. After about 5 seconds, cyanosis can be seen and the child loses consciousness. There may be a rigid opisthotonic posture, and sometimes a few clonic movements. Recovery is swift and complete. Differentiation from epilepsy and cardiac problems is made on the basis of a clear precipitant, a clear history of forceful crying before consciousness is lost, and the absence of confusion or drowsiness afterwards.

Consider whether the child has iron deficiency **anaemia**. If so, correction of the anaemia can abolish the behaviour. The mechanism is unknown.

Although parents are traditionally urged to ignore breath-holding spells, on the grounds that attention reinforces the 'habit', this is exceptionally difficult and the spells fade away as the child gets older, no matter how they are managed. What parents want to know is whether it is a dangerous habit (it is not), whether it is epilepsy (no) or may turn into it (also no), and how to terminate attacks when they occur. With respect to the latter, flicking drops of cold water on the baby's face sometimes works. (It is not necessary to provide a drenching with a tumblerful though!) The condition is benign and there is no risk of anoxic brain damage. Minimal intervention is the order of the day. Anticonvulsants and sedatives are useless. Should the above measures fail, the parents can be told to place the child in a safe place and carry on with what they are doing. They must avoid being manipulated by the child or becoming anxiously overprotective.

White (pallid) spells or reflex anoxic seizures are different.* Following surprise, pain or mild injury, such as bumping the head in a fall while learning to walk, the child falls to the ground limp and apnoeic. Robust crying does not precede apnoea, the breath is not clearly held in expiration, nor is cyanosis very prominent. The child's state reflects the effect of high vagal tone with bradycardia or even transient asystole.

An anoxic seizure may follow. This is aetiologically different from epilepsy since it is a consequence of cerebral ischaemia. (Words must be carefully chosen when explanations are given to parents so as to avoid unnecessary alarm.) Recovery is swift and uneventful unless a seizure has supervened, in which case some drowsiness is common.

It is sensible to check the cardiovascular system clinically, but there are no other investigations that are routinely helpful. Treatment is essentially reassurance and

---

* www.stars.org.uk is the parent support organisation.

advice to the parents to make sure the child comes to no harm during his brief spell of unconsciousness. They should not pick him up during an attack and place him in an upright position because of the risk of compromising cerebral blood flow and precipitating a seizure. No medication is required. The same dangers of overprotection or indulgence as mentioned previously are present. Medical over-enthusiasm may foster the development of such parental responses.

A sizeable minority of pre-school children with white breath-holding spells will go on to fainting in response to pain or surprise in later childhood and there may be a history of other family members who are prone to fainting. Otherwise the condition is benign and self-limiting within early childhood. The diagnosis can be made in primary care settings with confidence if (i) there is always a clear-cut painful stimulus immediately before the episode; and (ii) the attacks are infrequent and brief. However, in any other circumstances a specialist referral may be wise to confirm the diagnosis and to identify the very rare cases where some more active investigations or intervention need to be considered.

Febrile convulsions

Febrile convulsions[16] (FCs) are common in the second year of life. A child who has just suffered a first febrile convulsion should probably be assessed in hospital as there is a small risk of an underlying serious problem (*see* page 171). About one-third of children will have a recurrence. This is more likely if there is a family history of FCs, if the convulsion was associated with a relatively low fever or there was more than one convulsion within the same febrile episode. Prophylaxis, whether they are antipyretics or anticonvulsants, has not been shown to be effective in reducing recurrence. The risk of developing epilepsy after a febrile seizure is small (2–4%) and is associated with a family history of epilepsy, a complex initial febrile fit and the presence of a neuro-developmental disorder prior to the febrile fit.

The diagnosis of a first febrile convulsion is supported by the following:

▶ the child is between 6 months and 3 years of age (febrile fits can occur for the first time outside these limits but the diagnosis should be reviewed with extra care);
▶ there is a high fever, particularly if there is an obvious cause (earache, viral rash, etc.);
▶ the child has a brief convulsion (less than 10 minutes);
▶ the child rapidly recovers and has no further fits;
▶ there is a family history of febrile fits.

Beware of cases where:

▶ the child is under 6 months of age;
▶ there is only a slight fever or none at all;
▶ there are other major symptoms of illness (e.g. persistent vomiting, severe diarrhoea);
▶ the fit lasts more than 10 minutes;
▶ there are repeated fits in the same illness;
▶ the child does not recover full consciousness or there is continued marked drowsiness, or other unexplained disturbance of consciousness. In these cases, meningitis, encephalitis and meningococcal septicaemia should always be

considered as, although rare, they are devastating illnesses and early treatment may improve prognosis. In children under 18 months the absence of neck stiffness does *not* exclude these diagnoses.

Conversely, a child who is fully recovered, active and alert within an hour or two is most unlikely to have a serious underlying illness. A 4-hour observation period followed by re-assessment will usually resolves any doubts.

There are various points to remember:

▶ A first febrile fit is terrifying to the parents: they think the child is dying.
▶ True febrile fits have a very benign prognosis.
▶ For some children, the optimal management is to provide the parents (and if necessary nursery or playgroup staff) with emergency treatment options: buccal (0.4–0.5 mg/kg) or intranasal (0.2 mg/kg) midazolam or rectal diazepam (0.5 mg/kg) are effective and can be administered for a seizure lasting longer than 5 minutes. Long-term anticonvulsants should only be prescribed by a paediatrician and only in exceptional cases.
▶ Fever control by removal of clothes and paracetamol *might* help prevent febrile fits but will *not* stop them once they have begun.
▶ White breath-holding attacks can occur in febrile illnesses and are easily mistaken for a febrile fit.

Gratification phenomena

The term 'gratification phenomena' is preferred to 'infant masturbation', as it does not necessarily involve stimulation of the genitalia. The duration varies, but typically an episode might last around 10 minutes. Episodes may involve odd noises, rocking, sweating, giggling, shaking or going pale; they may end in going to sleep. The child can be interrupted or stopped and may look annoyed. It may be misdiagnosed as epilepsy or abdominal pain. It may occur in any situation; for example, while travelling in the car seat, going to sleep or in front of television. The average age of onset is 12 months and the frequency may vary from once per week to 12 times per day.[17]

Tantrums

Temper tantrums are a normal feature of development in the pre-school years. They become a problem when they are too frequent, too intense, when parents lose their authority over the child and cannot get him to do what they want, or when they fail to subside as the child matures.

Assessment: specific

Establish the ABC of one or two recent tantrums:

A What were the **a**ntecedents to the tantrum?
B What was the **b**ehaviour during the tantrum?
C What were the **c**onsequences that followed the tantrum?

Start with the **B**. What exactly constitutes a tantrum? Novice parents may have an exaggerated view of what ordinary children do. Next establish the **C**. What do they actually do during and after the tantrum? Do not be fobbed off with a claim that they 'ignore' the child; how do they do that exactly? Lastly find out the **A**. What were the immediate precipitants for a given tantrum? Not uncommonly, these include the parent having a tantrum at the child or otherwise behaving unreasonably. Few parents will tell you about this spontaneously or early in the consultation, so leave it until after establishing Bs and As for recent specific instances and ask them 'What exactly were *you* doing just before he started to shout . . .?'

Assessment: general

The following are points that need to be considered for a general assessment:

- **General health of child.** Is the child experiencing pain or other discomfort, fatigue (usually insufficient sleep)?
- **Delayed language development.** This is due to the frustration of the child at not being able to communicate his needs. Check his hearing.
- **Mental age of child.** A child who is intellectually immature for his age will be slow to grow out of childish practices and slow to learn tolerance, adequate communication, or postponement of gratification.
- **Consistency of parental discipline.** Parents who say one thing one day and another the next (or who disagree between themselves) have muddled and irritated children. Giving in to tantrums encourages them to recur.
- **Example provided by parents or older siblings.** No child who sees his elders and betters having tantrums will learn more acceptable ways of resolving frustration or conflict.
- **Medication.** Benzodiazepines, hypnotics, anticonvulsants and bronchodilators can all have adverse effects on the child's mood.
- **Mental state of child.** Check if the child is preoccupied, distressed at playgroup or school, has a depressed mood or other causes of irritability.

Management

The ABC analysis and the consideration of general factors may give you some guidelines for advice or action. In general terms, there are four components of management:

1 **Avoiding provocation.** This relates to the antecedents. Excitable children will need forewarning of events known to produce tantrums (bedtimes, etc.). Parents may need to learn how to express their wishes clearly and explicitly (saying what they want the child to do rather than telling the child continually what he must not do), not to tease their offspring, and not to set a bad example by throwing tantrums themselves.

2 **Withdrawing attention.** There is nothing wrong with the traditional advice to ignore a tantrum; it is just very difficult to put into practice. Simply telling parents to ignore it is not enough. More specific instruction is required. One possibility is for the **parent to remove themselves** from the room where the tantrum is taking place. For instance, they could grab a towel and a portable radio and go and have a bath, locking the bathroom door. To take things to such lengths is not always practical and often it is enough just to leave the room without talking to the child and refusing to answer his demands. The child should be left (ignored) for at least 3 minutes or until he starts to calm down, whichever is the sooner. This approach will only apply if the child can safely be left: having a tantrum in the

kitchen when pans are on the gas ring means that a toddler cannot be left there. Alternatively, the **child is removed** from the room to some uninteresting part of the house, such as the hall. The principle is the same as above and is often called 'time out' because the child is put out of the room. Actually, all withdrawal of attention represents time out since this is shorthand for 'time out from positive social reinforcement'. A similar time of 3 minutes or until the tantrum begins to calm is indicated (*see* page 340).

3 **Not giving in.** The child will learn that making demands in aggressive, threatening or histrionic ways is ineffective.

4 **Tuition in alternative ways of responding to frustration.** If the child does not have a tantrum, what can he do? This must be discussed with the parent with reference to the example elicited in the assessment. If the answer is that the child should comply with parental demands, then compliance without throwing a tantrum needs to be rewarded by pointed praise (e.g. 'Well done for not getting cross!'), perhaps in combination with a star chart whereby stars are earned for immediate compliance. Similar principles apply to frustration arising out of, say, motor clumsiness: the child needs to learn sober strategies for coping with frustration and disappointment. These have to be taught by parents who must explain, demonstrate and praise accordingly.

None of these approaches works immediately; they require several weeks to yield satisfactory results. In order to keep up morale and motivation, some form of charting helps. This may be a simple record, day by day, of the number of tantrums. A more informative system is to ask the parent to compile an ABC for each tantrum. This can then be discussed with the parent at weekly appointments. One twist is to ask the parent to enter the A and B *immediately* the tantrum occurs and ask for the record sheet to be kept permanently in a part of the house where tantrums are least likely to occur (such as the parents' bedroom). This has the effect of removing the parent from the child when a tantrum occurs and depriving him of attention.

Tantrums in public places, such as supermarkets, are more difficult since ignoring becomes impossible. One answer is not to take the child, but this may be unavoidable. Usually the tantrum arises out of a mixture of boredom and craving for displayed goods – the check-out queue is the worst place for both. Distracting the child with a toy, book, packet of raisins (press them down inside the box to make them less likely to spill) or, more realistically, a tube of sweets bought *beforehand* is one possibility. An older toddler may be able to hang on to the idea that not getting cross in the shop can be rewarded by being able to choose something from the check-out display at the end. The important principle is preventing the tantrum occurring in the first place and avoiding being coerced into giving into the child because the embarrassment of the tantrum is overwhelming.

Sibling jealousy

There may be some value in distinguishing between the response of a toddler to a new baby brother or sister and the feelings older siblings have towards each other. With the birth of a younger sibling, for example a sister, a young child may show overt hostility, crafty sadism or regression. On the other hand, he may be neutral or even welcome her. In the case of a negative reaction, the response is not to the baby as a person, it is a response to changes in the parents or altered relationships in the family. The parents may be preoccupied or exhausted; grandparents are primarily interested in the new baby; and so forth. The new baby is blamed by her brother for the changes in his world. He may also be jealous of her as an individual, but this is not necessarily so.

If sibling jealousy appears as a problem at this stage, it is too late for prevention as advised in so many childcare manuals. Certainly there is value in involving the child actively in the preparations for birth and providing him with a doll to care for. By the time the problem is manifest, a different approach is needed:

- The parents should consider what has changed in the older child's world and whether some things can be reinstated. In particular, they must ensure they are devoting attention to the child as well as to the baby. They must make time to play and talk to him on his own.
- They can involve the child in baby care: unfolding nappies, choosing clothes, brushing hair, etc., under supervision, so that he feels he has an active role in the newly enlarged family.
- When the baby is a little older, her responses to her older brother can be demonstrated so that he can see how she smiles at him.
- The parents should examine their own relationship with the child. Has father backed away from baby care and simultaneously removed himself from childcare?

Parents may sometimes prefer one child to another because of its gender, looks, or personality. It is very important that they keep these preferences to themselves: overt favouritism has very damaging effects on all the children in the family whether or not they happen to be the favoured one.

The situation with older children is likely to be different. Siblings may actually dislike each other. There is no law which says that they have to love each other, although it is reasonable to expect the older ones to bear some responsibility for the younger one's safety. Teasing between siblings is widespread and may reflect power relationships, rivalry for parental attention, or the way in which a younger sibling may remind an older one of how gauche, puny or naive he was himself at an earlier age. There is no reason why it cannot be treated as a disciplinary issue. If parents are in doubt as to who started it, separate both parties for a short time (15–30 minutes) turning a deaf ear to protests. It is preferable to run the risk of unfairness than to allow the teasing to continue.

Chronic teasing raises the question as to whether the parents are too preoccupied to offer the children a satisfactory ration of attention so that there is fierce competition for any parental response, positive or negative. Some parents respond to this by saying, in effect: 'I disapprove of both of you and will have nothing to do with you until you learn to get on together'. This just makes things worse. The correct principle is to devote more time to building each child's self-esteem by finding things that they can do that earn them praise and approval, *separate* from each other. These can include helping around the house, small tasks or errands, and constructive or creative play, which has an end product worthy of acclaim. All this requires a measure of active involvement of the parent. Leaving small (or large) children together in front of the television for hours on end is a recipe for squabbles.

Clinging

Many children pass through a phase of clinging somewhere between the ages of 1 and 4 years. This can get very wearing for parents, when, for example, the child hates to be separated from the parent even for a moment when they go to the toilet. It should be seen as a normal behaviour pattern. Parents worry about it because of embarrassment, fear that the child must have a weak or nervous personality, or sheer exasperation. Consider whether the child behaves like this mainly because of tiredness or anxiety; whether the parent has problems themselves that are making them more stressed and less tolerant; and whether other family members are being critical. The best approach is probably a gradual change with comfort objects being encouraged, and praise for self-sufficiency and coping during initially extremely brief periods of separation.

HEALTH EDUCATION TOPICS

There are a number of health education topics that parents need to be aware of.

Immunisations: are they up to date?

Nutrition and dental care: children should be under the care of a dentist for advice on dental care, fluoride, etc.

Injury prevention: as childen become more active and mobile between the ages of 12 months and 24 months, the variety of injury prevention increases (*see* Box 12.4).

BOX 12.4 Danger advice[*]

Road safety: keep child under constant control whenever near roads. Use a pedestrian safety harness if possible. Some toddlers are escape artists; check front door catches and garden gates.

Falls: restrict access to balconies and beware of low windows. Lock them if possible or fit devices to limit width of opening. Beware of widely spaced banisters or balcony railings.

Choking: reinforce previous advice (*see* Box 11.2). Beware of nuts, grapes, sweets, fragments of plastic, coins, beads, pen tops, bits of balloons. Keep such objects out of reach.[†]

Drowning: keep under constant control when near water. Most parents are aware of the risks associated with their own garden pond or pool. Drowning is more likely to happen at times of disruption to the normal routine, for instance on special occasions such as weddings; or on outings to parks or garden centres, or on holiday. Paddling pools left out are also a risk: a toddler can drown in a few inches of water. Water butts should have a lid. Being able to swim offers little protection for young children as they do not react promptly or appropriately if they accidentally fall into water.[18]

---

[*] *See Toddlers and up . . .* and *How Safe is Your Child in the Garden?* Available at: www.capt.org.uk

[†] *See* Factsheet: *Choking Accidents.* Available at: www.capt.org.uk

Poisons: medicine containers are at best child-resistant, not child-proof; dangerous substances should be placed in locked cupboards or otherwise out of reach.

Garden hazards: some garden plants are highly poisonous, for example, foxgloves and laburnum. Choose a greenhouse with non-breakable panes.

Dogs: children need to be taught how to recognise friendly, angry, or frightened dogs; how to approach dogs and owners before patting a dog; when to leave a dog alone (e.g. when it is eating).[19]

REFERENCES

1 Berk LE. *Child Development*. New York: Pearson education; 2005.

2 Duursma E, Augustyn M, Zuckerman B. Reading aloud to children: the evidence. *Arch Dis Child.* 2008; **93**(7): 554–7.

3 Juberg DR, Alfano K, Coughlin RJ. An observational study of object mouthing behavior by young children. *Pediatrics.* 2001; **107**: 135–42; *see also* Krakow JB, Kopp CB. The effects of developmental delay on sustained attention in young children. *Child Dev.* 1983; **54**(5): 1143–55.

4 Dunn J. Early friendships and children's social and moral development. In: Leavitt LA, Hall DMB, editors. *Social and Moral Development: emerging evidence on the toddler years.* New Jersey: Johnson and Johnson Pediatric Institute; 2004. 169–83.

5 Law J, Boyle J, Harris F, *et al.* The feasibility of universal screening for primary speech and language delay: findings from a systematic review of the literature. *Dev Med Child Neurol.* 2000; **42**: 190–200. *See also* Nelson HD, Nygren P, Walker M, *et al.* Systematic Evidence Review for the US Preventive Services Task Force: Screening for Speech and Language Delay in Preschool Children. *Pediatrics.* 2006; **117**: e298-319.

6 Gordon N. Iron deficiency and the intellect. *Brain Dev.* 2003; **25**: 3–8. *See* also Grant CC, Wall CR, Brewster D, *et al.* Policy statement on iron deficiency in pre-school-aged children. *J Paediatr Child Health.* 2007; **43**: 513–21.

7 Thorpe K, Rutter M, Greenwood R. Twins as a natural experiment to study the causes of mild language delay: II: Family interaction risk factors. *J Child Psychol Psychiatry.* 2003; **44**: 342–55.

8 www.mrc.ac.uk/Utilities/Documentrecord/index.htm?d=MRC002394 (accessed 4 January 2009). *See* also Baird G, Charman T, Cox A, *et al.* Screening and surveillance for autism and pervasive developmental disorders. *Arch Dis Child.* 2001; **84**(6): 468–75.

9 Happé F, Ronald A, Plomin R. Time to give up on a single explanation for autism. *Nat Neurosci.* 2006; **9**(10): 1218–21.

10 Robins DL, Dumont-Mathieu TM. Early screening for autism spectrum disorders: update on the modified checklist for autism in toddlers and other measures. *J Dev Behav Pediatr.* 2006; **27**: 111–19.

11 McConachie H, Diggle T. Parent implemented early intervention for young children with autism spectrum disorder: a systematic review. *J Eval Clin Pract.* 2007; **13**(1): 120–9. *See* also parent web sites: www.nas.org.uk; www.firstsigns.org

12 Dezateux C, Rosendahl K. Developmental dysplasia of the hip. *Lancet.* 2007; **369**: 1541–52.

13 Robson P. Shuffling, hitching, scooting or sliding: some observations in 30 otherwise normal children. *Dev Med Child Neurol.* 1970; **12**(5): 608–17. *See* also Robson P. Persisting head turning in the early months: some effects in the early years. *Dev Med Child Neurol.* 1968; **10**(1): 82–92.

14 Hirsch G, Wagner B. The natural history of idiopathic toe-walking: a long-term follow-up of fourteen conservatively treated children. *Acta Paediatr.* 2004; **93**: 196–9.

15 Sass P, Hassan G. Lower Extremity Abnormalities in Children. *Am Fam Physician.* 2003; **68**(3): 461–8. Available at: www.aafp.org/afp/20030801/461.html (accessed 4 January 2009).

16 Waruiru C, Appleton R. Febrile seizures: an update. *Arch Dis Child.* 2004; **89**(8): 751–6.

17 Yang ML, Fullwood E, Goldstein J, *et al.* Masturbation in Infancy and Early Childhood Presenting as a Movement Disorder: 12 Cases and a Review of the Literature. *Pediatrics.* 2005; **116**: 1427–32.

18 Kemp A, Sibert JR. Drowning and near drowning in children in the United Kingdom: lessons for prevention. *BMJ.* 1992; **304**: 1143–6.

19 Chapman S, Cornwall J, Righetti J, *et al.* Preventing dog bites in children: randomised controlled trial of an educational intervention. *BMJ.* 2000; **320**: 1512–13 (this study focused on children in school; however, the paper is relevant to pre-school children).

CHAPTER 13

2–5 years

CHAPTER CONTENTS

NORMAL DEVELOPMENT: 2–5 YEARS[1]

Language acquisition

By his third birthday, the child can usually join at least three words and many children are using sentences of four or five words or even longer. Comprehension is normally more advanced than speech production and many 3-year-olds can understand quite complex instructions involving three or four information words (e.g. 'put baby's shoes in the cupboard in the kitchen'). Almost all 3-year-olds can recognise and pick out (on request) one of a dozen or more objects. Articulation, vocabulary and grammar sometimes develop at surprisingly different rates. The ability to produce all the sounds of the native language is usually acquired within the first 3 or 4 years, although a few sounds may present particular difficulty and may not be perfected until 7 or 8 years of age. Some children may speak very clearly, yet have a poor vocabulary or very immature use of grammar. Others may have a great deal to say, using a wide range of words and grammatical structures, yet because of poor articulation they are almost unintelligible.

During the phase of very rapid language and vocabulary acquisition, many children copy whatever is said to them, as if mentally replaying a word or phrase out loud, which helps them to understand better. This is called echolalia. It is a normal finding in children up to 3 or 3.5 years of age, but if it persists much beyond this or if the child repeats words, yet shows no sign of understanding their meaning, there may be some difficulty with the overall comprehension of language.

In the normal course of language acquisition, over-generalisation is common; that is, the child applies a word to all objects in a class. For example, all fruits are bananas, all animals are dogs. Grammatical rules are also treated like this, resulting in words such as 'sheeps', 'hurteded', etc. He then refines these rules and learns the various exceptions. By the age of 4, the average child has almost mastered his native language except for some sophisticated grammatical constructions. Of course, he still needs to enlarge his vocabulary. There may still be a number of errors in pronunciation, but the great majority of his speech is intelligible. He can recount experiences, listen to a short story and tell it back to the reader.

Modes of thinking

Pre-school children think differently from adults. This is particularly important when asking or explaining reasons for things (like illness). They are likely to display the following:

Egocentric thinking (I'm tired, therefore it's getting dark). The child places himself at the centre of the world. This does not mean he sees himself as all powerful. If things go wrong (parents falling ill), he is likely to believe that it is because of him; something he has done or failed to do.

Events are interconnected and **all actions have a purpose** (a marble rolls downhill because it is going home). People and things **exist for a purpose** (the moon comes out at night to make it less dark; aunts exist to give you Christmas presents). According to **animistic beliefs**, inanimate things and animals can behave like people (a car hurts itself in a crash). In general, there is an intuitive, magical quality to thought rather than a logical approach. It is important not to overstate the case. For instance, small children are not entirely self-centred and can empathise; but there is a tendency to reveal such styles of thought frequently, without monitoring whether they are plausible in the way an older child would think.

Primary school-age children are less egocentric and more logical in their approach and are particularly adept at **classification and categorisation** (although they may have difficulty in realising that an object can have more than one characteristic at a time). They tend to be **rule-bound and rigid** having to think in terms of the here-and-now. Metaphors are not easily grasped and need careful explanation.

Only in mid-adolescence does it become possible for a child to think in an adult manner, using abstract concepts, metaphors, and being able to compare various hypotheses. Doctors are good at such thinking and so it is paradoxically difficult for them to communicate with young children who do not have such cognitive abilities and who are likely to resort to replying 'Don't know' to well-meant enquiries.

Play and skill development

In the third year of life, the child acquires various other skills, such as building models or structures with bricks or Lego, using a pencil (although rarely able to draw anything recognisable much before the age of 3), doing simple puzzles, playing games with rules, etc. Attention and concentration mature and play becomes more complex with routines and sequences and an increased ability to pretend, so that, for instance, a box can represent a car or a ship.

The child's ability to concentrate on a task and to accept suggestions while playing gives some insight into the way he is likely to respond in the classroom. If the child has not reached this level of mature concentration at the age when school entry is approaching, he may not benefit from the routines of ordinary school and some special provision may be needed.

By the age of 4, he can build recognisable models and draw pictures with at least some semblance of shape and form. Given adequate opportunity, it is not uncommon for him to be able to count, read some words and write his name.

Simple performance tasks are sometimes used to assess developmental skills, though their reliability and validity are limited (*see* Chapter 9) and they should not be used as screening tests. Bricks and drawing tasks are easy to use and need only a minimum of equipment, but they require concentration, coordination, adequate vision and understanding, so failure may have many causes. Box 13.1 summarises the most commonly used tasks and the wide age range at which they are achieved.

BOX 13.1 Common tasks in young children

Build a tower with bricks (1 inch cubes)
Method: The cubes are spread on the table and the child is shown and then asked to stack the bricks, with verbal encouragement if necessary.

- Some children can stack up to four bricks by 18 months; 90% can do so by 24 months.
- Some children can stack up to seven bricks by 18 months; 90% can do so by 30 months.
- Some children can stack eight bricks or more by 24 months; 90% can do so by 39 months.

Build models
Method: The model is made without the child seeing how it is done (e.g. behind a hand or sheet of paper), then the child is asked to copy it.

Build a bridge with three bricks

- Some children can copy the bridge by 27 months.
- 50% can do so by 36 months.
- 90% can do so by 45 months.

Build a train

- Some children can copy the train by 30 months.
- 50% can do so by 39 months.
- 90% can do so by 51 months.

Build three steps

- Some children can build three steps by 39 months.
- 50% can do so by 54 months.

Drawing shapes
Method: The shapes are drawn out of sight of the child and presented down one side of a sheet of paper; the child is asked to *copy* the shape. If he cannot do this, he is then shown how it is drawn and asked to try again (i.e. to *imitate* it). Imitation is easier than copying, but copying should be tested first. Accuracy improves with age and some judgment is often needed in deciding whether the child should be credited with the skill.

- A few children can copy a circle by 24 months; 50% by 36 months; nearly 100% by 36 months.
- A few children can copy a cross by 30 months; 50% by 42 months; 90% by 48 months.

- Some children can copy a square by 36 months; almost 50% by 48 months.
- A few children can copy a triangle (showing three corners) by 42 months; nearly 50% by 60 months.
- Some children can imitate a vertical line by 18 months; over 50% by 24 months; nearly 100% by 36 months.
- Some children can imitate a horizontal line by 18 months; about 50% by 24 months; over 90% by 36 months.
- Some children can imitate a circle by 18 months; over 50% by 24 months; nearly 90% by 36 months.
- A few children can imitate a cross by 24 months; around 75% by 36 months.

Draw a man
Method: The child is given a clean sheet of paper and asked to draw a man (or Mummy or Daddy). No help or advice should be given until the child has finished his first attempt.

- Children under 30 months either do not attempt the task or draw a very primitive man.
- Children between 36 and 48 months often draw a man with arms and/or legs but no trunk.
- Between 48 and 60 months the drawing is likely to show the head, body and limbs, often with other features.

Independence and self-help

With increasing emotional security the 3-year-old child can separate from his parents for increasing periods of time; for instance, to attend nursery or playgroup. He becomes more socially confident and able to cope with strange situations. Increasing understanding of daily routines coupled with greater motor coordination enable him to acquire increasing independence in daily activities, such as using the lavatory, washing hands, etc., and he can assist with household tasks. The 4-year-old has acquired considerable social poise and confidence although this may still crumble very quickly when faced with new situations. Given the opportunity, motor skill has advanced to the point where he may have learned to pedal a tricycle, catch a ball, swim, play the violin or ski!

HEALTH AND DEVELOPMENT REVIEWS BETWEEN 2 AND 5 YEARS
Policy

The Child Health Promotion Programme (2008) proposes a review of each child's progress between 2 and 2.5 years.[2] The main aims are to discuss the child's development and behaviour, and to provide health information and education, but the approach is flexible and is not specified in detail. The traditional school entrant physical examination has been discontinued in most parts of the UK because the yield of significant new findings is very small in a society with a well-developed healthcare system.

The most common developmental problem that worries parents between the second birthday and school entry is a delay in language acquisition. This may be accompanied by more general learning difficulties of mild or moderate severity, impaired social relationships or concentration and behavioural problems. It would be unusual for a child to present so late with an inability to walk, but other motor problems may need evaluation; for instance, excessive weakness, fatigue or clumsiness. Behavioural difficulties are common, though many are transient (*see* Chapter 14).

Summary of review

Any or all of the following may be relevant:

▶ Review worries, progress and development.
▶ Behavioural and emotional concerns.
▶ Growth and physical health.
▶ Motor ability.
▶ Language and ability to communicate.
▶ Social maturity; ability to cope with unfamiliar situations.
▶ Ask if parent has any concerns about vision or hearing; check for any high risk factors.
▶ Physical examination.
▶ Health education topics.
▶ Immunisations as indicated by schedule or, if necessary, catching up.

The review normally incorporates informal observation, history, developmental review and discussion of health promotion topics:

▶ Observe all aspects of the child's **behaviour** from the moment you introduce yourself to the parent.
▶ Offer the child a few toys, then ignore him while you talk to the parent.
▶ Give the child the option of sitting on the parent's lap or at a small table (the latter is encouraged).
▶ It is important to establish any worries, including **who is worried and about what**.
▶ Ask if the immunisation schedule is up to date.
▶ **Concentration and attention.** Consider the child's ability to **stay on one task** without being distracted. Can he **play with other children** and stick to the rules of a game? Are the parents worried that he is **hyperactive**? If so, what do they mean by this term? By the time a child reaches the age of 3, parents are beginning to think about school; therefore the child whose concentration is poor may cause them great worry.
▶ Is he able to **separate** from the parents without becoming unduly distressed? Some shyness and anxiety in a strange situation is, of course, perfectly normal, but if it is excessive it may become a real problem for both child and parent, and expert advice may be needed (*see* page 295).
▶ Ask about **hearing and language development**. Often the child's responses to remarks or questions from the parent within the first few minutes of a consultation are sufficient to assure you that language development is normal. If this does not happen, ask the parent if the child is talking well, and if in doubt, either refer the child or review the matter in more detail (*see* below). There are no easy screening tests for slow language development.
▶ **Behavioural disorders and emotional problems.** These are very common. Ask whether the parents have any such worries, and if so, whether they can cope or

whether they need advice (*see* Chapter 14 for detailed discussion).

▶ Evaluate **gross motor functions**. Ask whether there are any worries about the child's walking. Can he run? Is there any limp or asymmetry? Can he tackle stairs? Does he tire unusually easily compared to other children?

▶ Vision screening for all children is carried out between 4 and 5 years of age (*see* Appendix 2) but refer for **vision testing** if you or the parents have any concerns.

▶ A useful question is: **How do you think he's going to cope at school?** If there is any concern, consult with the community paediatric service or the Child Development Centre. They will arrange further assessment and will liaise with the Education Authority if necessary.

Consider **physical health** – the yield of *routine* physical examination at this age is very small but, if concerns have been raised, any or all of the following may be indicated:

▶ Measure and plot **height and weight**.

▶ Inspection of the **skin** (check for unusual marks; e.g. multiple café-au-lait patches suggestive of neurofibromatosis).

▶ Listen to the **heart** (*see* below).

▶ Listen to the **lungs** for wheezing. Ask the parent if the child ever **wheezes**; this is a useful indicator of possible asthma.

▶ Palpate the abdomen and check the descent of the **testes**. If in doubt about their descent, refer. If both testes were *definitely* descended at birth and at 6 weeks, it is very unlikely that they will re-ascend. This is why a careful check in infancy is vital and why a record must be made.

▶ Inspect the **spine** for evidence of dysraphism.

▶ Opinions differ on routine measurement of **blood pressure (BP)** in young children. Most authorities do *not* recommend whole population screening. However, the BP should be measured as part of a full evaluation in any child whose general health is causing concern. This will usually be done at a paediatric clinic. Do *not* measure the BP in children unless you have a selection of cuffs of various sizes. This is essential, otherwise substantial errors are inevitable. The cuff *must* be wide enough. The correct width is two-thirds of the distance between the shoulder and elbow. In practice, this means the largest cuff that comfortably fits around the arm. Figure 13.1 shows the normal BP range for different ages.

▶ **Innocent heart murmurs** are characterised by the absence of any other symptoms or signs of disease in the cardiovascular system; are often a soft and musical sound; there is a lack of radiation to the back or widely across praecordium; these change with position. They are *very* common; many children have a functional murmur if you listen carefully and particularly if the child is ill. Parents usually notice that you can hear something in the heart because you tend to frown and listen for longer! It is advisable to explain the concept of an innocent murmur, which is a normal noise made by the blood flowing through the heart and lungs. Do not recall the child for repeat examinations. One re-check is enough; it will not get any easier to decide! Either make up your mind that the murmur is innocent, or refer to a cardiologist or direct for an echocardiogram, depending on local policy. Parents can become very anxious if left in doubt about a possible heart complaint; they may restrict the child's activities and worry excessively over trivial ailments.

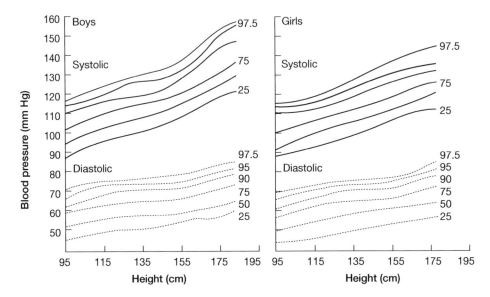

FIGURE 13.1 Relation of blood pressure to height in children. Figures are percentages of boys and girls. Reproduced from de Swiet, *et al.*[3] with the kind permission of BMJ Publishing Group.

COMMON PROBLEMS AGE 2–5
Worries about hearing

There is no universal screening programme for hearing loss between the newborn screen and the school entry hearing test, but continued vigilance is necessary as the newborn screen does not detect all cases of sensorineural hearing loss. In this age group, conductive hearing loss, due to otitis media with effusion (OME), is very common, but whole-population screening has been found to be impractical as the condition is episodic and transient in most children.

Hearing assessment is usually carried out in audiology clinics (often second-tier or community clinics). The methods used are summarised in Appendix 1. Assessment of hearing can be undertaken by primary care staff, but only if they have been adequately trained and have the necessary equipment and a quiet environment in which to test; any child who seems uncooperative, gives inconsistent responses or is hard to test for any reason, should be referred.

Primary care staff should not undertake hearing tests without proper training, equipment and facilities. If any concern has been expressed about a child's hearing, do not try to *exclude* hearing loss; arrange for assessment by someone with special training. However, the following may be useful, particularly when one needs to discuss the issue of a possible hearing impairment previously unsuspected by the parent(s):

▶ history;

▶ observing child's responses to simple voice stimuli;
▶ otoscopy.

History

Ask the parent these questions:

▶ What do you think about his hearing?
▶ Why do you think he can/cannot hear? Can he for example:
  — Listen to conversation?
  — Hear key in door?
  — Hear biscuit packet being opened?
  — Hear aircraft before parent?

(Note that all these sounds are mixed frequency, so the ability to hear them does not exclude a hearing loss affecting only part of the frequency range.)

▶ Does he respond better if:
  — You point or gesture?
  — You raise your voice?
  — You let him see your face while you speak?
▶ Does he say 'eh', 'what', 'pardon'?
▶ Do you often feel that he is ignoring you?
▶ Does he like the TV turned up loud? (This is not a reliable question on its own as many children do this!)

Simple stimuli

It is sometimes useful in primary care settings to observe and demonstrate how the child responds to voice. Use **simple, quietly spoken sentences** (*not* whispered) at 1 metre from the child: the speaker should hide the mouth behind the hand to prevent the child from lip reading. Ask 'Where did you put your teddy?' or a similar casual question. The ability to comprehend simple questions confirms not only functional (though not necessarily normal) hearing, but also gives information about language development.

Otoscopy

This can be useful, but otoscopy is often very difficult in young children and the drum is often partially obscured by wax. Furthermore, the physical signs of middle ear disease may be very subtle. The decision to refer a child is usually based on a history suggestive of a middle ear disorder, or on the presence of a hearing loss rather than otoscopic findings; but the latter may indicate whether a referral to the ENT department is appropriate as well as an audiological assessment. If impacted wax is seen, this should, if possible, be treated before the child is seen by secondary services (*see* below).

Otitis media with effusion OME (also called glue ear)

This is very common in children and particularly in those with cleft palate, Down's syndrome or Turner's syndrome. The most frequent complaint is of hearing loss, but there may also be pain and sometimes a disturbance of balance. Most children have a single attack, or repeated attacks with complete resolution between each episode, but a few have severe persistent OME and some of these may have poor language development.[4]

The **hearing loss** is typically of a modest degree and fluctuates from day to day and gets worse with colds. The parent may think the child is stubborn or disobedient and may also complain that the child turns the television up too loud. The **signs to look for through the otoscope are**: loss of the normal grey gunmetal sheen or translucency, with its light reflex (though this can be preserved in some cases), a blue, amber or inflamed appearance, and retraction indicated by change of the normal angle of the malleus (it becomes more horizontal). In suppurative otitis media, look for perforation and a discharge (in chronic cases, the odour may help you to distinguish between a discharge of wax and a true purulent discharge).

Treatment of OME

This is controversial. Time can lead to natural resolution in many children, but persistence of symptoms for more than 6 months indicates the need for active management. Medical management includes assessment of possible underlying factors, such as nasal allergy, poor immunity, chronic infection or exposure to cigarette smoke. Avoidance of allergens and use of intranasal cromoglycate or steroid sprays can be very useful if allergy is a factor. Decongestants do not help and have subtle but unpleasant side effects. Antibiotics have not been shown to be beneficial for OME.

For children with significant hearing problems, a thin and indrawn ear drum or repeated episodes of acute otitis media, myringotomy with grommet insertion may help, although the effect is short-lived as the grommets are extruded after only a few months and OME can recur. A limit is usually only two sets of grommets because this surgical procedure itself can scar the ear drum. Enlarged adenoids can block the Eustachian tube leading to OME and can also give rise to sleep apnoea (stopping breathing for 10–15 seconds followed by partial waking), which can be elucidated from the history. In such cases adenoidectomy or adeno-tonsillectomy may be indicated.

The use of hearing aids can be valuable, particularly in cases where grommets are contraindicated or are likely to have limited effect; for example, in children with Down's syndrome, children with additional medical needs, where two previous sets of grommets have already been used or when parents are reluctant for surgical intervention. The most common hearing aid used in this situation is a bone-conductor aid. The child usually 'grows out of' OME by the age of 7 years.

OME is very common and may co-exist with sensorineural hearing loss, so make sure that the child's hearing is tested before surgery and retested afterwards. Particularly in the first 18 months of life, careful and specialist hearing testing is needed to decide whether a hearing loss is entirely due to OME or has an additional sensorineural component. Parents are often all too willing to believe that an operation will solve the problem of hearing loss and fail to attend for a post-operative hearing test. Similarly it is often tempting to attribute language delay or global developmental delay to OME, but again this is unlikely to be the whole story.

Wax

Discharge from the ear is commonly due to wax. This is yellow or brown and odourless. The amount of wax produced varies widely and is genetically determined.

Many parents feel that the comment that the child has wax in the ear implies an accusation of poor hygiene, but they need to be reassured that this is not the case. They should never use cotton buds or other instruments to remove ear wax as this makes matters worse. Never attribute a hearing loss to wax until you have removed the wax and confirmed that the hearing has returned to normal. Wax can be removed in several ways:

▶ Soften the wax with one of the following:
  — olive oil, three drops, three times daily for 2 weeks; spend a couple of minutes massaging it down the ear canal while the child lies on his side;
  — sodium bicarbonate three drops three times daily for 1 week; this is recommended for impacted wax, but can be mildly irritating if used too long;
  — Cerumol® for 5 days; this may sting, so is best avoided in younger children;
  — Otosporin® may help if there is also otitis externa.
▶ After softening the wax, syringing with a gentle pulsing jet of warm water (Propulse III®), may be done by appropriately trained staff in children above the age of 5–6 years, but is more difficult in pre-school children. Contra-indications are a history of purulent discharge, previous chronic infection or perforation, grommets in situ, or pain.

Discharge
Purulent discharge accompanied by aural pain may be due to otitis externa. Meticulous aural toilet is indicated followed by treatment with antibiotic ear drops, such as Otosporin. Another cause of a purulent discharge with pain is acute otitis media, but the pain has usually subsided by the time of the discharge; no treatment is required and the discharge should settle within 3 days.

Purulent discharge without pain can indicate chronic suppurative otitis media, which needs careful ENT management. For this reason it is essential to get a good view of the ear drum after any complaint of discharge. Any defect in the ear drum, any wax or crusting adhering to the drum or any persistent infection needs an ENT referral.

Other risk groups
Children recovering from **bacterial meningitis** should have an **urgent** audiological assessment within 2 weeks of discharge from hospital. Children who have had **significant head injury, particularly with temporal bone fracture**, also need audiological assessment.

Vision problems
Serious congenital vision disorders have usually been detected long before the age of 3 years. The main aim of vision screening in this age group is to detect squint, refractive errors and amblyopia. Of these, amblyopia is the most important (*see* page 185). Colour vision defects ('colour blindness') are common and the majority are inherited. The most common type is a sex-linked impairment of red-green discrimination; it affects about 6% of boys, but only about 0.4% of girls. It does not seem to cause significant disability in the pre-school or early school years.[5]

Districts vary in their policy regarding pre-school vision screening.[6] The national recommendation is that the 'best buy' is for a community orthoptist to screen children in the pre-school age group (between 4 and 5 years). If this is not possible, those testing children should be trained and supervised by an orthoptist. Details of the methods are in Appendix 2. Screening of children younger than this is probably not cost-effective. Screening of children from deprived backgrounds has been emphasised; they are not necessarily more likely to have vision defects, but they are less likely to receive diagnosis and treatment.

Although it does not constitute a formal screening programme, the following approach will identify a significant number of problems: Ask parents:

▶ Have you any worries about his vision?
▶ Have you ever noticed a squint?

Ask the following as well if the parent is worried:

▶ Does he hold objects very close to his eyes?
▶ Can he recognise you at a distance (e.g. when you collect him from the nursery)?
▶ Does he feel for objects rather than look for them?
▶ Does he have particular problems seeing in poor light?

CHILDREN WITH SLOW OR ATYPICAL DEVELOPMENT

In this age group of 2- to 5-year-olds, the questions that often worry parents are 'Is my child slower than normal?' 'How will my child respond to the new demands of school?' and – if they are concerned about his progress – 'Might he need some form of special schooling?'. The task of health professionals is to respond to such worries and, where appropriate, identify conditions or circumstances that could affect a child's development.

A child whose progress is only slightly below average may well be perceived as slow by highly educated professional parents, whose standard of normality is an IQ in the superior range. Such parents are sometimes described in rather disparaging terms, such as 'pressurising' or 'over-ambitious' but their concerns are perfectly legitimate. In contrast, a child of below average ability may be regarded as normal by parents who live in a deprived area and whose education or intelligence is limited. It is the mismatch between their expectations and the child's actual ability and temperament that causes anxiety and disappointment to the parents; unfortunately this has knock-on effects on the child.

'Slowness' is generally taken to imply that the child's pattern of development is essentially similar to that of a younger normal child, but in some developmental disorders (e.g. autism) the pattern of behaviour and function is qualitatively different from that of the normal child.

Slow development can sometimes be attributed to inadequate stimulation in the home environment, or to major continuing stresses, due to marital violence, for example. Some children are less vulnerable than others to adverse circumstances and their development may remain within normal limits in spite of an impoverished home life. Nevertheless, they may well be performing far below their true genetic potential. It follows that simply measuring the level of development can never indicate whether intervention is desirable.

Movement problems

Developmental coordination disorder, also called dyspraxia or 'clumsiness', is a problem of motor coordination, which usually presents in the early school years. The child may have problems with gross motor activities (running, riding a bike, catching a ball) or with fine coordination (most often with handwriting). The child should be examined to exclude neurological disease but it is rare that any evidence is found of any specific disorder; in most cases dyspraxia may be regarded as a manifestation of limited motor abilities – just as some children have limited musical or artistic abilities. The possibility of a **vision** defect should also be considered in such children. A child with poor vision may, for instance, feel for steps with his foot before descending or bump into objects.

Management is aimed at helping his specific problems, i.e. it is education and therapy-oriented, rather than medical. Some so-called clumsy children have other learning difficulties as well. The term **dyspraxic** is sometimes used. Refer any such children for assessment at a Child Development Centre.[7]

Whenever there is concern about late walking, weakness, inability to run normally, excessive number of falls, difficulty on stairs, etc., in an otherwise healthy boy, it is vital to exclude Duchenne muscular dystrophy (DMD); this is the commonest type of inherited muscle disease and is sex-linked, i.e. affecting only boys. Observe the boy carrying out the Gower's manoeuvre (*see* Figure 13.2) and arrange a blood test for CPK (creatine phosphokinase). Some boys with DMD also have slow speech development.[8]

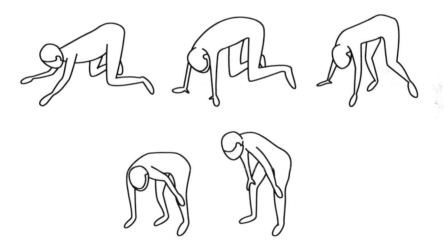

FIGURE 13.2 Gower's sign. This indicates weakness of the thigh and trunk muscles. The child is asked to lie on the floor and then to get up. He straightens by 'walking' his hands up his legs.*

Language development

The parents' account of what the child says (expressive language) often underestimates the child's speech output because of reluctance to credit him with a word if the

---

* For video clips *see*: www.youtube.com/watch?v=bI6utCce_3g&feature=related and www.youtube.com/watch?v=IpoT46EAuCU&feature=related

articulation is unclear. Parents worry most often about a lack of clarity in the child's speech. As a rough guide, a child's speech should be comprehensible to the family by the age of 3 years. However, from the prognostic point of view, isolated articulation difficulties are, in fact, rarely serious. More worrying is the child whose speech output is severely limited and who makes little effort to communicate or who, in spite of apparently normal hearing, grammar and vocabulary, frequently fails to understand instructions or stories. Inability to relate the theme of a simple picture at age 4 has been shown to be a warning sign of learning difficulties in primary school.

There are a number of uncommon disorders that cause serious problems in speech production in spite of normal comprehension, intellect and hearing. Diagnosis is difficult, but useful clues include persistent dribbling or problems with chewing and swallowing; expressionless face; severely restricted range of individual sounds; lack of progress over a period of time; motor disorders (e.g. DMD and ataxic cerebral palsy can present with speech disorders).

The crucial question: is there any impairment of comprehension? When assessing language, look first at comprehension (*see* Box 13.2). There are two reasons for this preference. Firstly, you can obtain clear information about expressive language from the parents, but they do not always find it easy to describe comprehension so precisely. Secondly, it is usually easy to test comprehension because the child does not have to give a spoken response to questions; comprehension can be tested by asking the child to respond by pointing. Every 3-year-old should be able correctly to select one from an array of a dozen common objects when asked to do so in a clear voice. Nearly all children of this age can recognise an object by function (e.g. 'Which one do you sweep with'?), and obey commands with two information carrying words (e.g. 'Give the doll to Mummy'). The older the child, the more comprehension he is expected to have.

The usual answer to the question: 'How much does he understand when you talk to him'? is 'Everything'. Parents tend to overestimate comprehension because children are good at recognising gestures and situational clues, such as preparations for meals or bedtime. It follows that if the parents have recognised the child's difficulty in understanding, it is almost certain that comprehension is seriously impaired.

Also consider the following:

▶ What do the parents feel about the child's **hearing**? (*See* above for more details.)
▶ **Does the child perform normally in other respects?** For instance, in play, self-help (washing, dressing, helping in the home). These are all activities that do not require language and can be learned by use of visual observation alone. A psychologist would designate these tasks as 'non-verbal abilities'.
▶ **Are the attention, concentration and social competence normal?** Does the child show attachment to the parents and have normal wariness of strangers?

Causes of impaired comprehension

A significant difficulty in comprehension is associated with four main groups of diagnoses:

1 If language is severely limited, but play, social behaviour and all other functions are normal, the diagnosis is **hearing loss** until proved otherwise. The diagnosis is

easily missed because both parents and doctors find it hard to believe that a deaf child can look and behave so normally in all other respects.

2   There are some children who, in spite of normal non-verbal intelligence and good hearing, fail to develop language normally. Opinions differ on the prevalence and precise definition of this group of developmental problems, which are collectively known as **language disorders**. The diagnosis is more likely if other family members also have isolated language problems.

3   If the child's non-verbal skills and the ability to concentrate or play constructively are also impaired, it is likely that the slow language development is a reflection of a more **generalised developmental delay**. The IQ is usually in the borderline range of ability or just below, now designated as 'learning disabilities' rather than 'mental handicap'. Many children with conditions causing severe delay are identified in the first year, but sometimes a child with an IQ of 50 or less may present at the age of 36–42 months for the first time, with language deficits as the presenting feature.

4   **Autism** should be considered when there is impairment of social functioning as well as delay in language development and is discussed in Chapter 12.

Referral guidelines

Assessment of developmental problems is usually undertaken in a specialist child development clinic; however, it is important to remember that some parents are less happy about referral. They may, for example, perceive the suggestion that their child needs help with his speech as a slur on their parenting ability and even as an accusation of neglect. If one fails to identify this concern, the parent may resentfully attend for the assessment only out of a sense of duty, or simply not keep the appointment.[9]

Health professionals have a duty to inform the Education Authority (with the parents' agreement) about any child who may have 'special educational needs'. The Education Act of 1981 uses this term in preference to 'defects or disorders'. Contacts with colleagues in the local education service are usually arranged by the child development or speech and language therapy service, but parents may ask primary care staff about how the system works. Local knowledge is essential as the structure, quality and availability of services vary widely. Health professionals can only *suggest* that the child may need an educational assessment or specialised education – it is not a medical decision.

A child may need further assessment IF:

▶ the parent(s) are worried about the child's development and primary care staff do not feel able to reassure them;
▶ at the age of 3 the child is unintelligible to the family OR is unable to produce a sentence of *four words*;
▶ at the age of 4 the child cannot be understood by strangers OR is unable to recount the theme of a picture;
▶ the child does not understand single words at 15–18 months, short instructions at 2 years (e.g. Get your coat) and longer instructions at 3 years (e.g. Get your coat and take it to Daddy);
▶ there is any abnormality of gait or other aspects of motor function;
▶ there is any suspicion of autistic behaviour patterns;

◗ there are behavioural problems that appear to be entrenched or are not resolving (*see* Chapter 14).

Problems of fluency: stammering and stuttering

Developmental stammering (also called idiopathic stuttering) affects between 1% and 3% of children. In spite of many theories the cause(s) are still unclear. Typically it begins around the age of 4. About three-quarters stop stammering by the time they reach their teens. About 40% stop stammering within a year of onset, but after this there is less chance of early remission, so early referral to speech and language therapy is recommended. There are two main approaches to management: (i) training in parent-child interaction (PCI), and (ii) the Lidcombe method, which has been shown to be effective in trials.[10]

BOX 13.2 Questions about comprehension: what the child understands

- *How much* does he understand when you talk to him?
- Does he look towards familiar people when named?
- Can you ask him to show you his nose, his feet, his eyes?
- Ask the parent to demonstrate by saying: 'Show me your hair/eyes/nose/mouth/feet/tummy (or dolly's hair, etc.).' There is wide variation at 18 months and some children are unable to point to any body part; but at 2 years the majority can correctly identify at least four parts.
- Does he understand if you ask him simple questions or ask him to do simple things; for instance, to get his coat or shoes?
- Ask the child (or ask the parent to ask the child) to carry out an instruction containing two information words; for example, 'Put the ball on the table', 'Give teddy to Mummy'. More than half of 2-year-olds can follow some such instructions.
- How much does he understand when you look at books together?
- Use pictures in a book or picture cards and say 'Show me the . . .' or 'Where's the . . .?'. At 18 months around half of all children can correctly point to a few items; at 24 months most can identify at least three and often many more. At 24-30 months, ask questions with verbs; for example, 'Which one is running/sleeping/eating?' or 'Which one do we eat with/sleep on/ride on?'.
- Use toys or pictures to see if the child can understand prepositions. 'In' and 'on' are understood early, by 24-30 months; 'under', 'behind' and 'in front of' come later, typically in that order, between 33 and 54 months.
- Could he still understand if you asked him when you were in another room, so that he couldn't see you or guess what you want? (This type of question helps to rule out the possibility that the child is actually responding to gestures or signs rather than speech.)
- Can you tell him a story? Does he follow it? Would he know if you changed the story or left something out?
- Remind parents that children aged 3 and upwards normally understand a great deal, so parents need to be careful of what they say in front of children of this age! You can ask parents to make a comparison with a younger sibling or with other children whom they know well. For example, 'If you said something a bit complicated, who would be more likely to understand, this child or the younger one?' A 4-year-old who understands less than his 2-year-old sibling probably has a serious problem.

- Abnormality of social behaviour, with a lack of interest in people and failure to show normal attachment to familiar adults, may suggest a diagnosis of **autism** (*see* Chapter 12).

Questions about what the child says
Until the child has relaxed, he should not be asked questions which *demand* a spoken response otherwise he may simply cry or refuse cooperation. For instance, if a child does not tell you the name of a toy, tell him, rather than wait for him to respond. By conveying to the child that it does not matter whether he talks, most will, in fact, be persuaded to do so.

How much does he say?

- How many single words that the child says can *you* understand as a parent? (You may find it helpful to prompt the parent – is it 2 or 3, 10, 20 or 50 or too many to count?)
- Are there a lot of words that cannot be understood even by those who know the child well?
- Are his words clear enough to understand? Do you understand him? Do strangers understand him?
- Are you mainly worried about *how much* he can say or is it the difficulty in *understanding* him that's the problem? Does he put two or three words together to make a little sentence, such as, 'Daddy gone'? Can you give an example?
- How well does he make his meaning understood?
- Can he tell you what he wants, what he's been doing? Can he relate a simple story?

Shy or autistic?
It may be difficult to decide whether a child is just unusually shy or has some more serious problem.

- Many young children are *extremely* shy with strangers, but they can respond normally to familiar people and most will gradually 'warm up' with people they do not know.
- Some pre-school children talk at home, but will not speak in nursery or in the first year at primary school ('elective' or 'selective' mutism). In many of these children, the problem resolves spontaneously, but some also have a speech or language disorder[11] (*see* Box 13.3).
- Autism is not an 'all-or-nothing' diagnosis (*see* page 262); there are varying degrees of language and social impairment, and the picture changes as the child gets older. Suspect autism if: the parents feel that the child does not relate to them in a normal way, or enjoy any form of communication, or show empathy (awareness of other people having feelings); or if the child does not pretend or play, or does so in a stereotyped repetitive way; or indulges in meaningless repetitive routines.

Differential diagnosis is not always easy: if there is no sign of improvement after a reasonable time, referral to a paediatrician, psychologist or child psychiatrist is advisable.

BOX 13.3 Selective mutism

Definition: A consistent failure to speak in social situations in which there is an expectation for speaking, despite speaking in other situations.

- The disturbance interferes with educational or occupational achievement or with social conversation, and is not better accounted for by a communication disorder (though the child may have some language problems) or by a lack of knowledge of the particular language.
- The duration must be at least 1 month and not limited to the first month in school. It is slightly more common in girls.
- It is said to affect less than 1 child per 1000, but the true figure may be higher, particularly in immigrant children.
- There may be a continuum between extreme shyness and selective mutism, and there is often a family history of either or both.
- There is often a long time-lag from first concerns – often after starting school – until referral, probably because both parents and teachers think they will 'grow out of it'. Early referral is wise.
- A home recording of the child having a conversation, and a talk to the schoolteacher, usually clinch the diagnosis (a one-way mirror is rarely needed).
- There are many different approaches to therapy, particularly behavioural therapy. A locally agreed referral pathway is desirable.

ASPECTS OF EARLY LITERACY

Literacy is a continuous process that begins early in life and is heavily dependent on environmental influence. Children become interested in picture books at 6 months of age. They enjoy the focus of attention associated with parents reading to them and this has several benefits:

- it provides language stimulation;
- it makes children familiar with the form and cadence of language;
- it gives them an understanding of books;
- it gives some positive associations and strong motivation around learning to read;
- parents use more language and more repetition when reading; the short sentences, repetitive phrases and limited vocabulary of picture books assist language processing.

There is a very wide social gradient in respect of how many books the child may have in their home, and how much and how often the parents read to them. There are several schemes designed to encourage parents; for example, in one approach, the child is given a book at each visit from 6 months to 5 years; the parent is given advice about how to use the book, and a volunteer acts as a model to show how it should be done (assuring the parent that it does not matter if the child puts the book in her mouth!). The benefits of such schemes are strongest among the poorest families. Early years librarians can be a great help.

Interest in environmental print should be encouraged. Every day there are opportunities to show children words, often in large print, such as labels on packets and the signs over shops or petrol stations. This helps to convey the concept that words carry meaning.

Box 13.4 summarises some of the important terms and concepts now thought to be important for all children when learning to read, and also for helping children who find reading difficult.[12]

Dyslexia/specific reading disability

Around 10–15% of children have difficulties with reading and with the sub-skills necessary for literacy, such as word identification and phonological (letter-sound) decoding. The terms 'dyslexia' or 'specific reading disability' are used when the child's difficulties are not obviously due to low intelligence, hearing or vision defects, or lack of opportunity. Problems with reading and spelling have a strong genetic basis: between one-third and two-thirds of the children of dyslexic parents have reading problems. These problems are more likely associated with difficulties in perceiving the *sound* structure of words rather than any fundamental dysfunction with their *visual* recognition. Dyslexia, if not recognised, has pervasive effects on educational achievement and therefore, ultimately, on the person's life course.

BOX 13.4 Reading: current concepts and terminology

- Phonological awareness: sensitivity to the sound structure of words. It includes:
  - Phonemic awareness: the ability to hear and manipulate individual sounds within words. For example, the word 'cat' has three phonemes: c/a/t/. Some children find it much more difficult than others to break down words into their phonemes and therefore to match letters to individual sounds.
  - Syllable awareness: for example, breaking down the name 'Timothy' into its three syllables and then blending then together again.
  - Rhyme awareness: the ability to identify rhyme, to say which pairs of words rhyme and to suggest rhymes.
- Phonics is the teaching of how letters and sounds correspond.
- Phonemic awareness is an important component and pre-requisite of phonics.
- Syllable awareness develops before phonemic awareness, which is seldom well-established in 3- or 4-year-olds.
- Early reading skills are acquired faster with training in phonemes, sounding out words letter-by-letter, than by learning whole words from start.
- Development of reading fluency, vocabulary and comprehension are other important aspects of mastering literacy.

Parents of pre-school children sometimes express concerns about possible dyslexia, either because of their own history or because they believe the child exhibits some of the features they have read about, which are said to be associated with, or predict, future problems. Such worries deserve to be taken seriously; unfortunately, the availability of local expertise varies widely and no single recommendation for referral can be made, except that professionals need to know whom to consult when parents request advice.

Expert assessment of such children may not be easily available either in the health service or in the education authority, but the community paediatrician or Child

Development Centre may be able to help. Parents may also find it useful to contact the Dyslexia Institute.[*]

Parents can be told that the emerging evidence about the acquisition of literacy applies equally to all children,[12] whether or not they are thought to be at risk of specific difficulties in reading.

HEALTH EDUCATION TOPICS

Nursery, nursery school or playgroup

Parents may need advice about meeting the child's needs for play, conversation and social learning. Some children are very happy to go to nursery or nursery school and separate from the parent without difficulty, but others get very upset and may take a long time to settle. Nursery nurses may suggest that the parent simply leave the child, in the belief that he will soon get used to being away from his parent. This may work, but sometimes the child becomes so distressed that the parent has to withdraw the child, often with serious consequences for their own job and income.

If the parent has a child who they think might react in this way, it is probably better to accompany the child to the nursery and stay with him, then after a short period leave with him before he has a chance to get upset. Each day, the parent should try to separate very briefly from the child; at first just across the room, then outside the door for a few moments, then coming back for him after a few minutes. This may take several weeks, but in the long run it will be worth it.

Some young and inexperienced parents need to understand that their responsibility to educate the child does not end when he goes to school! Their active support and interest is vital. For example, parents can improve their child's **reading level** by listening to the child read each day.

Television

A number of studies demonstrate a link between the amount of television watched by children and their level of aggressive behaviour.[13] Too much television appears to make children aggressive. The mechanism is obscure, but there are five possibilities:

1 The increase in the number of violent scenes they are exposed to, particularly when these depict real people in recognisable situations.
2 The passive nature of television watching, which allows fewer opportunities for developing concentration, forethought and experience in social interaction – all qualities required in social problem-solving through skills such as sharing, postponing gratification, and negotiation.
3 The amount of time taken up by watching television, which reduces the opportunities for active experience. There are fewer opportunities to learn self-occupational skills.
4 The amount of time parents spend watching television, which can remove them from active conversation and play with their children and each other.
5 Chronic tiredness from long evenings and late bedtimes.

Obviously there are times when television is a boon to a harassed parent, but the problems of excessive, inappropriate and indiscriminate watching are real. The

---

[*] www.dyslexia-inst.org.uk

ideal of only allowing children to watch a small number of particular programmes, chosen by them in advance in consultation with their parents, is almost impossible to achieve for some families. Most families can use a video-recorder or similar to regulate their children's selection of programmes. Others will have to manage their children's watching by sheer discipline. Stopping children switching the television on as soon as the parent leaves the room is difficult. One remedy is to interrupt the mains lead to the television with a three-pin connector so that there is a length of flex with a mains plug on one end and a connector socket on the other. This can be removed by the parent and put in a drawer or pocket so that the set is inoperable. It can be reconnected when appropriate.[*]

Other topics
Management of minor ailments
The good education and management of minor ailments by parents can make a difference. For example, admissions to hospital for wheezing can be reduced.

Immunisation
Pre-school booster and second dose of MMR should be given if they have not already been administered.

Dental care
It is important that diet (snacks, sweets, etc.) be checked. Bottle feeding should have stopped by now. Check tooth brushing, dental decay and attendance at the dentist.

Injury prevention
For this 2-to 5-year-old age group, parents still need to be vigilant regarding injury prevention (*see* Box 13.5).

BOX 13.5 Danger advice

2 years
Burns, fires: keep matches and lighters out of reach.
   Scalds: a young child can turn on the tap while sitting in the bath, scalding himself or a sibling sharing the bath. Check the thermostat setting or fit a thermostatic mixing valve.[†]
   Choking: reinforce previous advice (*see* Box 11.2 and Box 12.4); discourage young children from running around while eating.

3 years
Road safety: begin to teach traffic awareness and crossing safety.

5 years
Road safety: teach bicycle safety but children should not be cycling on the road or crossing roads alone yet.

---

[*] A more flexible approach is to use a parent-controlled timer: Google 'television viewing control timer' for examples.

[†] *See*: *Preventing Bathwater Scalds.* Available at: www.capt.org.uk

Drowning: teach principles of water safety and how to swim, if not already done but be aware that being able to swim does not prevent drowning in young children.

All ages
Drowning: reinforce previous advice regarding pools and ponds (*see* also Box 12.4).

REFERENCES

1 Berk LE. *Child Development.* New York: Pearson education; 2005.
2 Department of Health. *Child Health Promotion Programme.* London: DH; 2008. Available at: www.dh.gov.uk/en/Publicationsandstatistics/Publications/DH_083645 (accessed 31 December 2008).
3 de Swiet M, Dillon MJ, Littler L, *et al.* Measurement of blood pressure in children. *BMJ.* 1989; **299**: 497.
4 Lous J, Burton M, Felding J, *et al.* Grommets (ventilation tubes) for hearing loss associated with otitis media with effusion in children. *Cochrane Database Syst Rev.* 2005; (**1**): CD001801.
5 Cumberland P, Rahi JS, Peckham CS. Impact of congenital colour vision defects on occupation. *Arch Dis Child.* 2005; **90**: 906–8.
6 Carlton J, Karnon J, Czoski-Murray C, *et al.* The clinical effectiveness and cost-effectiveness of screening programmes for amblyopia and strabismus in children up to the age of 4–5 years: a systematic review and economic evaluation. *Health Technol Assess.* 2008; **12**(25): 1–194.
7 Dyck MJ, Hay D, Anderson M, *et al.* Is the discrepancy criterion for defining developmental disorders valid? *J Child Psychol Psychiatry.* 2004; **45**(5): 979–95. *See* also Dunford C, Street E, O'Connell H, *et al.* Are referrals to occupational therapy for developmental coordination disorder appropriate? *Arch Dis Child.* 2004; **89**(2): 143–7.
8 Smith RA, Sibert JR, Harper PS. Early development of boys with Duchenne muscular dystrophy. *Dev Med Child Neurol.* 1990; **32**(6): 519–27. *See* also Lundy CT, Doherty GM, Hicks EM. Should creatine kinase be checked in all boys presenting with speech delay? *Arch Dis Child.* 2007; **92**(7): 647–9.
9 Glogowska M, Campbell R. Parental views of surveillance for early speech and language difficulties. *Child Soc.* 2004; **18**: 266–77.
10 Ward D. The aetiology and treatment of developmental stammering in childhood. *Arch Dis Child.* 2008; **93**(1): 68–71.
11 Keen DV, Fonseca S, Wintgens A. Selective mutism: a consensus-based care pathway of good practice. *Arch Dis Child.* 2008; **93**(10): 838–44. *See* also Johnson M, Wintgens A. *The Selective Mutism Resource Manual.* Brackley, UK: Speechmark Publishing Ltd; 2001.
12 For a useful overview of recent research and its practical implications, *see* Shanahan T. *2005 National Reading Panel Report: practical advice for teachers.* Available at: www.learningpt.org/pdfs/literacy/nationalreading.pdf. *See* also www.nrcld.org/html/information/articles/ldsummit/jenkins.pdf, and Department for Education and Skills. *Learning and Teaching for Dyslexic Children.* DfES 1184–2005 CDI, DfES. 2005. CDROM. Available at: www.standards.dfes.gov.uk/primary/publications/inclusion/1170961/
13 Mitrofan O, Paul M, Spencer N. Is aggression in children with behavioural and emotional difficulties associated with television viewing and video game playing? A systematic review. *Child Care Health Dev.* 2009; **35**(1): 5–15.

CHAPTER 14

Common behavioural and management problems

THE IMPORTANCE OF FAMILY STRUCTURE AND RELATIONSHIPS

The common emotional and behavioural problems of early childhood are not always caused by parents. However, a good proportion are, either because the child responds in a particular way to aberrant parental handling or because the parents' response to a common variation in the child's developing behaviour has the effect of perpetuating and exaggerating it. It makes sense to advise good child-rearing practice and promote competent parenting.

Most parents are competent and fall within the general range of common sense parenting; they may fret about whether they are doing the right thing for their child, but the odds are that they are. It is the parents who fall outside the normal range who are likely to contribute to children's emotional and behavioural problems. Of course, they may be forced beyond the normal range by a difficult child and it is rarely correct to simply blame the mother (though this is often done). More usually the end-result is the product of an interaction between the child's individual characteristics, the personality and knowledge of each parent and the quality of relationships within the family generally. Within families, it is attitudes and relationships that influence psychological development rather than child-rearing practices alone. Often it is difficult to disentangle the two, but in the majority of families the emphasis should be on the quality of family relationships.

'Competent' parents can be defined by the following criteria:

- they protect their children from physical harm;
- they attend to their children's needs for shelter, food, affection, approval, information and advice;
- they keep adult business (sex, marital conflicts, major worries about money, etc.) separate from their children;
- they use authority so that they are in charge of their children rather than vice versa;
- they respect children's immature status and have a reasonable idea of what this is for each child;
- they set limits of acceptability on their children's behaviour;
- they use a *moderate* number of rules whose purpose can be explained to, and understood by, children;
- they are consistent from one occasion to another, between each other, and between children, according to their developmental status;
- they allow their child a measure of autonomy, tailored to developmental status, allowing him to experiment and learn from experience;
- they use praise focused on the child's achievements;
- they justify prohibitions (briefly) and use mainly non-physical punishments.

Competent parents avoid:

- threats that cannot be implemented;
- using fear as the only disciplinary weapon;
- protracted nagging or moaning;
- denigrating children;
- cruel punishments;
- excessive physical punishments;
- burdening children with worries with which they are not mature enough to cope.

These statements are derived from systematic studies, not a particular ideological approach, and are not advocating a liberal, open approach. Parents who are firm, kind and reasonable have children who are better adjusted than those who allow all emotions to be expressed to anyone, who have no rules, believe in arguing everything through, and who set no limits on children's choices and behaviours.

Questions to consider

The following checklist is useful when evaluating concerns about a child's emotional development or behaviour. The questions are couched in the male sex because psychological/developmental problems affect more boys than girls.[1]

- Are the parents competent in terms of their ability to protect the child, foster his socialisation and self-esteem? (*See* the section on *Fostering emotional and social development*, Chapter 3.)
- What is their attitude towards the child? (Positive or negative, overprotective, dismissive, etc.)
- What is the quality of the child's attachments? (Secure, insecure, avoidant or absent.)

- What is the overall quality of the relationship between child and parent? (Comfortable, tense, unstable, etc.)
- What is the child's temperament and how does it square with his parents' attitudes? (Easy, difficult, slow to warm up, boisterous, studious, sensitive, etc.)
- Are his parents mentally healthy? (Parental depression, personality disorder or alcohol abuse are risk factors for child mental health.)
- What is his capacity to learn? (General and specific cognitive development. Intelligence is a protective factor against the development of emotional and behavioural problems.)
- Is his language development satisfactory? (Developmental language delay may underlie aggressive outbursts or other behavioural problems; the child has to express himself in behaviour rather than words.)
- Is he learning appropriate ways of coping with challenges posed by development? (Such as separations, postponing gratification, having to give way to parental authority, etc. Many behavioural problems are manifestations of a failure to learn appropriate skills; the child is trying to solve a problem, but using the wrong techniques.)
- Can he form and maintain friendships? (Poor peer relationships are a poor prognostic sign.)

The answers to these questions can often be discovered by simple observation of parent and child during ordinary consultations and by a few conversational questions.

EMOTIONAL AND BEHAVIOURAL PROBLEMS IN CHILD HEALTH SURVEILLANCE

Emotional and behavioural problems are extremely common. For example, a study of the prevalence of emotional and behavioural problems in a random sample of 3-year-old children found that around 16% had 'poor' appetite, 14% frequently had difficulty in settling or woke frequently at night, 9% had fears and 8% had problems with siblings or peers.[2] Many of these problems are transient and self-limiting, but early active intervention to solve persisting or troublesome behavioural problems is worthwhile and is good preventive medicine. Involvement in child health surveillance means that the practitioner comes face-to-face with a host of questions and problems concerning a small child's behavioural and emotional responses. This can be puzzling to the novice since such topics are scantily dealt with in most undergraduate and vocational training programmes.

The first step in managing a child's emotional or behavioural problem is to obtain a description of the symptoms and their effect on the child and others. This should enable a decision to be made as to whether the complaint is about behaviour that is normal or abnormal for the child's age. If you judge the child's behaviour and emotional state to be essentially **normal**, the next question is: why should the parent complain about it? Several possibilities exist:

- The parents may be ignorant (first child), misinformed, or apprehensive because of similar symptoms in another child (or the childhood of someone they know) who became a problem.
- The behaviour may touch a raw nerve with them, because it reminds them of

part of their own experience or personality, which they are uncomfortable or upset about.

▶ They may be concerned about something else and are using the problem presented as an excuse for a consultation.
▶ They could be overstressed or mentally unstable.

This means that it is necessary to go beyond a simple reassuring statement that the behavioural or emotional state is normal – to ask what concerns the parent most about the problem: does it remind them of anything; is there anything else that they are worried about; and how are they coping themselves?

For some symptoms, such as babyish behaviour, clinging, misery or anxiety, the issue is also whether they can easily be understood as reactions to circumstances or whether they are so excessive or prolonged compared with what would be expected of an ordinary child that the reaction to adversity is abnormal.

When the presenting feature is an emotional problem in a child over the age of about 4 years old, it is useful to obtain the child's point of view and this may require a brief private interview. This can reveal private or secret sources of distress unknown to the accompanying parent as well as revealing the degree of inner emotional suffering.

The 'cause' of a problem is often a matrix of **predisposing, precipitating** and **perpetuating** aetiological factors. What originally caused a problem in a particular child may not be what is causing it to persist. When the complaint is about episodic abnormal behaviour, consider an analysis that includes an account of the:

Antecedents
Behaviour
Consequences

of a typical episode.

This should enable you to decide whether the child's response to general or particular circumstances is appropriate or excessive and what the impact upon the child is. Accordingly, you can decide if the child's reaction is abnormal. If it is not, then the appropriate action is usually to inform the parent of the cause of the child's distress (provided that the child agrees) and suggest what they might do to alleviate it.

If an abnormality of behavioural or emotional reaction seems to be present, then the next step is to estimate the prognosis. If this is thought to be good and the child is not suffering, then it may well be enough to **reassure** and offer a follow-up appointment that can be cancelled if no longer needed.

Good prognostic pointers include:

▶ good ability to get along with other children;
▶ reasonable family (use common sense to judge);
▶ good previous personality;
▶ an onset related to identified and reversible stress;
▶ brief duration of problem.

Should you consider reassurance and an expectant approach to be insufficient, or if matters have not improved within a few weeks, then a more **active intervention** will be required. Approaches within the capacity of many primary care staff include:

▶ counselling parents;
▶ counselling the child;
▶ simple behavioural programmes and contracts;
▶ medication.

Referral

If this is inappropriate or insufficient, consider **referral** to another agency (*see* also page 199). Many problems involving pre-school children or somatic complaints will be well dealt with in paediatric outpatients. If the local clinical psychology service has an experienced child psychologist they will prove a most useful resource, especially with behavioural problems of young children. Child and Adolescent Mental Health Services (CAMHS) are often at their best with serious cases or complex family problems and see more school-age than pre-school children. Very often, knowledge of local expertise outweighs any generalisation as to which agency should deal with a child's psychological problem.

Recognising emotional and behavioural disorders: the child

It is not necessary to get into an argument with yourself as to whether a young child has or has not got an emotional or behavioural disorder, is psychiatrically disordered or psychologically disturbed. All such terms overlap and none of them is absolute. If a child is doing something that is outside the range you would expect for his or her age and circumstances, and is either causing or experiencing distress, then there is a problem that merits attention. If what they are doing is getting in the way of living a reasonable life, similarly there is a problem. It is better to think in terms of problems, impaired functioning and suffering, rather than enter a sterile debate as to whether or not a disorder is present.

Psychological problems may be short-lived and understandable or chronic and perplexing. In many instances, working through the chart in Figure 14.1 will help. In particular, identifying factors that are associated with a poorer prognosis can help in prioritising interventions for the child.

Recognising emotional and behavioural disorders: the family

Parents and families may, by various vicissitudes, cause children's psychological problems, but not nearly as often as they think they do. Not all children's problems are the result of aberrant parenting and usually parents have less influence on children's *personality development* than they are commonly thought to have. Nevertheless, poor parenting, poor relationships between the child and other family members, unhelpful parental attitudes and practices, and deviant family functioning are the commonest causes of behavioural and emotional disorders in early childhood.

In order to make sense of parenting and family functioning and to identify problems early, some basic concepts are essential.

ISSUES IN NORMAL FAMILY FUNCTIONING

There are two concepts to grasp that relate to normal as well as abnormal families. The first is the idea of **identification** by which a child takes on himself the attributes

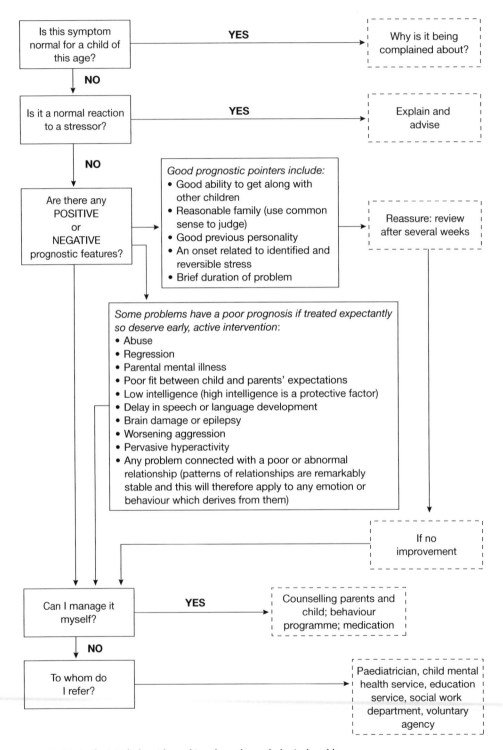

FIGURE 14.1 Chart to help with working through psychological problems.

of another person, particularly a parent. The second is the use of ideas derived from **systems theory** (i.e. boundaries and systems), which are used to describe the structure of the family as a functioning unit.

Identification

Early attachment behaviour (clinging and following) subsides during early development with the formation of interpersonal affectional bonds (*see also* page 46). These are emotions that form the foundations of close, loving relationships. They are characterised by a sense of affection, loyalty and an emotional security in the knowledge of being loved and cherished by the person with whom the bond is formed. These feelings survive geographical separation and therefore make separations possible so that clinging can be abandoned, but a permanent loss of contact with the loved person produces grief. The first relationships a child develops should be characterised by these feelings because they are immensely important in laying the foundations of future relationships, in enabling a secure sense of self to develop, and in learning how to manage anxiety and unhappiness.

Associated with these positive feelings is a strong tendency to take upon oneself the characteristics of the loved person; an identification with them. This aids socialisation and development of an adequate sense of self. Not all identification depends upon attachment formation, nor on warmth. It is a common observation that children, or indeed adults, are prone to adopt the characteristics of those who have power over them. Thus a child can identify with a parent who is aggressive to them, becoming aggressive in turn.

Boundaries and systems

One way of thinking about family functioning is to think about a family in terms of different patterns of role and relationship (**systems**). Thus there is always a parenting system (or **subsystem** if one thinks of the whole pattern of roles in the family as one system), which involves the parents in caring for and bringing up their children. In a two-parent family there will be a marital system, and when there are several children there will be a sibling system. Each system has business within it that is not part of other systems. Sex, for example, belongs within the marital system and should not leak out into the parenting system or incest could result.

Around each system and each person in the system is a **boundary** that is impermeable to a greater or lesser degree. Diffuse and inconsistent boundaries can cause problems as can inappropriate ones, as when one parent refuses to let the other parent become involved in looking after a child.

Risk factors for the development of disturbance
Maternal depression

This is a common problem in families of disturbed children, particularly pre-schoolers. Small children of a depressed mother may be uncontained and noisy. Older ones are more likely to be 'parentified' (*see* below). The mother herself may be irritable or inert or both and is likely to be self-preoccupied and inconsistent in her management of the children. Antidepressants may help, but often do not. As a rule, counselling, involving her partner or another relative in active support, building social links outside home and generally taking a social approach to the problem is more likely to succeed. Badly behaved children can exacerbate and perpetuate depression arising for other reasons, so it may be sensible to see if the mother can be spared the burden of care in some way by arranging playgroups, etc. Thus the involvement of a health visitor or social worker can be crucial.

Parentification

The child takes on the attributes of a parental role and comforts, reassures and looks after a sick, lonely or depressed parent, being solicitous and helpful to a remarkable degree. Obviously this can be appropriate when a parent is temporarily ill, but if the problem is longstanding it is likely to distort personal development as adult anxieties and responsibilities overwhelm the immature child (*see* also the section on young carers, page 86). This can be seen, for example, in many cases of maternal depression, incest and parental alcohol or drug abuse. Only a parent can relieve the child from such a role and many parentified children will not give up readily. Its abandonment by the child is often followed by temporary regression and deterioration in the child's behaviour. It is important to stress to parents that they should be in charge of children and not vice versa.

Overprotection

Although this is perhaps the most common criticism of parenting voiced by doctors, it is less common than many imagine. The overprotective parent infantilises their child. As a result, the child has a narrower range of experiences and fewer opportunities to experiment and solve social problems and feared situations by learning to master them. In consequence, he is likely to be less mature socially and more fearful. It may be coupled with parental indulgence with the consequence that the child becomes a spoilt brat who tyrannises the home by demanding behaviour, stubbornness and tantrums. The origins of parental overprotection are various:

- Precious child (parental sub-fertility results in the birth of a very long-awaited baby; a life-threatening illness in infancy has bred the notion of a fragile child).
- Affection is displaced to the child away from the husband because of marital estrangement.
- A mother who was deprived of affection in her own childhood is now compensating for this either by consciously deciding that the same deprivation of love and caring will not happen to her child, or by vicarious identification with the child whom she lavishes care upon, enjoying this at second hand.
- The child is actually resented by the parent who then overcompensates to assuage the guilt.
- The youngest child is usually the last to leave home and will thus leave the parents on their own with each other. They may not look forward to this and unconsciously hang on to him, keeping him a dependent child so that it will be difficult for him to leave.

It is usually wise to see both parents (possibly grandparents too) and explain how overprotection delays social maturation. As in many instances of advising parents, it is better to suggest what they *can do* (such as encouraging the child to make trips away from home to stay with friends) rather than repeatedly emphasise what they should *not* be doing.

Enmeshment

This is a family therapy term that refers to families with an over-close relation-ship with few boundaries and every member being over-involved with each other's business. In such families, members get upset or anxious on each other's behalf and there are often difficulties over whose feelings belong to whom. Understandably, it is difficult for members to feel themselves to be individuals.

Vicarious satisfaction

It is normal for parents to take pride in their children's achievements, but this can become a burden on the child. Parents may live through their children for the sake of excitement or achievement. Their own disappointments and shortcomings can thus be resolved at second hand. This may overtly or covertly encourage the child to do things he would not otherwise do. A more complicated variant is when a parent punishes a child for something that reflects an attribute or activity of their own that they are ashamed of and would like to punish in themselves. Such mechanisms are instances of the mental mechanism of **projection**.

Rejection

The child is disliked, even hated, and in serious cases the parents demand his removal from the family. As a consequence he may react in various ways:

- stealing from home;
- adopting a frantically ingratiating stance, writing letters to his parents with declarations of love; buying or stealing lavish presents for them;
- aggressive, limit-testing behaviour;
- depression.

Rejection is often associated with evidence of low self-esteem on the part of both parents and child. This seems to breed rigidity on both sides. Rejection is notoriously difficult to reverse, but counselling the rejecting parent(s) individually with a focus on their own childhood is often a helpful first move, since projection of unpleasant personal memories on to the child is a common underlying theme. This may have been made more likely by inter-current depression, which causes the parent(s) to brood on painful and unsatisfactory aspects of their life. Should a counselling approach to parents fail, consider a referral to a child psychiatrist.

Scapegoating

The child is seen, inappropriately, as the source of all the family's woes (and thus may be rejected). A whole family interview may allow the real causes of misery or failure to be identified. There is the problem that the child may act up to the label of troublemaker and be unwilling to give this up. However unrewarding it may seem to be, it is a role and way of behaving that he is used to and he may know no alternative. Formal family therapy is often indicated.

Discord

Open aggression, denigration and abusive disagreement between parents are impor-tant sources of psychological disturbance in the child, much more so than unspoken hostility. Parental separation or divorce may be preferable to an angry violent relationship, but nevertheless their impact on children is often underestimated.[3] As a rough rule, open discord is most likely to be associated with antisocial behaviour. The child is upset, will copy adult behaviour and is unsupported and uncontained by inconsistent, irritable parents. Occasionally, there can be threats to kill, commit suicide, abscond, etc., which are made during marital rows and overheard by a child who takes them literally, feels threatened and becomes insecure, anxious and clinging.

Triangulation

A marital dispute may not take the form of open confrontation between husband and wife, but be routed through the child, arguments between the parents being focused on each other's handling of the child or their respective expectations of him. Thus what is essentially a marital problem is concealed behind complaints about the behaviour of the child. The child may collude in order to keep the peace, but will experience torn loyalties and consequent misery. He may act the part of problem child, a role made easy by his confusion, especially if he is overtly asked to take sides with one parent against the other. Occasionally the child may be subtly encouraged by one parent to play the other one up, thus becoming a pawn in the contest between parents who have been unable to preserve an adequate boundary around their marriage, within which system the disagreement arises and needs to be resolved. Children should be kept out of marital disputes.

Displacement

A parent may find they have strong feelings, especially of resentment, towards a child. Although initially inexplicable, these may sometimes be traced to feelings that should more properly be directed elsewhere. Thus, a single mother may resent her small boy who presents an embodiment of the husband who deserted her. She may not be aware of this so that the simple question 'Does he remind you of anyone?' may be revealing.

Inconsistency

Parents who disagree between each other on handling or expectations or change their own stance from one minute to the next are likely to rear confused, anxious, angry or unsocialised children. It is the seriousness of the inconsistency that is the issue; most parents are somewhat inconsistent and it is frequently possible to blame inconsistency for behavioural problems merely because it is common. When inconsistency is obviously severe and undoubtedly contributes to a problem, it is often quite difficult to correct, if only because many wildly inconsistent parents are uncertain and unpredictable themselves. They may be depressed or have longstanding problems of personal inadequacy. Simple advice given to both parents as to what they specifically might do in certain situations is nevertheless a necessary starting point. A mere exhortation to 'be more consistent' rarely works.

Parenting programmes

Improving parent–child interactions in early childhood can improve long-term outcomes for children. This may involve individualised sessions for mothers, increasing her sensitivity to the infant's needs while taking into account her particular difficulties. Building supportive relationships with fathers, grandparents, and/or social support agencies is also important in some cases.

When parents are willing and able to become involved in parenting programs,[*] these have a good chance of affecting their behaviour.[4,5] The characteristics of programmes that work are now established (*see* Box 14.1), but there are often difficulties in engaging those parents who might benefit the most.

BOX 14.1 Parenting programmes

Parenting programmes in general are more favoured by parents if:

- they allow parents to share experiences;
- they make everyone feel included;
- they are easily accessible;
- they focus on educating parents so they can make their own choices and decisions;
- they are offered before the child is 3 years old;
- the programme is led by a parent.

Characteristics of parent training programmes whose effectiveness has been demonstrated in trials
Content:

- structured sequence of topics, introduced in set order over 8–12 weeks;
- subjects include play, praise, incentives, setting limits and discipline;
- emphasis on promoting sociable, self-reliant child behaviour and calm parenting;
- constant reference to parent's own experience and predicament;
- theoretical basis informed by extensive empirical research and made explicit;
- detailed manual available to enable replicability.

Delivery:

- collaborative approach acknowledging parents' feelings and beliefs;
- difficulties normalised, humour and fun encouraged;
- parents supported to practise new approaches during session and through homework;
- parent and child seen together in individual family work; just parents in some group programmes;
- crèche, good quality refreshments, and transport provided if necessary;
- therapists supervised regularly to ensure adherence and to develop skills.

Sources: Derived in part from Scott S.[5] Some material first appeared in and is reproduced from Hall and Elliman[6] with permission from Oxford University Press.

---

[*] Among the best validated parent-training systems is the one devised by Caroline Webster-Stratton. Its videos and other materials work best in groups, and are too expensive for most individual families. Available at: www. son.washington.edu/centers/parenting-clinic/interventions.asp The book *The Incredible Years*, also by Webster-Stratton, can be confidently recommended to parents wanting advice on the behavioural management of their children (up to about age 10).

BEHAVIOURAL AND MANAGEMENT PROBLEMS

The remainder of this chapter is concerned with common behavioural and management difficulties of pre-school children and those in their first year or two at school. Effective techniques for intervention can be mastered by primary care staff and the ability to deal with these common problems will be of benefit to the practice as a whole. The main disadvantage of the techniques described here is that parents must be properly counselled in their use, which takes time.

Success rates will improve with practice; therefore, it may be sensible for one particular member of the primary care team to develop their skills in this field as an area of special personal interest. Alternatively, the practice may choose to employ a clinical psychologist on a session basis to deal with these problems. However, few GPs will have access to such expertise and many staff, particularly health visitors, may derive considerable satisfaction from solving these common behavioural problems themselves and from the improved relationship with the parents that follows the elimination of a troublesome behavioural problem.

SLEEP PROBLEMS

These are common clinical problems of pre-school children with a prevalence of about 10–20%. Although apparently trivial, the stress on parents is severe, not least because the parents are sleep-deprived. Everyone seems to be an expert, but the problem persists. Although there are multiple causes, they can be readily managed according to Figure 14.2. The approaches have much in common with those

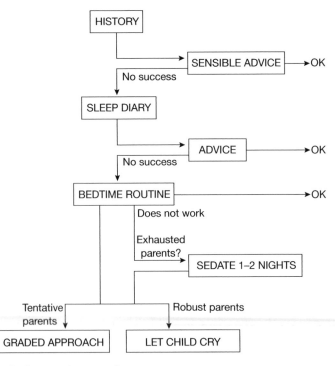

FIGURE 14.2 Difficulty in settling: overall management.

suggested for children age 6–24 months, but can be extended as children acquire more language and reasoning ability.

Difficulty in settling at night (see Figure 14.2)
See both parents, if at all possible, and tell them that:

▶ this is a common problem, and not usually a sign of bad parenting or a spoilt child;
▶ it is not always easy to deal with; there are no guaranteed short cuts;
▶ even adults find it difficult to fall asleep by effort of will;
▶ their first duty is to survive, not to win a battle.

Popular 'common sense' considerations when a small child will not go to sleep at the expected time include:

▶ not tired because he has had too long a sleep in the afternoon;
▶ not tired because he's not been given enough exercise during the daytime;
▶ not tired because he has been over-stimulated or excited just before bed;
▶ not tired because he customarily sleeps late in the morning (mother lets him sleep in because he got off to sleep late the previous night), thus his sleep period is displaced later than usual, but is of normal duration so that he is getting an adequate amount of sleep and is not tired at the early evening bedtime;

WEEK BEGINNING	Time awake	Mood on waking	Daytime naps (give times)	Time told to go to bed	Time in bed	Time asleep	Waking in night (give times)
Monday							
Tuesday							
Wednesday							
Thursday							
Friday							
Saturday							
Sunday							

FIGURE 14.3 A sleep diary.

- frightened of being left alone or abandoned (normal separation anxiety);
- anxious because of noises in the dark, parents having a row downstairs or because he knows he will eventually make his mother angry;
- confused as to what is required of him (mother puts him to bed before father gets home, but he knows father is pleased to see him when he gets in; different bedtimes every night, etc.).

Therefore, the first step is to obtain **a good account of the problem**. What exactly happens and why is it a problem for the parents (lack of privacy, tiredness, losing a power struggle, criticism from grandparents, lack of support from father)? You may be able to give **sensible advice**.

Next, establish what the child's **sleep pattern** is. This may lead to giving sensible advice straightaway. However, as parental accounts are not always clear, it is sensible to ask the parent to keep a prospective **sleep diary** over the next week. This should include:

- time awake in morning (and whether needed waking);
- mood on waking (many parents report no ill-effects of failure to settle until the problem is resolved, whereupon they comment upon the child's improved mood);
- times and duration of naps during day;
- the time he is told he must go to bed;
- the time he is known to be asleep;
- whether he wakes during the night (time, duration and parental action);
- other details may be included (but can be omitted in most cases), such as:
  — what time he is taken to bed;
  — which parent takes charge;
  — how they prepare him for bed (baths, stories, warnings, drinks, etc.);
  — whether/when he calls out or comes out of his room.

The diary can be drawn up on a sheet of paper (*see* Figure 14.3) rather than in a booklet and is best kept near the child's bed. Explain to the parent what it is that you want by drawing up columns and headings or by having a prepared sheet. This may establish something that you can give sensible **advice** about:

- unreasonable parental expectations;
- too much sleep during the day (think about getting him into a playgroup) but note that a *brief* early afternoon nap can improve the quality of night-time sleep;
- erratic bedtimes;
- displaced sleep cycle.

It is wise to **set a bedtime** (saves repeated ill-tempered negotiations each night) and establish a **bedtime ritual** with a fixed progression of events: from a warning that bedtime is approaching, through taking the child to his bedroom, undressing him, bath, tucking up, story, kissing goodnight and so on. This enables a small child who cannot tell the time to be aware of the approach of bedtime. The number of calls for glasses of milk, etc. should be limited in advance. The bedroom must be congenial and enhance falling asleep (nightlight, etc.). **The essential task is for the parent to help the child to learn how to fall asleep on his own** (*see* Figure 14.4).

Either setting a bedtime and routine is sufficient or further measures are needed. If the latter, pause for thought. If the parents are at their wits' end and exhausted, consider **medication** for the child for 1 or 2 nights. Trimeprazine tartrate as Vallergan Forte syrup in a dose of 45–60 mg about 2 hours before bedtime usually works, although the child may be irritable the following morning for a few days. It may take several nights to get the dose and timing right but a maximum of 2 weeks is a good rule for sedating a small child. Make sure the parents continue to use the 5 mL plastic spoon issued: domestic teaspoons can hold as little as 1.5 mL with consequent disappointing results.

Once the parents are feeling braver, discuss two options with them:

1 **Letting the child cry.** This is quick if the parents can manage it. Many parents will say they have tried it and it does not work. Closer questioning reveals that they could not stand the screams and gave up too soon. Advise them to make sure that the environment is conducive to sleep. A soft light (nightlight or landing light), toys in the bed (not exciting ones) and a tape recorder playing a story all help. The following steps are necessary:

▶ both parents must agree with each other that they are going to do it properly (both need to understand that being strict in this way is not harmful or brutal);

Helping a child fall asleep alone		
How long to wait before going in to child (in minutes)		
DAY	FIRST TIME	SECOND TIME	THIRD AND SUBSEQUENT TIMES
---	---	---	---
1	5	10	15
2	10	15	20
3	15	20	25
4	20	25	30
5	25	30	35
6	30	35	40
7	35	40	45

Shutting the door on a child who gets out of bed (minutes)		
DAY	FIRST TIME	SECOND TIME	THIRD AND SUBSEQUENT TIMES
---	---	---	---
1	1	2	3
2	2	4	6
3	3	5	7
4	5	7	10
5	7	10	15
6	10	15	20
7	15	20	25

FIGURE 14.4 Helping a child fall asleep alone.

▶ they *must explain* to the child what is going to happen: that once he has been kissed goodnight, they are not going to come in to him when he cries and that they want him to lie quietly in his bed and wait until he falls asleep;

▶ the child should not be able to get out of the door, but should be able to reassure himself that the parents are still around and have not deserted him (a burglar chain on the bedroom door or a stairgate in the doorway are useful ploys);

▶ the parents need to let the child know that they are still around (they should be urged to talk, sing, wash up noisily or have the radio or TV on; this is in contrast to the usual parental practice of creeping around silently to let him get to sleep);

▶ the parents must have something to do besides listening to the screams or they will not be able to stand it.

The parents may also have to warn the neighbours if they are geographically close. The total duration of crying before sleep should be recorded on a chart (*see* Figure 14.4). Both parents must understand that the crying *gets worse at first*. Like all behaviour intended to attract or be perpetuated for social attention, crying will initially intensify and last longer if attention is withdrawn. If the parents can last out for the first 4 nights, the crying should then gradually subside. The record kept will show this more clearly than the recollections of a fraught and somewhat guilty parent. Next morning the child can be praised for going to sleep on his own. With big smiles and congratulations, the parent supplies a star to stick on a chart or a bead to thread on a string at the foot of his bed.

Managing things gradually

This graded approach takes longer, but is more acceptable to many parents. The core programme is outlined below, but may require some preparatory work if the situation is out of hand. Again parents agree the procedure, tell the child and have a contingency plan for when the child screams.

▶ Parent (mother, for the sake of illustration) settles child briefly, *without letting him fall asleep* and leaves the room, telling him she will return in 5 minutes. The bedroom door is left ajar.

▶ She does not return for 5 minutes unless the child gets out of bed within that time, in which case she returns him and tells him that she will shut the bedroom door if he gets out of bed again.

▶ After 5 minutes she returns to the child and settles him briefly (about 2 minutes) and then leaves the room *before he falls asleep.*

▶ 10 minutes later she returns and settles him briefly again.

▶ 15 minutes later she visits again and subsequently visits at 15 minute intervals until the child is asleep. She must always leave the room before the child falls asleep since the object of the exercise is to help the child to learn how to fall asleep on his own. All she has to do is quieten him.

▶ Getting out of bed after the first warning is dealt with by the mother taking the child back to bed then going out of the door and holding it closed for a full minute. She can talk through the door to the child, telling him that if he goes back to bed, he can have the door left open. This can be repeated as often as necessary, gradually increasing the time the door is held closed. Talking through the door is allowed. Once he has returned to bed, at least 5 minutes should elapse before the parent returns to settle him.

▶ After the first night, the time intervals are subsequently increased by 5 minutes each night (i.e. for the second night, 10 minutes to the first settle, then 15 minutes, then 20 minutes). Similarly, if the child gets out of bed, the time that the door is held shut is lengthened progressively. Most children will be settling well by the end of a week. Nearly always the problem has resolved before reaching 45 minute timings.

Preparatory work

Some parents will have virtually lost control of the situation and be spending enormous amounts of time in the child's bedroom. If the child is used to a parent sitting by (or lying on) the bed or cot, start from there. Get the parents to take alternate nights on duty to share the burden. They must stop lying on the bed next to their child and move to sitting on the edge, then, over a number of evenings, to a chair by the bed, then moving the chair each evening nearer the door until eventually they are outside the door. They should have something to do other than watch the child: reading, knitting, crosswords, even listening to a personal stereo. If they have been singing the child to sleep for hours, get them to hum increasingly softly each evening. The principle is **very gradual change**.

Some children, mainly the 3-year-olds and over, can be encouraged by a simple **incentive scheme**. A string tied to the bed or hung next to it can be used to store large beads or buttons earned for completing certain tasks. These must start with the possible; for instance the child getting into bed himself once he is dressed in pyjamas. When that has been established for a week, a new task is set and different coloured beads are earned for the next stage, such as lying down while a story is read, then a new colour for lying quietly while mother goes downstairs for 3 minutes, and so on. Each stage is worked upon until it has been established for at least a week. It can, of course, be used in conjunction with the graded approach programme outlined above. If the problem is in coming out of the bedroom once well settled, the child can be rewarded for coming no further than the top of the stairs, then to the bedroom doorway, then for doing that without calling out and so forth. The ultimate aim is to have the child lying peacefully in bed, prepared for sleep, and staying there for an adequate amount of time.

Helping the child to fall asleep without a parent in the room is the aim of the exercise.

Waking at night

Most small children wake during the night, but only some make a fuss about it. There tends to be an association with settling difficulties because the child who cannot get to sleep in the evening without a parent present will have the same difficulty when he wakes in the night. In such a case, **treat the evening-settling difficulty first**. A variant of this is that the child may be able to fall asleep at bedtime with the landing light on, the television easily heard and the traffic outside. In the middle of the night it is dark and silent. It may therefore be a good idea to duplicate these conditions at bedtime (no lights, no noise from downstairs, etc.).

The child who settles comfortably in the evening yet wakes and cries in his own

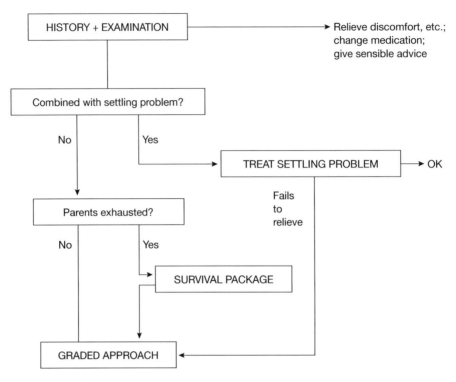

FIGURE 14.5 Waking at night: overall management.

room (or comes into his parents' room) at night should be examined to exclude a physical cause for discomfort: eczema, asthma, otitis media, glue ear (often overlooked as a cause of night time discomfort), teething, etc. The possibility of medication (especially bronchodilators) as a cause of insomnia should be reviewed. Other obvious problems, such as noisy neighbours (or parents) or recent stress may enable sensible advice to be given (*see* Figure 14.5 on management).

Some parents of frequent wakers will be too exhausted to implement a treatment programme straightaway. For such reasons the following advice (**survival package**) seems realistic as a medium-term measure over several weeks:

▶ Parents agree to take alternate nights on duty (saves the arguments and point scoring about whose turn it is); the child cannot insist upon the other parent dealing with him.
▶ If initial attempts to soothe the child or return him fail, then the parents can be given licence to take him into their bed.
▶ The parent not on duty moves out into any spare room or bed available for the rest of the night.
▶ If the child manages to stay in his own bed throughout the night without crying he is praised accordingly in the morning. He can earn stars for being found in his own bed in the morning.
▶ Medication (trimeprazine 60 mg at bedtime) can be added to take the edge off things, but should only be used as a short-term measure (1–2 weeks) to allow parents to overcome their own sleep deprivation. Earlier studies, which

suggested it was ineffective, have been overtaken by the demonstration that a dose of 45–60 mg provides a reasonable (although not complete) respite.

The risks of taking a small child into the parents' bed have been exaggerated. It is an extremely common practice and in most instances has no long-term sequelae. Taking the child into the parents' bed at the beginning of the night is a different matter if it interferes with their sex life, but this argument does not necessarily hold for the child who is taken in or allowed in during the night. Parents fear (or are told) that they will never get him out again, but in real life this does not seem to be a problem, particularly if the child is constantly reminded that staying all night in one's own bed is a sign of growing up. The cost is that the child will not learn to get back to sleep alone in the night, but it may be sensible to postpone having to teach him how to if the nights are cold.

The orthodox advice for managing children who come into their parents' bed at night is to return them straightaway and wait outside the door, calmly returning them to bed each time they emerge. However, this is arduous as it may have to be repeated 20 or 30 times a night. Therefore, parents who are ready to deal more definitively with the problem of a waking or wandering child should apply the **graded approach programme** in the section on settling difficulties, complete with the door-closing sanction. They return the child or go in to him and settle him briefly, returning after an initial 5-minute period, lengthening this gradually. It may be wise for the parents to arrange a strict alternate nights' rota to avoid arguments.

A child who wakes early (4:00–6:00 am) is difficult to manage. Sedation often will not work. If he wanders alone around the house at such a time and thereby puts himself at risk, the best that can be done is to ensure that there is an adequate supply of toys in his room and to keep him there with a stairgate in the doorway. If the problem is that he comes into the parents' room too early, tell them to put a time-switch on a bedside nightlight or suggest the use of a clock specially designed for the purpose.* If set for an appropriate time in the morning these provide the child with a visual indicator of when it is appropriate to come in to the parents. This can be linked with returning him if it is too early and, conversely, praise (perhaps with stars on a chart) for not disturbing them.

Parasomnias

Parasomnias are repetitive unusual behaviours or strange experiences that occur in relation to sleep. About 30 different types are known.[7] The most familiar are nightmares, night terrors, and sleep-walking and sleep-talking. A careful account of exactly what happens and when is important, as the significance and management are different for the various types of parasomnia.

Nightmares

Nightmares are bad dreams and occur during REM sleep. The child may cry out or wake, in which case he is clearly frightened and clingy. The contents of the dream can usually be recalled at the time or in the morning. Nightmares are common, particularly between the ages of 5 and 10 years and do not require any attention unless they are more frequent than once a week (as a rough rule) or unless there is

---

* Google 'children clock sleep' to find examples of suitable items.

a strong repetitive theme to the content, indicating a morbid preoccupation. It is possible to suppress them with a tricyclic antidepressant, such as amitriptyline or clomipramine (not trimipramine, which does not suppress REM sleep), but these are hardly ever necessary.

Generally speaking, preoccupations frightening enough to dominate ordinary dream content and produce essentially the same nightmare over a period of weeks merit psychiatric referral. The exception is recurrent nightmares following an identifiable traumatic experience, such as an assault or serious accident, in which case combine amitriptyline 50 mg at night for 1 month with attempts during the day to get the child to talk to a parent or a trusted adult about the incident in question and to play imaginative games or draw pictures related to it.

Some theories of the mind claim that dreams, as well as reflecting daytime experiences, assist their accommodation into memory, raising the question as to whether it is sensible to suppress dreams with medication. Formal studies of REM deprivation do not demonstrate any harm arising from dream suppression. While it is wise not to meddle unnecessarily with sleep, a short course of a tricyclic antidepressant can free the child from avoidable terror.

Night terrors

Night terrors arise out of one of the first phases of very deep (stage 4) non-REM sleep; in other words before midnight and often about 1–3 hours after falling asleep. The parents hear a loud shriek or loud burst of crying and run to the child who is found sitting up in bed or stumbling around the bedroom with open eyes. They may notice a racing pulse, dilated pupils and terror: signs of a very high level of psychophysiological arousal. The child may appear to be hallucinating, fending off invisible attackers with his hands, and may call out briefly to them. He will push his parents away and not cling to them. It is impossible to get through to him in spite of his appearing awake. After a few minutes he returns to sleep and has no memory of the episode in the morning.

Such attacks are much more common than most textbooks imply, although no formal prevalence figures have been established. They seem to be particularly likely in children under 7 years, although they can occur at any age. It used to be said that they indicated deep psychological disturbance, but there is no evidence for this in pre-school children, although their frequency will increase if the child is stressed. Nor is there any justification for the assertion that they reflect a disturbance in their parents' sex life, although given the timing of a typical night terror, it can certainly disrupt it. The myth persists because the sex life of many parents of young children is likely to be at a somewhat unsatisfactory stage in any case, for a number of understandable reasons.

There is an appropriate course to take with night terrors:

▶ **Reassure** the parents. They should be told that the phenomenon is a disturbance of sleep, which the child will grow out of. They should not try to wake the child during a terror.
▶ Get the parents to keep a prospective record of recurrent night terrors to identify the time at which they are most likely to occur. Once this is established, the parents should **fully wake the child 15 minutes before the projected time** each night for a week, subsequently allowing him to go back to sleep after

2–3 minutes (known as 'anticipatory waking'). This often abolishes the problem by encouraging the development of a different pattern of sleep stages. With good effect, it can often be extended to the treatment of other parasomnias. In the unusual instance of excessive frequency or resistance to the above method (e.g. more than 1 night in 3, for 1 month), night terrors can be abolished with diazepam 2–6 mg at bedtime since benzodiazepines inhibit stage 4 sleep. Although it might seem logical to use a short-acting benzodiazepine, this can merely postpone the terror until the final hours of the child's sleep, which is even more disruptive to parents' sleep.

▶ Continue this course for 3 weeks, then discontinue gradually.

Other parasomnias

Normal pre-school children are likely to show brief movements, such as face rubbing, squirming, muttering or moaning, and abrupt sitting up in bed about 1–2 hours after settling. These occur for a few seconds as the child emerges sharply from the first phase of very deep (stage 4) sleep. They are typical of older, mainly school-age, children and are all common. Usually there is a family history. They can be listed on a scale of increasing severity from brief, unsettled episodes, to dashing around the house in confused panic.

Sleep-talking

Sleep-talking rarely requires medical intervention beyond reassurance. It can be suppressed by anticipatory waking (if regular in its timing) or a benzodiazepine, but this is hardly ever necessary.

Sleep-walking

Sleep-walking is potentially dangerous; there is no truth in the adage that sleep-walkers come to no harm. The parents must ensure that the bedroom windows are secure and consider putting a gate across the child's doorway. It may be wise to move the child to the lower bunk bed where this applies. Older children may manage to reach the front or back door and these will then have to be locked or bolted with a high bolt. There is no point in waking a sleep-walking child; they will have no memory of the episode in the morning. Although obviously confused whilst walking, they are not basically psychologically disturbed and the best course of action is nearly always to steer them back to bed gently and play the whole thing down, ensuring that the child is safe.

If there is a regular pattern, waking the child 15 minutes before a likely episode each night for a week, as for night terrors, will usually work. If absolutely necessary, benzodiazepine suppression (diazepam 2–5 mg at bedtime for 3 months) can be implemented. This may be necessary if the disorientated sleep-walking child is prone to urinate in cupboards, or if night terrors and sleep-walking combine so that the child rushes around the house in confused panic. Even so, it is wise to obtain a prospective record in case a pattern can be established and anticipatory waking tried first.

Thrashing

Some children **thrash** around in bed in a confused, inaccessible state, which may occasionally go on for several minutes. They lack the apparent fear of a night terror, but usually respond to a week of anticipatory waking.

Tooth grinding

Tooth grinding in sleep (bruxism) seems likely also to be a parasomnia. However, the usual empirical remedy is dothiepin 50–75 mg at night rather than a benzodiazepine. If severe and protracted, a dental opinion may be necessary to check for enamel damage.

Night rocking, banging and head rolling

A number of small children develop rhythmic habits that seem to help them get off to sleep. These include sitting up and rocking backwards and forwards or side-to-side. They are harmless, even when quite alarming head-banging is involved, and nearly all children have abandoned the practice by the age of 4. The appropriate intervention is reassurance and practical measures to minimise noise (padding cot sides, putting foam under the cot legs). It may occasionally be possible to set a metronome to match the frequency of rocking and then gradually slow it, night by night, starting it off as the child settles to sleep.

Growing pains

Typically the child wakes at night with severe pains, usually in the lower leg. After 20 minutes or so, with parental attention and rubbing the affected area, the child settles back to sleep. The cause is not known, but the pains seem to be entirely benign. The parent may consult the GP because of unspoken fears about malignant disease (leukaemia, bone cancer). Investigation or referral is only necessary if:

- the pains are not in the legs;
- the pain is always localised to one spot;
- the pain is prominent during day time activity;
- there are other symptoms or positive physical signs.

Other functional pains: somatisation

The term 'somatisation' means that emotional problems become manifest as physical symptoms though it may be over-simplifying matters to say that the pain is *either* 'psychological' *or* caused by 'real' organic illness as both can play a part in some cases. It is widely understood by parents that pain may relate to stress or worry and, as they get older, may be used to avoid something the child finds difficult. Parents may worry that the child is not stoical enough or is too ready to give in to feelings of being unwell. Fathers in particular want to make sure that children do not see complaints of illness as a means of escape.

Most children with functional pains do not have any psychiatric disorder, but they may have an impaired ability to describe distress, simply due to immaturity or to difficulties in communicating emotional issues with other family members. The family may be dysfunctional or may have high expectations of the child, real health problems or preoccupation with illness. The first line of management is explanation, reassurance, management of the immediate presenting problems and behaviours, and where possible, the development of other ways of dealing with distress. Referral to a clinical psychology service may be worthwhile, both for immediate benefit and to reduce the risk of somatisation becoming a life-long problem-solving strategy.

HYPERACTIVITY

In general parlance, the term 'hyperactive' is imprecise. It may just mean a high level of motor activity or can include overactivity together with a short attention span, excitability or impulsivity (i.e. acting without adequate thought). It may be used variously to indicate a symptom, a syndrome or a disorder.

Many parents describe their child as 'hyperactive' without this necessarily meaning that he is, in fact, pathologically overactive. He may thus be:

▶ normally active for his age, but his mother may, in her turn, be a novice parent and does not realise the high activity level of young children; she may be chronically tired; she may have a quieter temperament than he; or she may be depressed;
▶ active at the wrong times (e.g. at meals and bedtime) or in the wrong places (e.g. in shops or the back of the car);
▶ disobedient (e.g. not sitting still when told);
▶ not overactive but noisy, uninhibited or distractible; qualities which affect the *style* of his behaviour.

This indicates the need for a good descriptive and developmental history, possibly with a home visit to observe the child on his own territory. A number of children can be boisterous at home or in a playgroup yet compliant and contained in a surgery or clinic. Check the mother's mental state, particularly for depression, which can make her an ineffective controller of children's exuberance, may alter her judgment so that she perceives a normally active child as overactive, and can induce provocative, high-amplitude behaviour on the child's part (i.e. he has to do more to obtain a response from her).

This initial assessment may suggest that:

▶ the child is not overactive, but there is a handling/behavioural problem with noisy non-compliance or abusiveness;
▶ the child is somewhat overactive and has not enough to do that is quiet and absorbing while extending his capacity to concentrate (often as a result of too much television);
▶ the child is overactive and has parents with inappropriate expectations of self-restrained behaviour;
▶ the child is overactive and has a parent who is depressed.

These problems need relevant advice or intervention. Bear in mind that the child may not be entirely normal; he may have an excitable, extroverted temperament. Some overactive children are **developmentally delayed**; their activity is commensurate with their mental age rather than their chronological age.

Overactivity can be **iatrogenic**: benzodiazepines (especially clonazepam), phenobarbitone, promethazine and metoclopramide have all been implicated as causes of inattentive restlessness. **Dietary constituents** are often blamed, yet they are only rarely a cause of overactivity (*see* page 115). Many parents will experiment with diets themselves. A tiny few succeed; the GP will see the failures. GPs should be wary of trying dietary manoeuvres without the advice of a dietician as malnutrition is a real risk. Remember that diets are expensive.

Once the above have been excluded, there are three main causes of serious overactivity, usually associated with inattentiveness in children:

1 **Anxiety** in those children who respond to their anxious mood by nervous overactivity. They may have multiple phobias or a history of a recent life-threatening event. There will be a history of recent acute onset rather than a story of overactivity 'since day one'. They should be considered for counselling on an individual or family basis and referred to a department of child psychiatry if there is no progress after a few weeks.

2 **Pervasive hyperactivity** (hyperkinetic disorder; i.e. *severe* attention deficit hyperactivity disorder (ADHD)) in which the child is, and always has been, overactive, restless and inattentive in *all* situations and is never still unless asleep. Many (but not all) have delayed development and some degree of learning disability. Severe cases are rare; but all cases need referral to a developmental paediatrician or child psychiatrist for a full neurological, psychological and educational assessment and consideration of medication (usually stimulants) or behavioural therapy.[8]

3 **Situational hyperactivity** in which the child is overactive in some situations (particularly the classroom) but not in others, and may appear quite normal when first seen. This is a milder version of the ADHD described above. It is a common problem, especially among boys, and often associated with such traits as impulsiveness, excitability, distractibility and fidgetiness. A considerable number are also naughty or even seriously antisocial. Not surprisingly, educational problems are frequent and may require an assessment by an educational psychologist.

Situational hyperactives are a heterogeneous group. Their overactivity will often respond to stimulative medication, but this is difficult to handle without experience and is essentially palliative. A sensible first line of approach would be to advise the parents to:

▶ adjust their expectations according to the child's capacity (e.g. shorten the duration of meals);
▶ provide structured, sedentary activities (puzzles, drawing, models, Lego) and actively encourage the child to carry them out by himself; note that allowing the child to run around to burn off excess energy does not work except *in extremis* when the child is ultimately too exhausted to do anything at all;
▶ reward such sedentary self-occupational activity by praise;
▶ respond to noisy outbursts calmly and firmly;
▶ maintain or build his self-esteem by finding behaviours or achievements to praise.

Failure of such measures should lead to referral to CAMHS or a developmental paediatrician, who will manage the situation similarly to hyperkinetic disorder.

Disruptive pre-schoolers

Disruptive pre-schoolers may come to the attention of community child health professionals because of concerns raised by early years staff. They have an increased risk of many problems in their school years and adulthood, including persistent aggression, peer rejection, drug abuse, depression, delinquency, and dropping out of school. Rejection by peers is important: to some extent it predicts poor performance at school, getting into trouble with the law, and some long-term psychiatric disorders. This is probably partly due to the rejection, and partly to the underlying factors that led to the rejection in the first place. Children who are rejected for their aggression or for their shyness and withdrawal have considerable risk of these problems persisting into adulthood.

Rejected aggressive children view others as unkind and hostile and in an ambiguous situation they are more likely to attribute hostile intentions to other children, perhaps because they have been exposed to more hostility than other children. Such children have a wide range of underlying difficulties, including hyperactivity, poor attention, and poor academic performance, and they are more likely to come from families with mental illness, criminality and substance abuse. Some have been exposed to violence at home, marital conflict, inconsistent or hostile parenting, or physical abuse.

AGGRESSIVE BEHAVIOUR [9]

It is usually sensible to think about aggression as a quality of behaviour rather than a drive or a trait in its own right of which the child has too much. This helps avoid suggestions such as punch bags, which are intended to help the child to 'get it out of his system' (but do not work).

The causes of aggression are multiple, but the following points may be useful to remember:

- Aggressive responses are likely to occur when a child feels threatened or **provoked** beyond self-restraint. A child who is repeatedly thwarted, taunted, hit or demeaned by parents, siblings or peers can strike back.
- Aggressive responses can be **learned**. A child may learn from the example provided by aggressive parents, whether angry, brutal or harsh. Aggressive acts may enable a child to get his own way or snatch toys, thus obtaining rewards for such a style of behaviour.
- There is a close link between aggression and **mood**, particularly anger, resentment, tension and irritability. A child in a bad mood is likely to behave aggressively.
- Aggressive responses are essentially **primitive** and are likely to be deployed when the child knows of no other response that will suffice. This means they are more common among younger children and those who have learned no other way of coping with provocation.
- Aggression that persists and worsens beyond the first few years of life is a remarkably **stable** characteristic of behaviour. If it becomes established as a general way of coping, it does not usually go away; reassurance that it will subside with time is likely to be wrong.

Commonly, several of these factors underlie the clinical problem of an excessively aggressive child. Families that are bad at teaching alternatives to aggression (such as self-restraint or negotiation) also tend to teach children how or when to be aggressive by using aggression to solve problems in personal relationships (e.g. employing harsh physical punishments, having rows, making physical or verbal threats). Therefore, aggression arises out of a mixture of learning unacceptable responses and a failure to learn acceptable ones.

Given a parental complaint about a child's aggressive behaviour, the first obligation is to review the general status of the child:

▶ **Mental age.** Is there any learning difficulty or any other impairment to learning more civilised behaviour? Does language impairment contribute to frustration?
▶ **General mood of the child.** For example, is the problem essentially one of unhappiness?
▶ **State of the family.** Is there justified hatred of a preferred sibling; teasing; expectation of a new step-mother to be loved; irritable and depressed parent?
▶ **Friends and school.** Are there sources of failure or sensitivity with friends or at school?
▶ **Physiological.** Does the child have chronic pain or fatigue? Check **hearing** in a toddler.
▶ **Pharmacological status.** Is the child taking benzodiazepines (sometimes given to the child by the parents from their own supply) or proprietary 'natural' or 'homoeopathic' remedies (some of which are quite strong)? A straightforward remedy may become apparent.

Secondly, it is important to understand how a typical episode occurs through carrying out an **ABC** analysis (*see* page 28). This may reveal unreasonable and unrecognised provocation in the eyes of the child; what constitutes aggression in the eyes of the parent; and how it may be being aggravated by the consequences. This approach will often indicate some areas of weakness, which can be remedied by straightforward advice or action.

Should matters appear less clear-cut, the following steps are necessary:

▶ Arrange to see both parents and persuade them that aggression indicates a **deficiency state**; something is missing because alternative and more mature ways of coping have not been learned sufficiently well.
▶ When their child does behave aggressively, they must tell the child that he is doing so and that it is unacceptable (**labelling**) using a sharp, brief interjection such as 'No – I won't have that'. (This must emphatically *not* be itself aggressive or become a nagging commentary on the child's actions such as 'You really ought to stop doing that . . . it's not at all nice to other little boys; they won't like you . . ..') They must tell him what he could be doing that is acceptable (**identifying desired alternatives**), such as waiting his turn or learning to negotiate a compromise.
▶ They should be encouraged to set up a **star chart** or other incentive scheme whereby the desired alternatives (pro-social actions that supplant aggressive responses) can be encouraged.
▶ Suggest that they demonstrate through their own actions and interactions how problems between people can be resolved without aggression. Failure of such an approach to yield results within several weeks is an indication for adding **time-out** (*see* page 340). If this fails to improve matters, make a referral to CAMHS earlier rather than later.

Aggressive behaviour in the playground

A child may be aggressive because he considers it a sensible way to solve an inter-personal problem (whether or not he knows of any other way) or because he is too angry or upset to deploy more considered tactics, such as negotiation. A complaint that a small child hits, pokes or bites other children, apparently without provocation, should therefore lead to **questions about the child**: can he participate in verbal (rather than non-verbal) exchanges? Does he know of other methods of resolving disputes and can he learn these? Impaired hearing and global learning disability need to be ruled out accordingly. A few children with secretory otitis media will intermittently have sufficiently impaired hearing to misinterpret what is said to them and react to what they wrongly perceive as hostile overtures from peers.

It is important to enquire about **the child's home life**. Do the parents habitually resolve their difficulties with him or each other by aggressive coercion or violence so that he has learned the wrong lessons? If not the parents, what about older siblings? Some children are upset and angry because of insecurities or injustices in their home life.

Advise carers to **intervene immediately** at any outburst of aggressive behaviour. Place the child in a corner (observed, but isolated from social interaction) for 5 minutes and, when he is receptive, describe to him more appropriate ways of behaving along the lines of 'What we do here is . . .'. Often this comes down to basic skills of sharing, turn-taking, asking nicely, and doing simple deals ('If you let me . . . then I'll let you . . .'). Moral remonstration along the lines of 'What would you think if someone did that to you?' or 'What if everyone did that?' are doomed to failure as the pre-school child cannot readily enter into that sort of hypothetical reasoning.

Helping the victim not to cry may be important. Patterson's classical study in a playgroup demonstrated that aggressive, coercive behaviours between young children are rapidly learned and that tearfulness when victimised provokes further aggressive attacks by others.[10] There are a few small children, usually with impaired empathic skills, who have a malicious interest in causing pain to others because they are fascinated by their overt distress or helpless fury. Even for them, the appropriate first line of management is supervision, prompt intervention for safety's sake, and tuition in alternative, civilised ways of managing disagreement or conflict.

Smacking

Health professionals may be asked for their opinion on smacking young children. The UK Government has been urged to make smacking illegal, but has so far stopped short of such a ban. In England, the Children Act 2004 makes it an offence to hit a child so as to cause grazes, scratches, abrasions, minor bruising, swelling, superficial cuts, a black eye or reddening of the skin that stays for hours or days (*see* Chapter 4 on safeguarding). The arguments against smacking are: it is usually inef-fective; it is often done in anger and therefore represents loss of control by the parent, which could lead to significant injury to the child; it sets an example of physical aggression as an acceptable way for individuals to deal with disagreements; and it can damage the relationship between parent and child. Parents must be equipped with other more effective ways of providing discipline and teaching children socially acceptable behaviours. The important questions to ask are what other strategies the parent is using (e.g. time out or loss of TV time), their consistency and severity, and whether the child can earn praise and affection.

EATING PROBLEMS

Eating problems sometimes begin in infancy with weaning (*see* Chapter 7 for further details of management in the under-2 year's age group). Pre-school children are often brought for professional advice by parents with the complaint that they will not eat and mealtimes have become a battleground. In most cases, at a casual glance, the child is well nourished and healthy. The first thing to do is **obtain a good account of what happens at a typical meal**. This may reveal that:

▶ meals are irregularly timed and there no consistent pattern;
▶ unsuitable or unacceptable foods are served (for some children, fish, potatoes, green vegetables, fried eggs or even all unfamiliar foods are genuinely nauseating);
▶ there are multiple opportunities for distraction (people coming and going; the television is on during mealtime, etc.);
▶ unreasonably large portions are served to the child.

Next, ask **what the parent is most concerned about**. This commonly reveals concerns about **nutrition** and **discipline**. The issue of nutrition can nearly always be dealt with in an entirely straightforward way by weighing and measuring the child and referring to a growth chart, then discussing the results with the parent. As far as discipline is concerned, first ask the parent whether they remember being upset by foods as a child, and what other people (particularly grandparents) have said about the child's eating and behaviour at meals. This helps place things in perspective. Thirdly, ask **how much the child eats between meals**. The initial answer is often 'nothing much', but persist. The child is getting food from somewhere.

Any doubt over these issues should lead to a request that the parent complete a **food diary for the child** for several days. All food eaten (including sweets, crisps and biscuits) is to be entered, as well as the food that is refused. If the child's eating goes in phases, the diary needs to continue long enough to get an overall picture. This usually enables you to make some common sense observations. As a first move there should be **absolutely no eating between meals**. No sweets as rewards, no snacks and care with high calorie drinks. They cannot force the child to eat – but in this way they can arrange for him to be hungrier at mealtimes. Warn parents about buying foods that they do not want their children to eat. Note that some foods are invisible to some parents who apparently do not regard crisps, sweets or chocolate as food. A variation on the theme is that the child does eat plenty of what the parents regard as junk food: baked beans, chocolate and crisps, but he will not eat 'healthy' foods.

The weight chart will confirm your statement that although it would be nice to persuade the child to eat a 'healthier' diet, he will certainly not fade away; beans, chocolate and crisps provide fat, carbohydrate and protein!

Only then move to giving advice about meals themselves. If a parent chooses mealtimes as the arena where discipline is to be imposed, they are likely to be unsuccessful. Nothing can coerce a stubborn child to eat except hunger. It is a battle no parent can win. In general terms, take the pressure off the child and the parent:

▶ Offer the child less to eat than usual.
▶ Some children are reluctant to face the sensory experience of eating; perhaps

fearing it will be disruptive or unpleasant. Promise to take the plate away if they just have one fork-full. After tasting a food they may want the rest.

▶ Some children want predictable foods; others want variety.
▶ Do not rush the child (within limits; there must be an end to the meal).
▶ If he refuses a particular food, take it away and offer an alternative.
▶ No nagging, coaxing, threatening, or blackmail and no urging 'one more mouthful'.
▶ No fuss about the order of courses, finger feeding or strange tastes and practices. They can be put right later.
▶ Involve the child in food preparation.
▶ Avoid too many drinks until the child has eaten a reasonable amount of food.
▶ Encourage anything that will defuse tension at mealtimes and make them more fun. It is usually helpful for the parent(s) to eat at the same time as the child, re-inventing the concept of a family meal. This gives him the opportunity to learn how to behave at mealtimes through observation.

Pica

Pica is the habit of **eating substances not normally regarded as food**. It should be distinguished from mouthing of objects, which is a transient developmental phase (*see* page 252). If mouthing is still occurring beyond the age of 2, it is likely to be associated with some developmental problem such as general backwardness. Toddlers sometimes experiment with eating undesirable substances, such as dog faeces or Plasticine. During this usually brief phase of development, it is very important that dangerous materials are kept locked away, and parents should check their garden for poisonous plants such as laburnum. Parents are most likely to seek advice in an emergency because the child has eaten a potentially hazardous substance; a poison centre may be contacted for information. Remember that while repulsive items like faeces rarely seem to do any harm, some apparently innocuous substances may be deadly; for example, crystals from a chemical set can be highly poisonous.

If the child persists in eating non-food substances and there has been no response to normal disciplinary approaches, there are a number of things to consider:

▶ The child may have some developmental disorder. If there is any evidence of backwardness or retardation of language development, consider referral to a developmental paediatrician.
▶ There is an association between pica and iron deficiency. The precise nature of this link is uncertain, but a short course of iron can do no harm and is occasionally very effective.
▶ If the child is eating *very old* paint or other potentially lead-containing substances, consider whether a blood lead estimation should be done. (**NB**: 'lead' pencils do not contain lead.)

Older children, usually boys, may acquire a dare-devil reputation by accepting challenges to eat increasingly repulsive items like slugs. The activity is quite difficult to eliminate and such reputations once acquired are guarded jealously. Serious harm is unlikely to result. The child may need some help in devising acceptable ways of declining these challenges without losing face.

BEDWETTING

All children wet the bed in infancy; progressively fewer do with advancing age. There is no absolute, fixed age at which ordinary bedwetting becomes the pathological condition of nocturnal enuresis, so the two terms are used interchangeably here. Clinicians vary as to when they routinely actively treat bedwetting. Many would do so from when the child is 7 years old, but if there is substantial distress and family concern, children as young as 4 can be managed effectively. The argument for not treating early as a routine is, firstly, that a (rather small) proportion of 4-year-olds and over will spontaneously acquire dryness and secondly, because 4- and 5-year-olds can be frightened by the sound of an enuresis alarm in the dark.

Management of enuresis is not difficult, but it is time consuming, since much depends on building rapport and confidence and explaining the method(s) being prescribed. For this reason, the best results may be obtained if the child is managed in a special clinic, which is often run by a nurse and supported by a paediatrician when required.

Relationship to developmental delay

Most enuretics seem to have an **isolated developmental delay** in acquiring nocturnal bladder control. In such cases, there are no clues as to causation beyond a family history of enuresis (which may not be obtainable unless both parents are interviewed). It is not uncommon for children with enuresis to have one or two other instances of specific developmental delay (speech, motor coordination, etc.). **Learning disability** is an obvious cause of delayed acquisition of nocturnal bladder control.

Relationship to psychological disturbance and stress

Most enuretics are psychologically healthy; only about 20% are psychologically disturbed, and in a number of children this is quite likely to be the consequence of bedwetting rather than its cause. The usual assumption is that secondary enuresis (that with an onset after a period of dryness) is most likely to relate to stress events or psychological disturbance. This is a generalisation and only partly true. Primary enuretics can be disturbed and secondary enuretics not so. In most instances of enuresis, there is no clear association with recent stress. Nevertheless, bedwetting *can* occur as a response to acute stress, such as bereavement or starting a new school and in such circumstances it is usually time-limited and does not commonly present as a clinical problem. If it does, provided that the stressor is clear-cut and the onset is within the last month, it can be treated expectantly.

More commonly there is **chronic stress** (such as an acrimonious parental relationship) and this is likely to reflect a more complex mechanism; the source of stress may also have interfered with the normal acquisition of dryness. In such cases, it makes sense to treat the enuresis symptomatically as a first move, not to delay treatment till the cause(s) of stress have been eliminated, since this is almost certainly a protracted process if it succeeds at all.

Physical causes

There are three possibly physical causes for enuresis:
1 **Urinary tract infection.** A small proportion of enuretics have demonstrable bacteriuria. Treatment of this may relieve the enuresis.
2 **Faecal soiling associated with faecal retention.** This is commonly associated

with enuresis, presumably in part because of a distortion of pelvic anatomy and consequent restriction of bladder volume and dysfunction of the basal plate and neck of the bladder.

3 **Polyuria secondary to diabetes (mellitus or insipidus) or renal failure.** This can exceptionally present as enuresis (nearly always with polydipsia and often associated with daytime wetting).

Three anatomical causes of enuresis are extremely rare:

1 **An ectopic ureter opening into the vagina in girls.** (This causes continual dribbling by day and night rather than bedwetting alone.)
2 **A neurogenic bladder.** (This also causes continual dribbling by day and night rather than bedwetting alone.)
3 **Epileptic seizures.** These could theoretically cause enuresis, but, in practice, enuresis is no more common among children with seizures.

It follows that assessment of the enuretic child will include a history and examination to rule out the above aetiological factors, even though most cases will not have an identifiable aetiology. It is wise to include a brief interview with the child, which may reveal sources of stress unknown to the parent and indicate whether the child is suffering from a depressed mood. The child's own reaction to his bedwetting can be documented.

Management

To manage enuresis, you should know the child's history and undertake an examination of the child.

To ascertain the child's history, find out:

▶ the duration and course of enuresis with relationship to obvious life events;
▶ if there is associated daytime wetting;
▶ if the child has excessive thirst, sufficient to wake the child for drinks at night;
▶ if the child experiences dysuria;
▶ if there is associated soiling;
▶ the general level of the child's development;
▶ any associated emotional and behavioural problems;
▶ if there is any family history of enuresis;
▶ who sleeps where;
▶ past and present methods of dealing with it;
▶ the attitude of the child to wet beds;
▶ the attitude of the parent to the child and to wet beds.

Examination is unlikely to reveal anything, but indicates that the problem is being taken seriously. Undertake:

▶ a general inspection of abdomen and back to exclude palpable bladder and spina bifida occulta or other spinal lesion;
▶ an examination of genitalia;
▶ an examination/testing of mid-stream urine for sugar; proteinuria; many white cells; infection.

Treatment

The above steps will have effectively ruled out conditions to which enuresis is secondary and the following require management in their own right:

- ▶ learning difficulty (mental handicap);
- ▶ acute stress;
- ▶ urinary tract infection;
- ▶ faecal retention;
- ▶ anatomical lesion;
- ▶ diabetes (mellitus or insipidus);
- ▶ chronic renal disease.

These can be dealt with appropriately. Assuming that there are no clues in the history to suggest infection and a stick test reveals no excess protein or sugar, the mid-stream urine specimen can be despatched to the laboratory and the child and parent attended to.

Reassurance is the first step. The child can be told that bedwetting is quite common and that there will be at least one other person in his class at school who is bedwetting. If there is a family history of enuresis, he should be told that too. His parents should be told in his presence that it is something he cannot help. **Punitive practices should cease and the problem made easier to live with.** Newspapers and a plastic sheet could go into the bed underneath the bottom sheet. Nylon sheets dry more quickly. A duvet filled with artificial fibre is more easily washed. Wet sheets are stripped in the morning and can be washed and dried so that the child has a warm, dry bed to get into each night. The child should wash in the morning rather than be sent to school smelling. Any urinary dermatitis can be treated with a barrier cream: Drapolene, Siopel, etc. Fluid restriction in the evenings rarely reduces urine production sufficiently to avoid night time wetting; but it is worth checking that the evening intake is appropriate (i.e. drinking just a small proportion of the day's fluid then, with more in the first half of the day; and avoiding caffeine-containing beverages such as Pepsi and Coke).

Promote social learning and self-esteem. Suggest that the parent deal with wet beds in a matter-of-fact way and meet dry beds with exaggerated approval and pleasure. There is an argument for getting them to say 'That's terrific' or 'How wonderful' rather than 'Well done', as the latter implies that the dryness is achieved by conscious effort. If the child has been creeping into the parents' bed after wetting, this should be stopped as it may function as an unintended reinforcement for wetting.

A star chart with stars for dry nights must be kept by the child and can be put on open display unless the child is embarrassed, in which case it can go inside a cupboard door. The parents keep the stars. A common practice is to award a gold star when three consecutive dry nights are achieved. This should be continued for 4 weeks. There is no need for the parents to back the stars up with any tangible reward. At 4 weeks, review the chart with child and parent. Show approval for successes; this pleases and motivates the child and can provide a demonstration to the parent of good praising technique. It will either show a decreasing frequency of wetting (in which case continue, and review at 2-week intervals) or a reasonably stable pattern, which forms a baseline for the next stage.

A star chart is effective in its own right in about one-third of cases. If it is not, proceed to an **enuresis alarm** (previously known as the bell and pad). This must be given to the child as his alarm and demonstrated to him and his parents. Alarms are not available on prescription; parents can buy their own from manufacturers at a cost of about £30–£40, but a better system is to keep a couple or so in the surgery, purchased by donated funds. The local department of community child health, paediatric out-patients or CAMHS will all have their own stock and referral can be made to them if all else fails. Nevertheless, it is preferable to keep your own supply and move smoothly from star chart review to adding the alarm without loss of therapeutic momentum. Alarms can be booked out on loan.

Alarms operate on the principle that voided urine completes an electric circuit (by bridging a gap or by linking dissimilar metal pads, which then act as a battery), and sounds an alarm (or activate a vibrator, which is useful for children who share a bedroom or who are hearing impaired). There are three main types of alarm:

1 The alarm is the size of a matchbox and is pinned to the child's pyjama top. It contains a tiny battery and emits a penetrating buzz, which may be pulsed. It connects to a small square of plastic on which are two concentric electrodes. This sensor is placed inside a perineal absorbent pad (Vespre® or similar) which is, in turn, put inside the child's underpants so that it is held next to the urethral orifice. There is some evidence that this type of alarm achieves dryness more quickly.
2 The alarm is a box (commonly the size of a half pound box of chocolates) that goes on a chair by the bed, just out of arm's reach. It contains a battery and emits a loud buzz. Two wires lead to two large wire-mesh or aluminium foil pads, which are placed, one on top of the other, in the child's bed under the part where the child sleeps. They are separated from each other by a sheet and from the child by another sheet.
3 A similar alarm connects to a single PVC pad on which are two separate, concentric, adjacent metal ribbons. The pad is covered by a single sheet upon which the child sleeps.

Demonstrate the alarm to the child in his parent's presence. He is then asked to explain it himself all over again to his parent. The small alarms can be set off with a wet finger on the electrode. Demonstration of the larger alarms will involve making a mock-up on a chair using the mesh pad(s) and old sheets or kitchen paper between and over them. Sit the child on the pad(s) and pour some salted water between his legs onto the pads, triggering the alarm. In the presence of his parent show him how to turn it off and demonstrate all the ways in which he can stop the apparatus working. This lessens the chance of covert sabotage later. Give the alarm to him and consider putting his name on it with a sticky label to emphasise the point that it is his for the time being. Point out that the alarm cannot give him an electric shock.

If asked, you can reassure them regarding safety. There is no risk of psychological trauma in a 7-year-old, and 'buzzer ulcers' no longer occur. The buzz of the alarm must wake the child or it is useless. In order to ensure this, the larger alarm boxes can be fitted with a separate booster or, more simply, put in a biscuit tin. The parents will need to get up the first few times it sounds to check that the child wakes and gets out of bed when it sounds. He should go to the toilet, then strip the bed or remove the small alarm. There is no need to reset the alarm for the rest of the night; he can go back to bed. For simplicity, two layers of bedding can be used separated by a plastic sheet which is stripped with the wet sheet.

In the morning, dry beds are rewarded by a star on the **star chart which is continued throughout the alarm treatment** as a record. The parents should telephone you after the first night to ensure all went well. Thereafter, contact should be every 2 weeks or so, preferably by appointment or home visit to see the child, praise progress, and check the alarm is still in working order. Full dryness is likely to take at least 8 weeks to achieve, maybe longer, and the child must be told this. Unfortunately, all alarms are technically unreliable and the parents must be told to notify the surgery or clinic immediately a fault arises so that a replacement alarm can be provided. It is wise to telephone or visit the home after the first night to sort out any difficulties. If excessive sweating sets off the alarm, try using less bedding (or try cotton sheets which are more absorbent than nylon, though harder to dry).

Mesh pads usually need replacing every 4 weeks or so; once they have become lumpy they are less efficient and broken wires can penetrate sheets causing short circuits. Aluminium pads may be reduced to pulp very rapidly and are less popular than mesh. Pads made of copper braid are robust in themselves, but are commonly vulnerable at the point where the wires to the alarm are connected. It is not absolutely necessary to treat every single night, in fact there are grounds for not doing so since this cuts down the chance of relapse.

Other ways of minimising the chance of relapse include **overlearning**, whereby the child, once dryness has been achieved for 2 weeks, starts to drink a glass of water before going to bed. He is warned that this is likely to result in a wet bed or two, but the alarm will teach his bladder to hold on to this extra load. When dryness has been re-established for a week, he is asked to drink two glasses of water at bedtime. Once dryness has been established under this regime, the alarm and the extra bedtime water are both discontinued simultaneously.

The alarm, coupled with a star chart, is a highly effective treatment provided that the child and parents are satisfactorily engaged in the process and technical faults are dealt with promptly. About one in five children will relapse after dryness has been achieved; sometimes after a delay of several weeks. The alarm is reinstated until dryness is achieved. A second relapse is extremely unlikely. Although the alarm might seem to be contraindicated in families where the enuretic child shares a bedroom, in practice, the others in the room quickly learn to sleep through the buzz. Should this not occur (or if the child is deaf) a vibrator alarm can be used. However this has the disadvantage of not alerting the parents.

Desmopressin, a synthetic anti-diuretic hormone (ADH) analogue, is available as a tablet (200–400 micrograms), which should be taken before bedtime and may also be a sensible short-term intervention, though there is a high relapse rate. To minimise the risk of water intoxication and hyponatraemia, fluid intake should be restricted in the evening when it is to be used and children should avoid swallowing large amounts of water when swimming. It should be stopped if the child has vomiting or diarrhoea. The treatment should be stopped for a week and reviewed every 3 months. For children who cannot take tablets, the sublingual preparation (120–240 micrograms at bedtime) can be used; the nasal spray can cause nasal congestion and is no longer recommended.

When there is an urgent need to establish dryness, **imipramine 25–50 mg at night** will stop bedwetting in most children; but there are a number of concerns that limit its use. In nearly all studies, when it has been used alone the relapse rate during the months following discontinuation of the drug has been very high and it cannot be considered an effective treatment in its own right. Most clinicians who believe that it works well use it in conjunction with a star chart, which begs the question of which is the active treatment? There is a risk of accidental overdose (and ingestion by the enuretic child's younger siblings); it may disturb sleep, usually produces hypertension and the anticholinergic side effects can be unpleasant. It is best reserved for first aid measures, such as staying overnight with friends or going to cub or scout camps, and followed up by an alarm treatment. There is no point in combining it with an alarm.

PROBLEMS WITH DEFECATION

This subject is bedevilled by lack of any uniform terminology. The following definitions are used in this chapter:[11]

▶ **Constipation** means difficulty, delay or distress in defecation. Chronic functional constipation in pre-school children can be defined by the presence of at least two features, present for at least 1 month, from the following list: two or fewer defecations per week, painful or hard bowel movements, a large faecal mass in the rectum, very large stools that obstruct the toilet and stool retention.
▶ **Soiling** refers to frequent passage of small amounts of stool, often liquid, usually without the child being aware of this; it is also known as **overflow faecal incontinence**.
▶ **Encopresis** is the passage of stools in socially inappropriate places.
▶ **Faecal impaction** means retention of large amounts of faeces such that spontaneous evacuation is unlikely to occur. It may result in a **megarectum** – a stretched or high capacity rectum.
▶ **Withholding** is a pattern of conscious behaviour intended to avoid defecation. (Constipation in infancy is discussed on page 215.)

Defecation problems in toddlers and older children[11]

Parents may use the word 'constipation' to describe delayed defecation, painful defecation, or the appearance or degree of hardness of the stool. Often they become concerned about delay in acquiring faecal continence. Anxiety about potty training or excessively coercive or laissez-faire attitudes may cause difficulty and call for sympathetic advice and explanation. Children with learning difficulties are likely to acquire continence in line with their mental age rather than their actual age. Sudden upheavals and life events may cause temporary loss of continence.

SOILING

Young children sometimes resist defecation for various reasons. An unusually firm or hard stool that is painful to evacuate may be the result of illness, dehydration or lack of opportunity; for instance feeling insecure when sitting on an adult-sized toilet, long journeys or dislike of the toilets at nursery or school. A fissure may result from passing hard stools or may be the primary cause of pain. Perianal streptococcal skin infection and rectal prolapse are other less common but important causes of painful defecation. Constipation and fissures set up a vicious circle, but its origin may have been forgotten by the time the child presents.

Some children adopt a typical posture when trying to resist the urge to defecate, for fear of pain. They stand on tiptoe with straight legs and an arched back. Parents may be convinced that the child is trying hard to pass stool whereas in fact he is doing the opposite.

Over time, the rectum and anal canal become chronically loaded and distended so that the child loses sphincter control, has habituated to distension and no longer receives a call to stool. He may have so much loss of rectal wall tone or such hard faeces that voluntary evacuation is impossible. There may also be a problem with daytime wetting because of the distortion of pelvic anatomy secondary to acquired megarectum and megacolon. Incontinence arises because of mechanical displacement of rectal contents by descending colonic contents or as a result of physical exercise. Obstruction of the rectum by hard faeces can result in liquefactive fermentation of faeces proximal to the blockage and consequent spurious diarrhoea.

FIRST STEPS: DEFINING THE PROBLEM

General history allows exclusion of systemic causes of constipation and assessment of development:

▶ Is there any evidence that the child has other health problems, or developmental or learning difficulties? (Rare causes include anal and sacral anomalies, hypercalcaemia, hypothyroidism, cow's milk allergy, coeliac disease, disabling conditions, such as cerebral palsy).
▶ How did the problem begin? Has the child ever been continent?
▶ What is meant by 'constipation' and 'soiling'? What is the frequency and nature of episodes?
▶ What have the parents done so far?
▶ What are the attitudes of the parents and child to the problem?
▶ Is there any associated abdominal pain, anal pain or wetting?

EXAMINATION

The child should be examined to assess the nature of the problem:

▶ Abdomen: are there faecal masses?
▶ Anus: check position; are there visible fissures, infection, rectal prolapse?
▶ Rectum: the presence of faeces, whether hard or soft, is abnormal but rectal examination is best avoided whenever possible.
▶ Is the child otherwise well and growing? Plot the weight and height on a growth chart.
▶ A plain abdominal x-ray will indicate the presence faecal masses in the abdomen or rectum, but is not needed as a routine.

MANAGEMENT

It is vital to establish rapport with the parents and the child and give them confidence that the problem will be resolved. The **first step** in treatment is to **explain** to child and parent (with the aid of a diagram) how soiling happens. The parents of a soiling child do not usually realise that he may be retaining faeces and will view the prescription of laxatives with suspicion unless their rationale is explained. Secondly, it is imperative to **empty the child's rectum**. Current opinion and trials favour the use of polyethylene glycol (PEG 3350, 1–1.5 g/kg/day for 3 days), which is superior to lactulose. A stool emulsifier such as docusate can also be used. Softened faeces can usually be evacuated by stimulant laxatives such as Senokot syrup. It is often sensible to give the dose at night to avoid crises at school. Sodium picosulphate can be tried if Senokot is not successful.

Failure to respond to these approaches is an indication to consider use of suppositories or a phosphate micro-enema, or higher doses of PEG by naso-gastric tube, but these are potentially distressing treatments and most primary care teams may prefer referral to a paediatrician or paediatric gastroenterologist, preferably one who has a special interest in the problem and is supported by a specialist nurse.

Recovery of rectal tone and normal defecation habits takes a long time and treatment may need to be continued for many months; stopping too soon may result in relapse. Once the rectum has been cleared, a **maintenance dose of laxative and softening agents such as PEG** should be continued in conjunction with a **diet rich in fruit and fibre**. Many children will not eat cereals with a very large content of bran because they dislike the taste, so parents will often need to include baked jacket potatoes, vegetables and wholemeal bread in the child's diet. In conjunction with this, the child will need to learn to keep his rectum empty by **defecating in the lavatory daily**. He may be unwilling to do this at first because of anxieties he has about lavatories and defecation but will usually respond to encouragement and sympathetic support from the parents. Children who are frightened of falling in the lavatory are often reassured by having a box or a pile of telephone directories to rest their feet on. Those with a fissure may benefit from a local anaesthetic cream, but this should be used only for short periods as it may sensitise the skin.

The child attending nursery will need free access to the lavatory, particularly at times of the day when he is most likely to soil, and should spend adequate time on the lavatory once there. Success in having produced a stool should be witnessed by a parent or carer who must respond with praise and provide a reward in the form of a star on a **star chart**. Further soiling episodes are treated as accidents and noted, with minimum fuss, on the same chart, which then provides a record.

For children who have started school, it is often sensible to send an explanatory letter to the school health service who can, if parental permission allows, discuss arrangements to cope with accidents at school. These may include sanction to be excused class without question, to use the staff lavatory, and to keep a clean change of clothing at school.

The star chart should initially be reviewed every 2 weeks. It is difficult to maintain children's enthusiasm for star charts over a long period of time and it may be necessary to tie in some back-up incentive such as money, bearing in mind that this can cause its own difficulties. Unfortunately, a chronically distended rectum will take months to shrink back to normal size so that protracted treatment is nearly always necessary; therefore, it is wise to continue treatment for months and sometimes years. A return of the child's feeling that he 'wants to go' is a good sign.

Failure of such a regime may occur for the following reasons:

- the rectum is not completely emptied at the beginning of the regime or not kept clear subsequently;
- instead of promoting defecation in a lavatory, the parents have rewarded clean pants; this may drive the child back into retention;
- the child is so apprehensive that he denies the problem to himself and will not fully cooperate; alternatively it may be the case that he is so miserable or

anxious that he just does not concentrate on his treatment programme;
- the child is so low in self-esteem or the parents are so fed up that the will to succeed is feeble; the child's nursery or school may prove unsympathetic; humiliation there can also undermine motivation;
- the soiling, although having primarily a physical basis, is also maintained by psychological factors such as secondary gain or masked protest.

Faecal soiling is a serious complaint. Everyone despises and shuns a soiler. It needs to be taken seriously and treated enthusiastically in order to maintain the motivation of the child and parents. Either party can become disastrously exasperated and demoralised. Specialist referral should be arranged as soon as it becomes clear that the situation is not improving.

Children who are wetting as well as soiling usually become dry when the rectum has been emptied and pelvic anatomy returns to something like normality. Should this not occur, then the wetting will need investigation and treatment in its own right.

ENCOPRESIS

Typically, the child is **intentionally defecating** in a place that is chosen to offend a parent or other caregiver. The stool is well-formed with a pointed end and well placed; for instance in the parent's shoe or bed. This is different from the practice involuntary soilers often adopt, of trying to conceal soiled pants or their contents by tossing them under the bed or wrapping them in newspaper and putting them out of sight in a cupboard. Rather similar principles apply to smearing; some disturbed children will smear aggressively and may write insults with fingers dipped in faeces. However, more commonly, the smearing of a wall or curtains is the result of a child trying to clean his fingers after he has put them into soiled pants, or results from 'finger-painting' by a learning disabled young child who has just defecated on the floor or in a nappy that has been taken off. In contrast, intentional placing or smearing is obvious and hostile, and indicates a serious problem in the child's relationship with his parents. It merits referral to a child psychiatrist.

INCENTIVE SCHEMES

The simplest incentive scheme is the star chart, but ticks on a chart, beads on strings, beads in a jar and so forth are all alternatives. Star charts have a rather dubious reputation for being impotent, but, if carefully implemented, are remarkably powerful agents for promoting changes in behaviour. Typically they are used to build compliance or otherwise get the child to do something that is already in his repertoire, but not done often enough.

Perhaps because they are often effective in their simplest form, star charts in particular are likely to be applied casually. This underlies a frequently heard objection that they work at first, but the child loses interest quickly. When systematically applied, this is not a particular problem. An advantage of star charts or ticks on a calendar over devices like beads in a jar or on a string is that they provide a written record of day-by-day achievement, which may reveal whether, for example, weekends are particularly difficult.

The term 'star chart' is used here for simplicity; the principles are the same for all schemes. To obtain maximum value from a simple points scheme, such as a star chart, the following steps are crucial:

- **Establish, ideally with both parents in the presence of the child, exactly what has to be done to get a star.** Avoid being vague about goals ('Be good') or attitudes and relationships ('Be more helpful'); adhere to observable behaviour that everyone can recognise and agree upon. This is likely to take the form of: 'If you get dressed by yourself in the morning you will get a star for your chart. You have to put on all the clothes that are put out on your chair and do up all the buttons.' The behaviour earns the point, not the manner in which it is carried out unless this can be quantified (e.g. within 1 minute of being asked). The child should, at the end of this operation, be able to specify what he has to do to get a star.
- **Agree with parents and child how the stars and chart are going to be kept.** The parents keep the stars and, when these are earned, dispense them promptly, together with praise. The chart may be displayed prominently or privately (in an exercise book or pinned inside a wardrobe door). Wherever it is, the child must be able to see it when he wants to. To maximise the chances of success, encourage the parents to promote conditions that make the desired behaviour more likely to occur. Frequent opportunities to learn that a desired behaviour is rewarded by a star and praise means rapid learning. There should be early opportunities to succeed; early goals should be within the child's reach and stars be frequently and promptly dispensed. When these are given to the child they should be paired with specific (pointed) praise such as 'well done for getting dressed'.
- **Clarify whether stars or points can be cashed in for tangible rewards.** It is not necessary to back up stars with rewards if the programme is to last less than 1 month. Beyond that, interest wanes and it may then be necessary to arrange for them to be exchanged later for something such as a toy, money or a privilege once a specified number of stars has been earned. The conditions for dispensing such a reward need to be agreed. Some parents want rapid results and insist on ambitious and unrealistic targets coupled with huge rewards ('a bicycle if you have no more fights with your brother'). Failure is inevitable, rapid and bitter. The general rule is small rewards, preferably privileges, dispensed immediately and contingent upon small improvements. Success is encouraged by making it as easy as possible for the child to achieve; nothing succeeds like success.
- **Examine how the scheme could go wrong.** Ask the parents what will happen if the child does what is required but grumpily; whether they will give stars for other desired, but unspecified behaviour or if they are going to take stars away for subsequent bad behaviour (usually a bad idea). If stars ultimately earn money for the child, what happens to ordinary pocket money and what happens if Granny gives him £5? If the programme succeeds and he earns rewards, what about jealous siblings? If the child earns enough stars for a particular privilege within a few days, what happens for the rest of the week?
- **Specify how the programme should be reviewed.** With the above principle in mind, frequent reviews to examine how reinforcement and behaviour links

are necessary. Ask the child to bring the chart in for you to see and spend some time looking at it with him.

▶ **Change the plan after a week if it isn't working.** If the child is not winning stars, then either the task is too difficult or the reward isn't big enough. Reduce the task to make it easier, and combine the star with lots of hugs and attention.

▶ **Agree what constitutes ultimate success.** Parents often have a less ambitious view than clinical professionals about what a suitable conclusion of treatment should be. For instance they may want the behaviour brought under control rather than abolished. This may save time and demoralisation caused by attempts to achieve a 'cure' that exhaust family and child.

Such a programme is considerably more sophisticated than the simple instruction to 'put him on a star chart for good behaviour' and is vastly more durable and more effective. It is clear that a number of mechanisms underlie this apparent effectiveness. The establishment of such a programme facilitates the use of praise by parents, enhances parent–child communication, increases parental sensitivity to their child's behaviour, establishes a culture of success and so on. More than just simple learning is involved.

Response cost

For some problem behaviour, where it is more difficult to specify exactly what the desired behaviour is, a 'response cost' scheme may be indicated. The simplest form is to tell the child he is to be issued with a supply of points at the beginning of a time period and specify the behaviour that will lose him points. At the end of the period, points that remain can be exchanged for rewards, such as food. This is only really suitable for children with some grasp of numbers and works best for short periods of time, such as shopping trips or car journeys. Such schemes often go wrong, particularly because the child gets angry at being fined. There is also the problem of what happens when the child has used up all the points allocated.

Time-out

'Time-out' is the common abbreviation for an American term '**time-out from positive social reinforcement**'. Unfortunately, it is commonly misunderstood as meaning enforced confinement in a small room, which is not always the same thing at all. The principle is that behaviour, particularly bad behaviour, may be maintained by social attention, which is rewarding to the child. Removal of social attention when bad behaviour is exhibited will thus, it is argued, lead to the behaviour becoming less frequent. Though the psychological mechanisms of time-out are probably more complicated than this,[12] the *effectiveness* of time-out has been demonstrated in thousands of studies.

Not all behavioural problems are maintained purely by attention; in most cases there are other contributory factors as well. A history of the problem is therefore an essential preliminary. Following this, several possibilities for intervention exist:

1 If there is a link between the problematical behaviour and parental (or sibling) attention, encourage the parent to provide **more attention** (i.e. praise and interest) generally and especially **for desired behaviour**. It is quite often the case that the nagging or criticism dealt out by the parent for bad behaviour is

effectively the only attention available to the child. In this case, discuss how the parent might **ignore** the child's bad behaviour.

2   **Avoid** the situation that led to the problem (e.g. sleepiness, hunger, or noise).
3   Provide alternatives (e.g. football, Playstation, or other **distractions**).
4   Draw up a plan whereby the child is **removed** (or told to remove himself) from the parent's presence when he misbehaves.

The usual course of action will be to combine one or more of the above. A star chart is one instance of how a parent's attention may be brought to bear on positive behaviour. It is better to structure parental behaviour by explaining exactly what to do rather than give general exhortations to be more consistent. Choosing between ignoring or removing the child is essentially based on practicalities. A large child cannot easily be manhandled, which may mean it is impossible to remove him from the presence of a parent without a battle (which would invalidate the whole procedure). Under such circumstances the parent may have to remove herself from the room or merely turn her back and refuse to say anything *at all* for a few minutes (known as 'structured ignoring'). Most parents will prefer to remove the child from their presence because this is a measure that can be instituted when other people, such as siblings, are present; otherwise the siblings may pay attention to the child while the parent is ignoring him.

It is necessary to give some thought as to what might be an unstimulating place (socially or otherwise) where the child can be sent. Bedrooms and bathrooms, although often used, may be quite interesting places even when socially barren. The hall is, for many houses and flats, the most boring room. Valuable fragile objects should be put somewhere else and the front door locked as a precaution.

Setting up a time-out programme needs some planning. The child should be told what will happen. This is based on a **1-2-3 rule**:

1   When he misbehaves he will be told to stop.
2   If he does not stop, he is warned he will have to go to time-out (or be ignored).
3   Continued misbehaviour leads to him being put into time-out (or experience structured ignoring).

A reasonable guide for setting the duration of time-out is **1 minute for each year of age**. It is also important to **avoid releasing a child from time-out when he is at the height of a tantrum**, otherwise he may learn to scream in order to obtain release and attention. Wait until the tantrum has started to abate; it is not absolutely necessary to wait until it has completely subsided.

A record of the number of times time-out is instituted each day, with the duration of each episode, is valuable. Such a progress record can demonstrate several things and illuminate reasons for lack of progress:

▶ An **extinction burst**. Following the withdrawal of attention, any behaviour that is maintained by attention will initially worsen as if the child is striving to regain the attention that has been lost. The usual duration of this is only a few days, but it is the most common reason for parents giving up ('It made him worse'). Warn them beforehand and they should welcome it if it starts to happen; it is a sign that time-out will work because it indicates that the behaviour is responsive to attention.

▶ The child's behaviour may be improving (fewer episodes of time-out) even though he is not contrite or apologetic when released. Time-out need not be a weapon in a power game to be effective; tell parents not to expect contrition at first. If the child blusters ('I don't care; I like it'), they should take no notice. It is not meant to be a maximally aversive punishment but a treatment intervention, which needs to be repeated many times. It does not work instantaneously.

▶ The child may be spending too much time in time-out so that he is being generally starved of opportunities for involvement and positive family attention. He will then continue to misbehave in order to stimulate involvement, even when this is negative. Failure of a time-out programme indicates the need to reconsider:
— Is the child misbehaving because of reasons such as emotional confusion or communication breakdown, which need sorting out first?
— Is he misbehaving because he lacks the knowledge or skills to act more positively (fights with sister because he has not learnt to take turns)?
— Is time-out really time-out from social reinforcement?

REFERENCES

1 Costello EJ, Mustillo S, Erkanli A, *et al.* Prevalence and development of psychiatric disorders in childhood and adolescence. *Arch Gen Psychiatry.* 2003; **60**: 837–44.
2 Richman N, Stevenson J, Graham PJ. *Pre-School to School: a behavioural study.* London: Academic Press; 1982. *See* also Crowther JH, Bond LA, Rolf JE. The incidence, prevalence, and severity of behavior disorders among preschool-aged children in day care. *J Abnorm Child Psych.* 1981; **9**(1): 23–42.
3 Tripp JH, Cockett M. Parents, parenting, and family breakdown. *Arch Dis Child.* 1998; **78**(2): 104–8.
4 Grimshaw R, McGuire C. *Evaluating parenting programmes.* London: National Children's Bureau; 1998.
5 Scott S. Parent Training Programmes. In: Rutter M, Taylor E, editors. *Child and Adolescent Psychiatry.* 4th ed. Oxford: Wiley Blackwell; 2005. pp. 949–67.
6 Hall DMB, Elliman D, editors. *Health for All Children.* 4th ed. revised. Oxford: Oxford University Press; 2006.
7 Stores G. Aspects of parasomnias in children and adolescents. *Arch Dis Child.* 2009; **94**(1): 63–9.
8 National Institute for Health and Clinical Excellence. *Attention Deficit Hyperactivity Disorder. NICE guideline 72.* London: NIHCE; 2008. Available at: www.nice.org.uk/guidance/CG72
9 Tremblay RE, Gervais J, Petitclerc A, Early childhood learning prevents youth violence. Montreal, Quebec. Centre of Excellence for Early Childhood Development; 2008. Available at: www.excellence-earlychildhood.ca/documents/Tremblay_AggressionReport_ANG.pdf
10 Patterson GR, Littman RA, Bricker W. Assertive behaviour in children: a step towards a theory of aggression. *Monogr Soc Res Child Dev.* 1967; **32**(5): 1–43.
11 Rubin G, Dale A. Chronic constipation in children. *BMJ.* 2006; **333**: 1051–5. *See* also Clayden GS, Keshtgar AS, Carcani-Rathwell I, *et al.* The management of chronic constipation and related faecal incontinence in childhood. *Arch Dis Child Educ Pract Ed.* 2005; **90**: 58–67.
12 Leitenberg H. Is time-out from positive reinforcement an aversive event? *Psychological Bull.* 1965; **64**(6): 428–41.

CHAPTER 15

Families and children with special needs

CHAPTER CONTENTS

INFANTS BORN PREMATURELY

Premature and low birth weight infants requiring special or intensive care have additional needs to those of full-term healthy infants. After discharge from the hospital, the family is often supported by an outreach nurse from the neonatal unit and the neonatal paediatricians and their colleagues, but the family may also need and welcome the support and advice of the local primary care team on a number of topics:[*]

Kangaroo mother care (KMC). KMC originated in services for poor families in Colombia, but is now used in the Western world as well. Babies weighing 2000 g or less at birth and unable to regulate their body temperature are attached to mothers and other carers' chests in skin to skin contact, wearing only a nappy and a baby bonnet, and are kept upright 24 hours a day. The carer sleeps in a semi-sitting position. Exclusive breastfeeding is the goal. KMC continues to around 37 weeks post-conception age and is a safe and effective method of care.[1]

Sudden infant death. There is an increased risk of sudden infant death syndrome (SIDS) in infants born prematurely. The standard advice should be reinforced with particular reference to the hazards of exposure to cigarette smoke and the importance of babies sleeping on their backs (even if they had been nursed prone in the intensive care unit).

Infections. Premature babies may be at increased risk of infections, in particular, respiratory syncytial virus (RSV), which is the main cause of bronchiolitis. It is an important cause of re-hospitalisation for premature babies. Debate continues about the role of giving monoclonal antibodies (Palivizumab®) to reduce the risk of RSV infection for the most vulnerable babies.[†]

---

[*] Valuable further information is available on the BLISS web site for staff and parents managing premature infants: www.bliss.org.uk

[†] *See* www.hta.ac.uk/execsumm/summ1236.shtml

Stress. Parents have additional stresses with a premature infant. Longer spells of hospital care add to the financial burden for the family. The mother (and perhaps also the father) is more likely to be depressed and feel inadequate. They will be getting to know their baby at a more difficult stage than usual. Compared to term babies, he is likely to be less responsive and predictable, to smile less and make less eye contact.

Long-term problems. Premature babies have an increased risk of long-term problems.[2] There is a high rate of permanent disability in infants who were very premature and of extremely low birth weight. Many of those without obvious disability have subtle learning and attention deficits that come to light when they start school and often have a significant educational impact. The baby may be affected by the underlying reason(s) for his prematurity, by any complications occurring in the special care or intensive care unit, and by nutritional deficiencies at a time when in utero brain growth should be rapid. Hearing impairment is more common and should be detected by the newborn hearing screening programme, which is modified for these babies. Retinopathy of prematurity similarly should be identified in the neonatal unit. In spite of these concerns, however, the majority of premature babies do well and the reported quality of life for most of these children as they grow up is satisfactory.[3]

Twins and triplets. In multiple births, babies are likely to be smaller and born prematurely; they are also more likely to result from assisted conception. Caring for two or three very small babies is particularly demanding and many parents will need a lot of support. There is also a significant risk with multiple births that one or more babies may have died in utero or in the neonatal unit. (*See* below for bereavement issues.)

Technology dependence. Some low birth weight infants have chronic lung disease and need oxygen; some have tracheostomies, require tube or gastrostomy feeding, or have other major medical and nursing needs.[4]

Developmental support programmes. Some studies have suggested that intensive family support through home visits, during the first 3 years, produce gains in IQ, vocabulary, and behaviour, with benefits persisting to at least age 8, mainly in the heavier low birth weight children; however, other researchers report little benefit. Whatever the actual measured gains, parents do feel more vulnerable if their infant was premature and most appreciate easy access to expert professionals.[5]

Immunisations. These should be given in accordance with uncorrected chronological age. Some premature children may require influenza immunisation. *See* Chapter 8 for more details.

Development and growth. Correct the chronological age by the appropriate number of weeks before interpreting any developmental observations or plotting head circumference, height and weight on the growth chart. Do not automatically assume that slow growth is solely due to prematurity or low birth weight. *See* Chapter 7 for more details.

CHILDREN WITH DISABILITIES AND LONG-TERM PROBLEMS

The majority of disabling or long-term health problems in infants and children are diagnosed by hospital paediatricians and their colleagues; nevertheless, much can be done by primary care teams to support the parents. When talking to parents who have recently been faced with some major problem in their child, remember the following points about sharing information, which are emphasised by those who have been through the experience. Parents say that they want to be told:

▶ as soon as the health professional has any suspicions – even if there is still uncertainty;
▶ what can be done to resolve uncertainty;
▶ in privacy;
▶ without interruptions: this may mean handing bleeps/pagers/mobile phones to someone else;
▶ with both parents together, or with grandparent or friend if they're an unsupported parent;
▶ simply; not too much talking without a pause;
▶ at least twice, because they do not take in what they are told the first time;
▶ in writing as well as verbally.

Having a child with long-term problems is a highly stressful experience. Learning to cope with stress is facilitated by support and by appropriate information.[6] A written report and/or literature often help. In particular, guidance on parent support groups and on the use of the internet are appreciated (*see* page 33).

Follow-up

Ensure that appropriate follow-up has been arranged for the parents; this will usually be the responsibility of the paediatrician, but may sometimes be undertaken by the GP, health visitor or social worker. Fellow professionals who meet the parents in varying settings may have good opportunities for identifying a variety of worries; listen to colleagues or the specialists involved, who can tell you what the parents are really worried about. Suggest that parents should write down their questions in anticipation of any consultation. If the parents of a disabled child were educated in a different culture, a good interpreter is important to ensure that information is passed on correctly and to warn you about potentially damaging worries that families in that culture may have. For example, there may be a belief that the cause of a defect must be in the mother, or confusion or anger about the role of consanguinity, or a fear that the mother's siblings might become unmarriageable.

If parents want to discuss their concerns with you, do not burden them with your own solutions to their problems; good counselling is about helping people to find solutions that are right for them. Listen for the unspoken questions, such as: 'Will the child die?' 'What is the life expectancy?' 'Is it inherited?'. Having a disabled or chronically ill child can be regarded as a form of bereavement – 'the death of the perfect child the parents had hoped for and his replacement by the real imperfect child they have'.* Figure 15.1 illustrates this concept. There is a wide range of human response to grief; do not try to persuade the parents that they feel guilt when they do not or be surprised when they fail to exhibit emotions in an orderly sequence.[7]

Information is vitally important to parents of a disabled child; without detailed knowledge and understanding of the issues they have great difficulty in handling their sadness or planning ahead. Primary care staff can sometimes help by using a

---

* This quote is from a lecture by Professor Joan Bicknell, St George's Hospital, London.

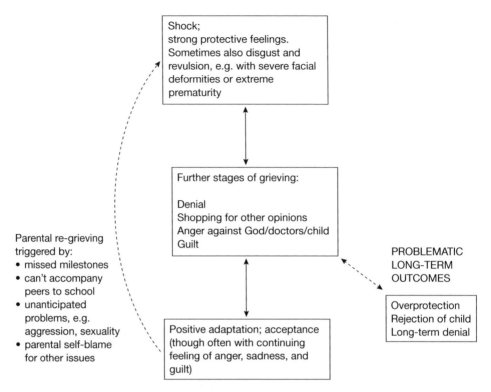

FIGURE 15.1 Grieving for a child's disabilities is complex, difficult and recurrent. Bereavement is the reactions experienced by parents (also siblings, grandparents and other close family members). Having a disabled or seriously ill child may elicit the same reactions as the death of a child, but is repeated each time his outlook is revised downwards, or he falls behind his peers.

checklist to ensure that the parents have received all the information and services that the child may require (*see* Box 15.1).

Parents may ask the advice of primary care staff on a number of issues outlined in the following paragraphs.

Practical help. Generally it is best to consult the specialist team responsible for the child's care. In the case of disabling conditions, this is usually a child development centre or team. Their aim is to help the child to make the most of his abilities, however severe the condition, and to help the family to come to terms with and live with, their problems.

Therapy. It is difficult to prove that early therapy intervention changes the outcome in terms of improved function in the child, but it is certainly effective in reducing the impact of disabling conditions. Early physiotherapy and occupational therapy do not cure physical defects, such as cerebral palsy, but therapists often become the parents' main advisers on how to handle and care for the child. Speech therapists may offer advice on feeding and general communication issues as well as more formal interventions involving spoken language. The quality of the advice and the ability of the parents to put it into practice on a daily basis are often more important than the number of sessions provided by therapists but, understandably, parents often feel that more therapy must equal better outcomes.

Coordination of care. Parents can be overwhelmed with the number of people they have to relate to and the appointments they are expected to keep. Unresolved difficulties with the key worker role include insecure funding and insufficient parent involvement in planning and management. Other ways of improving coordination of services include shared premises, multidisciplinary intake meetings, and single-appointment, multi-specialty assessments.[8]

The 'Team Around the Child' is an evolving 'model of service provision in which a range of different practitioners come together to help and support an individual child. It places the emphasis firmly on the needs of the child, rather than on organisations or service providers. Unlike traditional models of the "Child Development Centre", it does not imply a multi-disciplinary team that is located together or who work together all the time but is a virtual team, providing the flexibility needed so that services can meet the diverse needs of every child."

A second opinion. This is a perfectly reasonable request, but it is important to choose someone who is really knowledgeable about the particular problem! If a paediatrician first broke the news to the parents, he/she will greatly appreciate a telephone call in this situation, so that the most constructive second opinion can be selected. If relationships with local services are damaged right at the outset, it will be difficult to offer optimal care for the child.

Dental care. The principles of preventive dental care are the same as for any child, but dental care of children with complex health problems is best undertaken by someone with a particular interest in this field. Some of these children have orthodontic problems and a high risk of gum disease and they may also have the distressing habit of bruxism (grinding their teeth).

Immunisation. The principles are the same as for other children (*see* Chapter 9).

Respite care. This is vital for many families, but availability varies widely. Information should be available locally and guidance can be obtained from Contact A Family.[†]

Emergency healthcare. Common minor medical conditions can usually be dealt with by their GP as with any other child, although it may be harder to make a diagnosis. However, children with complex problems often bypass primary care when they are acutely unwell. Children with disabilities are more than usually prone to respiratory illnesses, seizures, vomiting and reflux, and unexplained distress. A fast track arrangement that allows direct access to the paediatric ward helps to reduce the stress of repeated visits, waiting and history-taking at the A&E department. The disadvantage of such hospital-based arrangements is that the primary care team may not get to know the family very well, which can cause problems for the GP as the child grows up and comes to rely more on his local services.[9]

Education. Parents often feel that the child would benefit from early educational input. 'Early Support'[‡] is a programme designed to simplify and coordinate the provision of relevant information and services. Communication between health and early years or education professionals is vital. It is facilitated by joint meetings,

---

* www.everychildmatters.gov.uk/ *See* also Siraj-Blatchford I, Clarke K, Needham M. *The Team Around the Child: Multi-agency Working in the Early Years.* Stoke: Trentham Books Ltd; 2007.

† www.cafamily.org.uk

‡ www.earlysupport.org.uk/

a philosophy of sharing information and documentation with parents' permission, not relying solely on parents to transmit information, and a clearly defined role for the Special Educational Needs Coordinator (SENCO).*

In desperation, some parents seek specialist private assessments and treatments. The assessments are often useful in obtaining additional help (e.g. through a Statement of Special Educational Needs). However, private treatments rarely achieve much more than treatments and educational interventions available in the state sector. Parents should be counselled to obtain *impartial* expert advice before going heavily into debt to obtain new or unusual interventions.

Nursery and school provision. Early Years Development and Childcare Partnerships (EYDCP) bring together private, voluntary and independent settings in receipt of government funding to provide early education.† They coordinate work with local education authorities, social service departments, health services and parent representatives to plan and provides services. The SENCO provides advice and support to other practitioners and ensures that appropriate individual educational plans are in place.

The 1996 Education Act and the Code of Practice.‡ This Act, with its accompanying Code of Practice, is intended to rationalise and improve the process of assessing and supporting children who need extra help to cope with education. It emphasises a child's educational needs rather than his medical or diagnostic 'label'; it calls on health authorities to notify the Education Department when they suspect that a child may have special educational needs, and to tell the parents about the relevant voluntary organisation; it gives the parents more say in their child's school placement; it encourages integration of handicapped children into mainstream school whenever possible.

The Code of Practice sets out a staged approach to children who are thought to have special needs.§ The simplest intervention is to provide special attention within the normal school budget; such a programme is called 'School Action'. If this proves insufficient to meet the child's needs, the next step is 'School Action Plus' which involves calling on expert assistance and advice. If the child is still having major difficulty, the next stage is a Statutory Assessment, resulting in a Statement of Educational Needs. This is needed for about 3% of all children. In some boroughs, many requests for Statements, and disputes about what provision should be made, are only settled after parents appeal to the Special Needs Tribunal. The most common interventions stipulated by a Statement are that a child can attend a special school or can have increased one-to-one attention (anything from 10 extra hours for the subjects the child finds hardest, to full-time).

Type of schooling. The question of whether a special or a mainstream school would be preferable often causes parents much anguish. There are arguments for both solutions. Fortunately 'specialist units' resolve the problem for some children. Health professionals should generally be cautious in offering opinions on school choice as these arrangements are primarily the responsibility of the local education

---

* *See* www.tda.gov.uk/teachers/sen/nationalstandards.aspx for role and training of SENCOs.

† *See* www.surestart.gov.uk for details of EYDCPs.

‡ *See* www.teachernet.gov.uk/docbank/index.cfm?id=3724

§ A parents' guide to special education is available at: www.direct.gov.uk/en/Parents/Schoolslearningand development/SpecialEducationalNeeds/DG_4000690

authority (LEA). Contradictory advice from multiple sources exacerbates their difficulties and sometimes leads to conflict between the LEA and the parents, which adds to their stress and does not help the child.

The first option, **mainstreaming**, has several benefits: the child grows up with his local peers; he has access to the full curriculum; he is more likely to take pride in what he can do than focus on his limitations; other children (and therefore ultimately society as a whole) become more accepting of disability.

There are also some difficulties with mainstreaming. Misery and social isolation are common when children are so far behind that they are unable to join in any normal peer relationships or are being 'mothered' by other children and doing lessons that have no connection to the topics studied by their peers. Children with a wide range of developmental difficulties have increased risk for a wide range of psychological problems including low mood, anxiety, hyperactivity and aggression. Children with physical and sensory impairments face additional disadvantages, including negative attitudes of peers, restricted social opportunities, complicated parent–child interactions, and often other subtle difficulties. The net result is that they often have special difficulty mastering the social tasks of gaining entry into peer groups, maintaining play, and resolving conflicts. Not surprisingly, disabled children are often the least preferred play partners of other children. Social skills training can sometimes help, as it does in typically developing children. Play environments and games can usefully be adapted to encourage interactions.

The second option, **special schools**, offers more specialist expertise in the staff, many of whom have specially requested and trained for work in the area. The emotional benefit of not being bottom of the class is important for many children; in contrast, some of the more able children in a special school lack the benefit of competition. In addition, some children learn maladaptive behaviours from their peers, though the damage from this is much less than many parents fear. Each special school typically specialises in one of these areas: moderate learning disability, severe to profound learning disability, autism, physical disability, hearing impairment, and visual impairment. These schools are regularly visited by specialists from the Department of Health as well as the Department of Education. Special schools have high staff:pupil ratios so extra one-to-one attention is usually not provided.

A third option, the **specialist unit** attached to a mainstream school, often combines the strengths of both types of school. This allows a child to have specialised help and social support when he needs it, and to attend mainstream classes in his strongest subjects.

Social skills training. This can sometimes help, as it does in typically developing children. Play environments and games can usefully be adapted to encourage interactions. Specialist knowledge of specific disabilities and local resources is invaluable. As with other children, it is important that failures be attributed to situations or mistakes, rather than blamed on the children.

BOX 15.1 Checklist for parents of special needs children

- Do the parents know precisely what is wrong with the child? Do they have a report in writing, to show relatives, etc.?
- If the child is on medication, do they know what, how much and why? Have they a record card?

- Do the parents and the primary care professionals fully understand the diagnosis? If necessary, check with the relevant specialist. Remember that in many conditions there can be additional complications as well as those that are obvious when the diagnosis is first made.
- Do the parents know about the local register of children with a disability (as a means of improving services for all children)?
- Has the child had a hearing test and a vision test, if indicated (there is an increased risk of hearing and vision defects with a wide variety of long-term paediatric conditions).
- Are they in touch with the appropriate individuals in the local education department?
- Do they want any day care from a playgroup, nursery school or social services nursery?
- Do they want any help from a social worker, psychologist, therapist, teacher, housing department, etc.?
- Do they want books or leaflets on the child's problem? Contact A Family* can put them in touch with appropriate groups and can provide leaflets about common problems in disabled children.
- Do they know about the parent organisation(s) relevant to the child? (If not, ask the above sources.)
- Would they like to meet another family with similar problems? This can be very useful, but can also be counter-productive if the family is not adequately prepared – for example, if the child they meet has distressing complications or his parents are not coping.
- Financial help: the Disability Living Allowance is valuable. Social Services and voluntary organisations can provide up-to-date advice.
- Don't neglect routine child health promotion: is the child growing? Have the parents had the usual advice that would be given for every child?
- Have they had advice on the genetic implications of the child's disorder?
- Have they had dental advice for the child?
- Discuss whether respite care would be useful. Some parents are initially upset about this suggestion, but after they have become used to playgroups and after-school 'respite', longer periods should be considered, especially if the parents are exhausted and sleep-deprived.

Hearing and vision impairments

The parents of a hearing impaired child should receive the following:

▶ an assessment of the type and severity of the hearing loss as soon as this is possible;
▶ advice on what can (and cannot) be achieved by various approaches to communication, including Makaton, British Sign Language, hearing aids and cochlear implants;
▶ a paediatric assessment and investigation to determine the cause of the hearing loss;

---

* www.cafamily.org.uk

- an ophthalmalogical assessment; it is important for the deaf child to have good eyesight; furthermore, some forms of hearing loss are associated with eye disorders;
- genetic advice where appropriate;
- an introduction to educational services, including support from the peripatetic teacher specialising in deafness;
- introduction to social services and voluntary organisations such as the National Deaf Children's Society.

Children with impaired vision

Severe visual impairment reduces the rate of early development and may also result in some undesirable secondary phenomena. Social smiling, reaching, hand regard, grasping objects, localisation of sound, sitting, the development of object permanence and stranger awareness, the urge to crawl and walk in pursuit of interesting objects are all dependent on vision in the normal infant and are slow to emerge where there is visual handicap. Language development is also delayed in many cases, because the baby is at a disadvantage in learning the association between the objects he perceives and their names. The older child may show excessive echolalia and a tendency to inconsequential chatter as a means of maintaining social contact.

Blind babies sometimes adopt an unusual posture, with the hands inert and resting beside the shoulders. Parents may feel that the child is somewhat slow and unresponsive; indeed they may feel rejected and therefore find it difficult to give the attention that is needed. Lacking the social contact and attention that he needs to make sense of the world around him, the infant may withdraw into self-stimulating procedures, such as rocking, head banging or eye poking. Good early counselling and management help to reduce or avoid these various secondary disabilities is advised.

Primary care staff would not normally be involved in the management or developmental examination of a child with poor vision, but the following points may be helpful to those who have a **child with visual impairment in their practice**:

- Few paediatricians see enough children with severe visual impairment to acquire much expertise or to build up an expert team and referral to a regional child development centre may be necessary.
- Paediatric ophthalmology is a highly specialised field, and a second opinion regarding the diagnosis may be worthwhile. The clinical geneticist may have particular skill in recognising unusual syndromes, which may be important from the genetic point of view.
- Assessment of hearing in the infant with poor vision is crucial, but clinical tests are particularly difficult because turning and localising responses are impaired or absent. The child may respond to a sound only by smiling or by cessation of bodily activity.
- The child is likely to perform considerably better in familiar surroundings and with his own toys and possessions. Lighting and colour contrast may affect the ability to make use of residual vision.

Disability register

Each local authority is obliged to maintain a register of all children with disabilities. It is not easy to do this to a high standard.[10] Professionals may forget to discuss this with parents and parents may refuse to allow their child's name to be recorded on the register, so most registers are far from complete or accurate. Nevertheless, while refusal should not deny any resources to the child, the recording of the name gives a number of potential advantages, such as receiving mailings of information on various disorders, resources, welfare rights, etc.

BEREAVEMENT
Sudden unexpected death in infancy

The term 'sudden unexpected death in infancy' (SUDI) includes all infant deaths that were not anticipated because of congenital abnormalities or previously diagnosed illness. When comprehensive investigation fails to reveal any cause, the term 'sudden infant death syndrome' (SIDS) is used. The term 'cot death' is widely used colloquially. In the UK in 2005 there were around 0.4 such deaths per 1000 live births (or less than 1 in 2000). The rate of SIDS fell substantially after parents were advised to put babies to sleep on their backs; however continuing falls in the last few years are probably due to more precise diagnosis of the cause of infant deaths, since overall mortality has not changed. (*See* page 229 for more details about SIDS.)

A baby who dies unexpectedly is often taken directly to a hospital casualty department. Sometimes the GP may be called to the home or the baby rushed to the surgery. GPs should ensure that coroners, hospitals and out-of-hours services would inform the family doctor immediately of an unexpected infant death.

A post mortem examination is usually required by the coroner. Infant post mortems should be done by a pathologist with paediatric training, since the death may be due to conditions that are outside the expertise of a pathologist who deals only rarely with infant deaths; for example, conditions such as heart disease or metabolic disorders. The coroner's officer should explain the procedure and discuss the issue of tissue retention.

From 1 April 2008, Local Safeguarding Children's Boards must review **all** deaths in childhood. In the case of unexpected infant deaths, the best practice is for a home visit to be undertaken as soon as possible after the death,[11] by a paediatrician with appropriate training, together with an officer from the police child protection team. A careful review of the scene of the death and any available evidence, though seeming intrusive, is in the parents' best interests. Sometimes this approach offers clues to the cause of death and eliminates any concerns that a death may have been unnatural.

The role of community child health and primary care services in the event of cot death

The role of the different help services in the event of cot death will vary according to circumstances, but it important that at some stage all of the following are addressed:

▶ As soon as the primary care team hear of the baby's death, a member of the team should contact the family to express sympathy, by a home visit if possible. Early support prevents later misunderstandings.
▶ Unless there is obvious injury, a history of illness or the parental attitude arouses suspicion, the parents will be told that the likely diagnosis is a cot death,

but that a post mortem examination will be necessary to establish the cause of death. If death remains unexplained, it may be registered as SIDS. Some parents want to see or hold their child after death is confirmed, but before the body is taken to a mortuary.

▶ Whoever sees the parents should: explain the coroner's duty and the possibility of an inquest; warn parents that they or relatives may be asked to identify the body; advise the parents that they will be asked to make a statement to the coroner's officer or police, and that bedding may be taken for examination to help establish the cause of death; give advice on registering the death and making funeral arrangements (the coroner's officer may need to know the parents' choice of burial or cremation).

▶ If considering offering parents a drug to alleviate the initial shock, it is known that many do not want anxiolytics or antidepressants, but prefer something to induce sleep.

▶ If the mother was breastfeeding, she may need advice on suppression of lactation and relief of pain. There is very little good evidence on the optimal methods.[12] Options include breast binding, ice packs, cabbage leaves, and use of a breast pump sufficient to relieve tension in the breasts, gradually reducing the frequency and amount removed over several days.

▶ Take particular note of siblings. Twin babies may carry an extra risk of cot death and some believe that a surviving twin should be hospitalised for observation, though there is little evidence of any increased risk unless the death was due to a specific cause (i.e. not SIDS). Give guidance on emotional needs of siblings, who may be neglected or overprotected; reassure parents that older children are not at risk. Do *not* advise parents to have another child as soon as possible. Loss of a twin is doubly distressing as the survivor constantly reminds the parents that there should be two babies instead of one.

▶ Advise parents of likely grief reactions, such as aching arms, hearing the baby cry, distressing dreams and strong positive or negative sexual feelings, but reassure them that these and other symptoms, such as loss of appetite and sleeplessness are normal. Anger, sometimes directed towards the GP, guilt and self-blame, especially on the part of the mother, are common grief reactions for which doctors should be prepared.

▶ Offer parents copies of the Foundation for the Study of Infant Deaths (FSID) leaflet *Information for the Parents Following the Sudden and Unexpected Death of their Baby*. The Foundation offers further support and information and can put parents in touch with others who have suffered a similar bereavement.*

▶ Make sure that parents have a relative or close friend near them during the 48 hours after the death, and offer explanations to them and, if so desired, to the minister of religion. Make sure the family's health visitor and other members of the primary care team know of the baby's death and are prepared to give continued support.

▶ A subsequent meeting with the parents is desirable to discuss the cause of death. Make sure the coroner informs you of the initial and final post mortem findings and consult with the pathologist and/or paediatrician if any

---

* The Foundation for the Study of Infant Deaths: Artillery House, 11–19 Artillery Row, London SW1P 1RT. Helpline: 020 7233 2090; General: 020 7222 8001.

clarification is needed. If not already arranged, the primary care team should offer parents a later interview with a paediatrician both for themselves and the siblings. An independent opinion, based on the post mortem results, may be beneficial to the parents and sometimes also to the GP, restoring parental confidence in the primary care team and sharing some of the load of counselling, particularly concerning future children.

▶ The message from the primary care team is: we care about you; we will listen; we will talk about your baby if and when you want to.

The follow-up meeting after a child has died

The ideal timing of a follow-up meeting seems to be between 8 and 12 weeks. Often this will be undertaken by a designated paediatrician, but sometimes the primary care team may undertake this task as well as, or instead of, the specialist. The time-lag gives the family time to think about the questions they want to ask and for the post-mortem results to be available. New information should be shared and explained; support for siblings and professional help for the family may need to be offered; and sometimes parents may want to visit the ward or intensive care unit where the child died. An information pack with factual material may be helpful.

There are some things you should *not* say to the parents: 'I know how you feel' (you don't); 'You'll get over it' (they won't, though they will learn to cope with their grief); 'Your other children will be a comfort' (they might not be); 'You're young enough to have another baby' (babies cannot be replaced).

Warn parents that their friends may avoid them and will certainly avoid talking about the baby who died; the baby's birthday and the anniversary of the baby's death will always be painful times.

Miscarriage, stillbirth, and deaths affecting twins or triplets

Parents may be profoundly distressed after a miscarriage and memories may re-surface after subsequent live births, whether or not there are any problems with the baby. The Miscarriage Association provides information and support.[*]

Stillbirth similarly causes intense grief and most hospitals now have procedures in place that support parents in this situation. A long delay between diagnosis of intra-uterine death and the delivery unsurprisingly seems to be particularly upsetting. Because of the belief that confronting parents with the reality of stillbirth facilitates healthy mourning, some staff may apply this as a dogma, demanding that every woman should inspect and hold her stillborn baby. This can have unfortunate results. There are no absolute rules about how long the parent(s) should have with the stillborn baby, or when or how many times. Many parents value tokens of remembrance; such as ultrasound scans, locks of hair, photos, footprints, etc. Primary care staff should be sensitive to these and anticipate that parents may wish to talk about them or seek reassurance that this is not strange or macabre. The Stillbirth and Neonatal Death Society has useful information for parents and professionals.[†]

The perinatal loss of a twin or triplet requires similar care to that expected for the death of a singleton. Photographs are important, separately and together, even if parents say that they don't want this at the time. They may be unable to celebrate

---

[*] www.miscarriageassociation.org.uk

[†] www.uk-sands.org

the surviving bab(ies); for example putting off a christening date. Mothers who have multiple births resent re-labelling if one dies (e.g. if one triplet dies, do not refer to the surviving babies as twins). Well-meaning but deeply hurtful remarks reported by parents include: 'At least you have one healthy baby' and 'Three would have been too much to cope with'. A helpful parent organisation is the Twins and Multiple Births Association Bereavement Support Group.*

Care of next infant

Parents who have lost a baby unexpectedly will need extra attention and support with their subsequent children from their obstetrician, paediatrician, general practitioner and health visitor. In particular, they will inevitably be very anxious that subsequent children may die from SIDS. The CONI (Care of the Next Infant) scheme is designed to help allay this anxiety.[†] It is organised at local Trust level. When the mother is pregnant with her next child and books in at the maternity clinic, she is put in touch with her local coordinator. After delivery, she will be offered advice and support with a combination of frequent health visitor visits, regular weighing to confirm that the baby is well and thriving and/or an apnoea alarm.

There is no conclusive evidence that these measures reduce the risk of a second unexpected death, but they undoubtedly reduce the parents' anxiety. Further details can be obtained from the community paediatrician, the Director of Nursing Services for health visiting, or the Foundation for the Study of Infant Deaths.[‡]

The expected death of a baby or child

The action to be taken for the expected death of a baby or child should be planned in advance, as far as possible, by the paediatrician and/or GP. For example:

▶ What paediatric palliative care services are available?[§]
▶ Should the child be at home, in a hospice, or hospitalised in the terminal stages?
▶ Are any tissues or organs needed for diagnostic or research purposes?
▶ Do not be afraid to use appropriate medications as for terminal care in adults.
▶ Do not assume that the parents will be relieved 'because it is all over'. This mistake is often made when the child is severely disabled. There may be some relief, but also great sadness.
▶ If the child dies at home under the care of primary care or community-based staff, inform the paediatrician.
▶ Consider who else needs to know (e.g. if relevant, ensure that others are to be informed: playgroup, nursery, school, etc.).

REFERENCES

1 Charpak N, Ruiz JG, Zupan J, *et al.* Kangaroo Mother Care: 25 years after. *Acta Paediatr.* 2005; **94**(5): 514–22.

---

* www.tamba-bsg.org.uk

† www.fsid.org.uk/coni.html

‡ www.fsid.org.uk/coni.html

§ The Association for Children's Palliative Care: www.act.org.uk

2 Cooke RW, Foulder-Hughes L. Growth impairment in the very preterm and cognitive and motor performance at 7 years. *Arch Dis Child.* 2003; **88**(6): 482–7. *See* also Cristobal R, Oghalai JS. Hearing loss in children with very low birth weight: current review of epidemiology and pathophysiology. *Arch Dis Child Fetal Neonatal Ed.* 2008; **93**(6): F462–8. *See* also DiBiasie A. Evidence-based review of retinopathy of prematurity prevention in VLBW and ELBW infants. *Neonatal Netw.* 2006; **25**(6): 393–403.

3 Cooke RW. Health, lifestyle, and quality of life for young adults born very preterm. *Arch Dis Child.* 2004; **89**(3): 201–6.

4 Kirk S, Glendinning C. Developing services to support parents caring for a technology-dependent child at home. *Child Care Health Dev.* 2004; **30**(3): 209–18.

5 Jacobs SE, Sokol J, Ohlsson A. The Newborn Individualized Developmental Care and Assessment Program is not supported by meta-analyses of the data. *J Pediatr.* 2002; **140**(6): 699–706.

6 Davies S, Hall D. Parents and professionals in partnership. *Arch Dis Child.* 2005; **90**: 1053–7.

7 Foy E. Parental grieving of childhood disability: a rural perspective. *Australian Social Work.* 1997; **50**(1): 39–44. *See* also Godress J, Ozgul S, Owen C, *et al.* Grief experiences of parents whose children suffer from mental illness. *Aust NZ J Psychiat.* 2005; **39**(1–2): 88–94.

8 Sloper P, Greco V, Beecham J, *et al.* Key worker services for disabled children: what characteristics of services lead to better outcomes for children and families? *Child Care Health Dev.* 2006; **32**(2): 147–57.

9 Mahon M, Kibirige MS. Patterns of admissions for children with special needs to the paediatric assessment unit. *Arch Dis Child.* 2004; **89**(2): 165–9.

10 McConachie H, Barry R, Spencer A, *et al.* The challenge of developing a regional database for autism spectrum disorder. *Arch Dis Child.* 2009; **94**(1): 38–41.

11 Foundation for the Study of Infant Deaths. *Recommendations for a Joint Agency Protocol for the Management of Sudden Unexpected Deaths in Infancy.* 2005. Available at: www.fsid. org.uk/editpics/202–1.pdf (accessed 10 December 2008). *See* also Fleming PJ, Blair PS, Sidebotham PD, *et al.* Investigating sudden unexpected deaths in infancy and childhood and caring for bereaved families: an integrated multiagency approach. *BMJ.* 2004; **328**: 331–4.

12 Busta Moore D, Catlin A. Lactation suppression: forgotten aspect of care for the mother of a dying child. *Pediatr Nurs.* 2003; **29**(5): 383–4. Available at: www.medscape.com/viewarticle/464568 (accessed 10 December 2008).

APPENDIX 1

Hearing tests for young children

CHAPTER CONTENTS

TERMINOLOGY AND DEFINITIONS

▶ The intensity of a sound is measured in decibels (dB).
▶ Loudness is the subjective impression of intensity.
▶ Thresholds: 0 dB is the hearing threshold of the average person (*not* the absence of sound); minus 10 up to 20 dB is the normal range of hearing thresholds; 50–60 dB is the intensity of a conversational voice; 100–105 dB the intensity of a shout; and 115–140 dB the threshold of pain. A person with impaired hearing only hears sound when it is raised above the normal threshold of 20 dB. The threshold of hearing is the quietest sound an individual can hear at a specified frequency. A person with thresholds of 80 dB is said to have a hearing loss of 80 dB. Degrees of hearing loss are defined as follows:
  — mild: thresholds are greater than 20 dB
  — moderate: thresholds are greater than 40 dB
  — severe: thresholds are greater than 70 dB
  — profound: thresholds are greater than 95 dB.
▶ Hearing loss is measured with an audiometer.
▶ Intensity is measured using a sound-level meter (dBA scale).
▶ Frequency is measured in cycles per second or Hertz (Hz).
▶ Pitch is the subjective impression of frequency. The human ear can detect sounds of between 16 Hz and 20 000 Hz, but in clinical practice tests are confined to the speech frequencies, usually 250–8000 Hz. Vowel sounds tend to be low frequency sounds (250–1000 Hz) and consonants are usually high frequency; the ones with the highest frequency are ss, sh, f and v. A whisper has a frequency range above 1000 Hz whereas a voice, however quiet, contains low frequency components of 250–1000 Hz.

PRINCIPLES OF TESTS

It is now generally agreed that hearing tests for pre-school children should be carried out only by staff who have been adequately trained and working in suitable premises with proper equipment. For this reason, we no longer include detailed descriptions of the various methods in this book, but they can be accessed at www.healthforallchildren.co.uk/.

The Infant Distraction Test

The Infant Distraction Test is now not used for whole-population screening in the UK as it was difficult to maintain high standards of testing and there were many missed cases as well as a high false positive rate. However, it remains a useful tool if correctly used.

The test relies on the ability of the child to turn and locate a sound made outside the field of vision. The distraction test is most valuable between the ages of 7 and 12 months. For a detailed description, *see* www.healthforallchildren.co.uk/.

Hearing tests for children age 2–5 years
Speech discrimination tests

The ability to discriminate between similar speech sounds provides a valuable indication of hearing. The toy test can be used as a screening test of hearing, but does not replace the need to test a child's hearing properly if there is concern. The technique is easily learnt and is capable of detecting even quite minor degrees of hearing loss. The most convenient test for testing pre-school children is the McCormick toy test. This consists of 14 toys, each with a single syllable name. The toys are paired so that they sound similar; for example, plane and plate, shoe and spoon. Very young or immature children may have difficulty with the small toys, but can sometimes be tested, albeit less accurately, using four or five large common objects (cup, spoon, shoe, duck, cow). For a detailed description, *see* www.healthforallchildren.co.uk/.

Performance tests

The hearing of children between 2 and 5 years of age may also be checked by means of performance tests. These require the child to make some form of response to a sound signal, usually involving a toy; for example, placing a brick in a basket or a wooden man in a boat. Performance tests provide a useful way of estimating hearing thresholds when a hearing loss has been suggested by the results of the speech discrimination test. The sound stimulus can be either voice or an electronically generated signal produced by a portable audiometer. The latter method is, of course, more precise and rather surprisingly some children seem to respond better to these artificial sounds.

Impedance measurement (tympanometry) is a technique of estimating the mechanical properties of the middle ear. The stiffness or impedance of the eardrum and middle ear structures is altered by the presence of fluid or negative pressure in the middle ear cavity. It is therefore a very sensitive way of detecting the presence of otitis media with effusion ('glue ear'). Impedance measurement does not provide a direct means of detecting hearing loss; its main value is in investigating the site (middle ear versus cochlea or nerve) of a hearing problem already demonstrated by the tests described previously.

Examination of the eyes

CHAPTER CONTENTS

EXAMINING EYE MOVEMENTS

This section outlines the procedures used in a more detailed examination of the eyes; however, these techniques are not easy and anyone undertaking them should seek tuition from an orthoptist. Note that the procedures used to assess visual function in children under the age of about 3 years can determine whether the eyes are functioning normally as a pair, but do not give a detailed measure of visual acuity. This requires a degree of subject cooperation (with the exception of specialised techniques mainly used in major referral centres or research studies).

Although several methods have been used to identify vision defects in pre-verbal children, none has so far been found to meet the criteria for a community-wide screening programme. Current recommendations are for a vision test of all children between the ages of 4 and 5 years; by the age of 4 the majority of children can cooperate sufficiently to give reliable results, whereas younger children often have to be recalled for a second test because the test cannot be completed. Ideally the screening programme should be undertaken by orthoptists, who are trained to assess visual function in young children, but if this is not possible the staff who undertake testing should be trained and the quality of their work checked by orthoptists.

The next section summarises the procedures most likely to be used in vision screening, though for many staff the screen will be confined to a test of visual acuity.

Observe

Observe whether there is any **head tilt**. This posture is sometimes adopted by the child to compensate for a squint and in itself is sufficient indication for referral. (There are other causes of head tilt, such as sternomastoid tumour, vertebral anomalies or – very rarely – brain tumours.)

Check the eye movements

1 Various forms of squint may be demonstrated by testing **eye movements**.
2 If the child is hypermetropic (long sighted), he may squint when looking at very close objects, so **test convergence** by bringing a target (a small toy is

ideal) to within 15 cm of his nose. The eyes may fail to move together in a conjugate fashion, or they may separate on upward or downward gaze. Any such abnormality calls for expert examination.

3 **Shine a small torch** with a fine beam on the child's eyes from about 40 cm distance. Check whether the reflections are symmetrical in the two eyes. They may not be *central* in the cornea because the eyes may be converged if the child is looking at the light. This is a useful test in cases where you are not sure whether the child has a squint or a pseudosquint.

4 Elicit the full range of horizontal, vertical and oblique eye movements by moving a small target in front of the eyes, at about 40 cm distance. A light can be used but a small, interesting toy often holds the child's attention more effectively. Small children usually move the whole head rather than the eyes alone when tracking a target so it may be necessary to restrain the head gently with one hand, or ask the mother to do this. The eyes should move smoothly together in all directions. One or two jerks at the extreme lateral range of gaze can be accepted as normal and should not be interpreted as nystagmus.

5 Persistent **downward deviation** of the eyes is often called the 'sunset sign' because the white rim of sclera above the pupil gives the appearance of the sun going down behind the horizon. It may be a sign of raised intracranial pressure (e.g. in hydrocephalus) and is an indication for urgent referral. However, transient 'sun-setting' may be seen in normal babies.

6 Carry out a cover test and an alternate cover test (*see* Figure A2.1).

Orthoptists also use a number of other procedures but none of these has so far been adopted for screening in the UK.

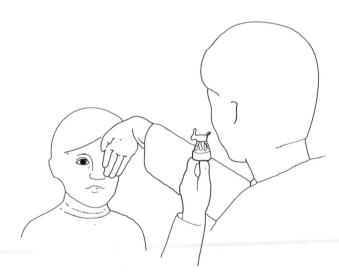

FIGURE A2.1A The cover tests: these should be performed with the child fixing first on a near object and then, if possible, on a distant object.

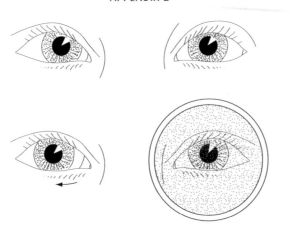

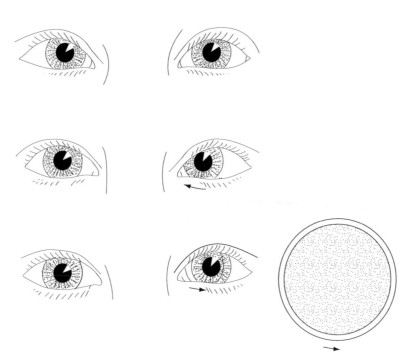

FIGURE A2.1B The cover test. The examiner suspects a squint in the right eye (top picture). When the left eye is covered, the right eye is seen to move outwards to assume fixation. The diagnosis is a right manifest convergent squint.

FIGURE A2.1C The cover-uncover test for latent squint. In the top picture, no squint is apparent. In the middle picture, where the left eye is covered, it is unable to maintain fixation and deviates medially behind the cover. In the bottom picture, the cover is briskly removed from the left eye which is observed to move outwards to resume fixation. The diagnosis in this example is left latent convergent squint. NB: This test is more difficult than the cover test and may need to be repeated several times.

VISUAL ACUITY TESTS

The precise measurement of visual acuity requires tests that examine the ability to separate adjacent visual stimuli – the **minimum separable** tests. With these it is possible to detect the minor impairments of vision that are associated with refractive errors or amblyopia. (In contrast, **minimum detectable** tests, such as those using small rolled balls or 1 mm sweets can only identify children with severe impairment of visual function.)

The standard method of measuring visual acuity is the **Snellen** test type. The child is asked to read a series of letters displayed at a distance of 6 metres. A person with normal vision is said to have 6/6 vision. The largest letter on the Snellen chart can be read by the person with normal vision at a distance of 60 metres. A person who could read this letter only at a distance of 6 metres would be described as having 6/60 vision. Note that this is a pseudo-fraction; it does not mean that the vision is one-tenth of normal.

The Snellen test type method of measuring visual acuity has been modified in various ways so that it can be used by young children who do not yet read letters reliably. It can be simplified by reducing the number of letters and by using a selection of letters that children seem to cope with most easily, such as V, T, O, H, X. The **LogMAR** charts use the same principle, but incorporate a number of improvements with regard to the letter sizes, spacing and layout. They are now the method of choice and should replace Snellen charts.

SINGLE-LETTER TESTS

The **Stycar test** consists of five or seven letters, mounted on individual cards. Alternatively, the **Sheridan Gardener test** can be used; this has a wider range of letters of each size and because it is presented on matt rather than shiny card, it is easier for the child to identify the letters. These tests include a letter of 6/3 size. If it is essential to carry out the vision test at a distance of only 3 metres (as is often the case in primary care premises), the child must be able to read this size of letter to pass the test at a true 6/6 level.

Although single-letter tests have the merit of simplicity, they are not an ideal method of testing visual acuity because they underestimate, or even fail to identify, amblyopia. This is because of the so-called 'crowding phenomenon', which means that the child has considerable difficulty in identifying the individual letters in a line, even though he may be able to do so quite adequately when the letter is displayed on its own without distracting adjacent visual stimuli. For example, a child may appear to have 6/12 vision when tested with single letters, but 6/36 when tested with the LogMAR or Snellen chart. Since the detection of amblyopia is perhaps the most important justification for pre-school vision screening, single-letter tests can no longer be regarded as a satisfactory screening technique.

The **Sonksen Silver test** (Figure A2.2) has been devised to overcome these problems. It uses a line of letters with a matching card, and can be used at 3 metres. It is probably the best available test for pre-school screening for visual acuity defects. However, many children lack the maturity to perform any kind of matching test and this remains the limiting factor in the screening programme and leads to many re-tests.

Whether one is using the LogMAR chart or a single-letter test, it is essential to **check each eye separately**. One eye may be occluded by an eye patch with an elastic headband, or a sticky patch; alternatively, a folded tissue in the parent's hand may be used. The child should not be allowed to occlude the eye with his own hand as he will certainly peep through his fingers if the vision with the other eye is unsatisfactory. Although some very young children will tolerate occlusion at any age, many object strenuously. By the age of 39 months, most children will tolerate occlusion with a little persuasion (*see* Figure A2.2).

The test procedure

It is important to make sure the child understands the task. Seat the child at the table with the parent beside him. Set out the matching card or plastic letters on the table. Using the single-letter teaching book, teach the child the concept of matching, saying 'Can you find me one like this?' As soon as he understands the task, retreat to 3 or 6 metres (you will lose rapport with many young children at the longer distance) and tell the child you are going to repeat the task.

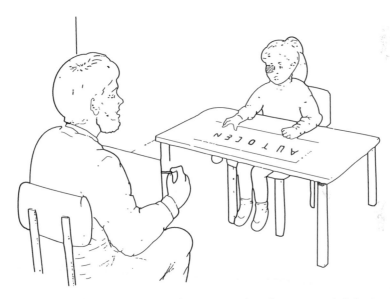

FIGURE A2.2 Sonksen Silver test – testing each eye separately with one eye occluded using a patch.

Near vision

Near vision can be measured using the reduced Snellen chart, but this is not usually necessary as part of a routine assessment of vision in the pre-school child.

Referral

It is sometimes difficult to decide when to refer a child for further examination. If there is a persisting difference in visual acuity between the two eyes, amblyopia may be present and detailed examination is advisable. Using linear LogMAR tests a child should be referred if he does not achieve 0.2 in either eye (roughly equivalent to 6/9 on a Snellen-based linear chart).

Index